Effect of Nutrition on Maternal Health, Fetal Development and Perinatal Outcomes

Effect of Nutrition on Maternal Health, Fetal Development and Perinatal Outcomes

Guest Editors

Themistoklis I. Dagklis
Ioannis Tsakiridis
Michael Chourdakis

MDPI

Basel • Beijing • Wuhan • Barcelona • Belgrade • Novi Sad • Cluj • Manchester

Guest Editors
Themistoklis I. Dagklis
Third Department of Obstetrics and Gynecology
Aristotle University of Thessaloniki
Thessaloniki
Greece

Ioannis Tsakiridis
Third Department of Obstetrics and Gynecology
Aristotle University of Thessaloniki
Thessaloniki
Greece

Michael Chourdakis
Laboratory of Hygiene, Social & Preventive Medicine and Medical Statistics
Aristotle University of Thessaloniki
Thessaloniki
Greece

Editorial Office
MDPI AG
Grosspeteranlage 5
4052 Basel, Switzerland

This is a reprint of the Special Issue, published open access by the journal *Nutrients* (ISSN 2072-6643), freely accessible at: https://www.mdpi.com/journal/nutrients/special_issues/HKW773MA29.

For citation purposes, cite each article independently as indicated on the article page online and as indicated below:

Lastname, A.A.; Lastname, B.B. Article Title. *Journal Name* **Year**, *Volume Number*, Page Range.

ISBN 978-3-7258-4729-7 (Hbk)
ISBN 978-3-7258-4730-3 (PDF)
https://doi.org/10.3390/books978-3-7258-4730-3

Contents

About the Editors

Themistoklis I. Dagklis

Themistoklis Dagklis, is an Associate Professor of Obstetrics & Gynecology—Maternal-Fetal Medicine at the Third Department of Obstetrics and Gynecology, "Ippokrateio" Hospital, School of Medicine, Faculty of Health Sciences, Aristotle University of Thessaloniki, Greece. He has received the Fetal Medicine Diploma after completing a two-year fellowship at the Fetal Medicine Foundation, London, UK.

Ioannis Tsakiridis

Ioannis Tsakiridis, is an Assistant Professor of Obstetrics & Gynecology at the Third Department of Obstetrics and Gynecology, "Ippokrateio" Hospital, School of Medicine, Faculty of Health Sciences, Aristotle University of Thessaloniki, Greece. He has received the title of "Subspecialist in Maternal-Fetal and Perinatal Medicine", after completing a two-year clinical fellowship according to the European Board and College of Obstetrics and Gynecology and European Association of Perinatal Medicine.

Michael Chourdakis

Michail Chourdakis is a Professor at the School of Medicine, Faculty of Health Sciences, Aristotle University of Thessaloniki (Hygiene—Medical Nutrition), at the Laboratory of "Hygiene, Social & Preventive Medicine, and Medical Statistics."

He founded the Postgraduate Program at the School of Medicine titled "Applied Nutrition and Health Promotion," and is the director of the WHO Collaborating Center for Quality of Life and Wellbeing.

Preface

Nutrition in pregnancy is a major contributor to fetal development, as well as perinatal outcomes. Macro- and micronutrient requirements increase in pregnancy, thus a healthy nutrition or the use of supplements may be indicated. To date, several discrepancies exist globally on the nutrition of pregnant women, mainly attributed to different guidelines and cost-effective studies.

Themistoklis I. Dagklis, Ioannis Tsakiridis, and Michael Chourdakis
Guest Editors

nutrients

Editorial

Effects of Nutrition on Maternal Health, Fetal Development, and Perinatal Outcomes

Aikaterini Apostolopoulou [1], Antigoni Tranidou [1], Ioannis Tsakiridis [2,*], Emmanuella Magriplis [3], Themistoklis Dagklis [2] and Michail Chourdakis [1]

[1] Laboratory of Hygiene, Social & Preventive Medicine and Medical Statistics, School of Medicine, Faculty of Health Sciences, Aristotle University of Thessaloniki, 54124 Thessaloniki, Greece; katapost@yahoo.gr (A.A.); antigoni.tranidou@gmail.com (A.T.); mhourd@gapps.auth.gr (M.C.)
[2] 3rd Department of Obstetrics and Gynecology, School of Medicine, Faculty of Health Sciences, Aristotle University of Thessaloniki, 54642 Thessaloniki, Greece; dagklis@auth.gr
[3] Laboratory of Dietetics & Quality of Life, Department of Food Science and Human Nutrition, Agricultural University of Athens, Iera Odos 75, 11855 Athens, Greece; emagriplis@eatsmart.gr
* Correspondence: iotsakir@gmail.com

1. Introduction

The early life theory states that the first 1000 days of a person's life are highly influential, as lasting health impacts can be attained during this period [1–3]. Growing evidence has shown that optimizing maternal nutrition prior to pregnancy, including micronutrient adequacy both in the preconception period and during pregnancy is crucial for later-life health [3]. This Special Issue, "Effect of Nutrition on Maternal Health, Fetal Development, and Perinatal Outcomes", brings together pivotal studies that address these points, shedding light on the multifaceted nature of nutrition and its implications for perinatal outcomes.

Despite certain controversies, there is an overall agreement regarding nutritional requirements during pregnancy and a focus on a balanced diet, in line with guidelines on healthy eating, to ensure the adequate intake of energy and macro- and micro-nutrients during this period [3,4]. Moreover, guidance on appropriate weight gain during pregnancy is included in the recommendations; it is generally agreed that weight gain during pregnancy should be monitored as it affects maternal and child health during and after gestation [5]. High-fat and carbohydrate diets are related to inflammatory processes that may be harmful to children's brain development, increasing the risk of impaired cognitive function and neuropsychiatric disorders, such as depression, attention deficit hyperactivity disorder (ADHD), autism spectrum disorder (ASD), and anxiety [6,7]. In addition, the overconsumption of nutrient-poor foods may lead to another form of malnutrition due to micronutrient deficiencies [8,9] despite energy overconsumption. This condition, known as hidden hunger, is common throughout the world, mostly in high-income countries [10]. Recent evidence shows that young pregnant women are more vulnerable to this condition and could develop iron, iodine, and vitamin D deficiencies, which, in turn, are related to several pregnancy complications [10]. In adjunction to this form of malnutrition, ultra-processed food consumption has also increased in recent years and has been related to oxidative stress [1], and this may further affect pregnancy outcomes.

According to a recent meta-analysis, higher adherence to a healthy diet, characterized by high intakes of fruits, vegetables, whole grains, low-fat dairy products, vegetable oils, and fish reduced the risk of gestational hypertensive disorders, maternal depression, low birthweight, and preterm delivery [11]. On the contrary, higher maternal adherence to an unhealthy diet, characterized by refined grains, foods high in saturated fats, red meat, processed meat, fast foods, and high sugary foods or a mixed diet (combination of both healthy and unhealthy foods) was associated with a higher risk of gestational hypertension [12]. Higher intake of sugar-sweetened beverages and lower intake of oily fish were most prominently associated with higher glycemic results on the test of glucose tolerance among high-risk women [13].

Several systematic reviews have pooled together interventional studies to increase the understanding of a diet's role in pregnancy [11,12] and indicated the importance of women's nutrition before and during the first trimester of pregnancy. Another systematic review assessed the effects of healthy diet and exercise interventions during pregnancy and revealed a possible lower risk of gestational diabetes and cesarean section, while no clear differences were identified between groups for hypertensive disorders, perinatal mortality, or large-for-gestational-age neonates [13]. Regarding overweight or obese pregnant women, diet and/or exercise (regular aerobic exercise) interventions initiated at <21 weeks of pregnancy may reduce gestational weight gain but have no effect on the risk of hypertensive disorders of pregnancy [14]; diet interventions included dietary advice or related interventions in pregnancy that aimed to optimize health outcomes, which might include controlling excessive gestational weight gain or improving glycemic control.

2. An Overview of Published Articles

A Greek study developed a model to be used as an early prediction tool for gestational diabetes mellitus (GDM) risk, combining maternal characteristics, obstetric and medical history, and early pregnancy-specific biomarker concentrations, readily available in healthcare settings (Contribution 1). The model can be used for the proactive management of GDM, allowing for timely nutritional and lifestyle interventions that can significantly alter the course of pregnancy and fetal development, as well as the perinatal outcomes.

In addressing the broader spectrum of maternal health, a cross-sectional study in Poland emphasized the importance of physical activity both before and during pregnancy, highlighting its positive impact on reducing adverse perinatal outcomes (Contribution 2). The key discoveries from this research indicate that engaging in physical activity both before and during pregnancy, along with maintaining a normal pre-pregnancy body mass index (BMI), can have a positive impact on pregnancy outcomes. This influence is manifested in a decreased risk of preterm birth rates and a lower likelihood of delivering children with low birth weight.

Another critical area of concern, as highlighted in a study focusing on Romanian women of reproductive age, is obesity (Contribution 3). The study provides a comprehensive analysis of BMI trends over 12 years, revealing a worrying increase in overweight and obesity rates. The findings indicate that, during the first-trimester morphology scan evaluation, 29% of the participants were either overweight or obese, while the rates of overweight and obese women exceeded 40% in the second trimester of pregnancy. In this study's population, the association of obesity with other risk factors showed an elevated risk of obesity among multiparous individuals, those who smoked or were ex-smokers in the second trimester, and participants who did not take folic acid or multivitamin supplementation.

Furthermore, in Indonesia, a mentoring program implemented throughout pregnancy as an intervention yielded superior outcomes in terms of fetal growth and neonatal birth weight (Contribution 4). Notably, women who participated in the program exhibited a significantly higher weight-for-length Z-score (WLZ) for their newborns, although there was no significant difference in the length-for-age Z score (LAZ) compared to those who received standard care alone. This innovative approach, focusing on preconception and pregnancy care, demonstrates significant improvements in fetal growth and neonatal birth weight, offering a promising strategy for enhancing maternal and child health in low- and middle-income countries.

3. Conclusions

The ongoing pandemic of "hidden hunger", characterized by excessive consumption of ultra-processed and nutrient-poor foods, is prevalent in Western countries, particularly among young individuals. While evidence on maternal nutrition predominantly focuses on low-income countries, emphasizing the detrimental effects of malnutrition on fetal growth, research examining the impact of "hidden hunger" on fetal development remains insufficient and lacks robustness to significantly influence medical decisions and interventions for young pregnant women. This Special Issue has the potential to significantly contribute to filling these existing gaps.

In conclusion, this Special Issue captures the diversity and complexity of research on nutritional impacts on maternal health, fetal development, and perinatal outcomes. The range of methodologies and subjects covered in these articles reflects the dynamic nature of this field. From predictive modeling to practical interventions, these studies significantly contribute to our understanding and management of maternal and fetal health. This compilation not only provides valuable insights into current research but also sets the stage for future investigations in this vital area of public health. More research is needed to explore personalized nutritional strategies grounded in contemporary scientific knowledge for enhancing maternal health and optimizing perinatal outcomes.

Conflicts of Interest: The authors declare no conflicts of interest.

List of Contributions

1. Tranidou, A.; Tsakiridis, I.; Apostolopoulou, A.; Xenidis, T.; Pazaras, N.; Mamopoulos, A.; Athanasiadis, A.; Chourdakis, M.; Dagklis, T. Prediction of Gestational Diabetes Mellitus in the First Trimester of Pregnancy Based on Maternal Variables and Pregnancy Biomarkers. *Nutrients* **2024**, *16*, 120. https://doi.org/10.3390/nu16010120.
2. Szablewska, A.W.; Wierzba, J.; Santos-Rocha, R.; Szumilewicz, A. Can Pre-Pregnancy Body Mass Index and Maternal Exercise Affect Birth and Neonatal Outcomes—A Cross Sectional Study. *Nutrients* **2023**, *15*, 4894. https://doi.org/10.3390/nu15234894.
3. Ursache, A.; Bujor, I.E.; Cristofor, A.E.; Zelinschi, D.O.; Nemescu, D.; Matasariu, D.R. Maternal Body Mass Index Trends and Weight Gain in Singleton Pregnancies at the Time of Fetal Anatomic Survey: Changes in the Last Decade and New Trends in the Modern Era. *Nutrients* **2023**, *15*, 4788. https://doi.org/10.3390/nu15224788.
4. Hadi, H.; Nurunniyah, S.; Gittelsohn, J.; Alfiana, R.D.; Fatimatasari Lewis, E.C.; Nurdiati, D. Preconception Maternal Mentoring for Improved Fetal Growth among Indonesian Women: Results from a Cluster Randomized Controlled Trial. *Nutrients* **2023**, *15*, 4579. https://doi.org/10.3390/nu15214579.

References

1. Hsu, C.N.; Tain, Y.L. The First Thousand Days: Kidney Health and Beyond. *Healthcare* **2021**, *9*, 1332. [CrossRef] [PubMed]
2. Agosti, M.; Tandoi, F.; Morlacchi, L.; Bossi, A. Nutritional and metabolic programming during the first thousand days of life. *Pediatr. Med. Chir.* **2017**, *39*, 157. [CrossRef] [PubMed]
3. Koletzko, B.; Godfrey, K.M.; Poston, L.; Szajewska, H.; van Goudoever, J.B.; de Waard, M.; Brands, B.; Grivell, R.M.; Deussen, A.R.; Dodd, J.M.; et al. Nutrition during pregnancy, lactation and early childhood and its implications for maternal and long-term child health: The early nutrition project recommendations. *Ann. Nutr. Metab.* **2019**, *74*, 93–106. [CrossRef] [PubMed]
4. Adair, L.S. Long-term consequences of nutrition and growth in early childhood and possible preventive interventions. In *Nestle Nutrition Institute Workshop Series;* S. Karger AG: Basel, Switzerland, 2014; Volume 78, pp. 111–120. [CrossRef]
5. Aoyama, T.; Li, D.; Bay, J.L. Weight Gain and Nutrition during Pregnancy: An Analysis of Clinical Practice Guidelines in the Asia-Pacific Region. *Nutrients* **2022**, *14*, 1288. [CrossRef] [PubMed]
6. de Rooij, S.R.; Wouters, H.; Yonker, J.E.; Painter, R.C.; Roseboom, T.J. Prenatal undernutrition and cognitive function in late adulthood. *Proc. Natl. Acad. Sci. USA* **2010**, *107*, 16881–16886. [CrossRef] [PubMed]
7. Torres, N.; Bautista, C.J.; Tovar, A.R.; Ordáz, G.; Rodríguez-Cruz, M.; Ortiz, V.; Granados, O.; Nathanielsz, P.W.; Larrea, F.; Zambrano, E. Protein restriction during pregnancy affects maternal liver lipid metabolism and fetal brain lipid composition in the rat. *Am. J. Physiol.-Endocrinol. Metab.* **2010**, *298*, E270–E277. [CrossRef] [PubMed]
8. Mathur, P.; Pillai, R. Overnutrition: Current scenario & combat strategies. *Indian J. Med. Res.* **2019**, *149*, 695–705. [CrossRef] [PubMed]
9. Godfrey, K.M.; Reynolds, R.M.; Prescott, S.L.; Nyirenda, M.; Jaddoe, V.W.; Eriksson, J.G.; Broekman, B.F. Influence of maternal obesity on the long-term health of offspring. *Lancet Diabetes Endocrinol.* **2017**, *5*, 53–64. [CrossRef] [PubMed]

10. Sok, A.; Antony, C.; Vora, R.M.; Karmarkar, S.J. The silent tragic reality of Hidden Hunger, anaemia, and neural-tube defects (NTDs) in India. *Lancet Reg. Health-Southeast Asia* **2022**, *6*, 100071. [CrossRef]
11. Abdollahi, S.; Soltani, S.; de Souza, R.J.; Forbes, S.C.; Toupchian, O.; Salehi-Abargouei, A. Associations between Maternal Dietary Patterns and Perinatal Outcomes: A Systematic Review and Meta-Analysis of Cohort Studies. *Adv. Nutr.* **2021**, *12*, 1332–1352. [CrossRef] [PubMed]
12. Lindsay, K.L.; Milone, G.F.; Grobman, W.A.; Haas, D.M.; Mercer, B.M.; Simhan, H.N.; Saade, G.R.; Silver, R.M.; Chung, J.H. Periconceptional diet quality is associated with gestational diabetes risk and glucose concentrations among nulliparous gravidas. *Front. Endocrinol.* **2022**, *13*, 940870. [CrossRef] [PubMed]
13. Ramakrishnan, U.; Grant, F.; Goldenberg, T.; Zongrone, A.; Martorell, R. Effect of women's nutrition before and during early pregnancy on maternal and infant outcomes: A systematic review. *Paediatr. Perinat. Epidemiol.* **2012**, *26*, 285–301. [CrossRef] [PubMed]
14. Shepherd, E.; Gomersall, J.C.; Tieu, J.; Han, S.; Crowther, C.A.; Middleton, P. Combined diet and exercise interventions for preventing gestational diabetes mellitus. *Cochrane Database Syst. Rev.* **2017**, *11*, CD010443. [CrossRef] [PubMed]

nutrients

MDPI

Article

Evaluation of Polyphenol Intake in Pregnant Women from South-Eastern Spain and the Effect on Anthropometric Measures at Birth and Gestational Age

Daniel Hinojosa-Nogueira [1,2,†], Desirée Romero-Molina [2,3,†], Beatriz González-Alzaga [2,4,5], María José Giménez-Asensio [2], Antonio F. Hernandez [2,5,6], Beatriz Navajas-Porras [1,2], Adriana Delgado-Osorio [1,2], Antonio Gomez-Martin [2,4], Sergio Pérez-Burillo [7], Silvia Pastoriza de la Cueva [1], Marina Lacasaña [2,4,5,*,‡] and José Ángel Rufián-Henares [1,2,*,‡]

[1] Biomedical Research Center, Department of Nutrition and Bromatology, Institute of Nutrition and Food Technology, University of Granada, 18071 Granada, Spain; dhinojosa@ugr.es (D.H.-N.); beatriznavajas@ugr.es (B.N.-P.); adrianadelgado@ugr.es (A.D.-O.); spdelacueva@ugr.es (S.P.d.l.C.)
[2] Biosanitary Research Institute ibs.GRANADA, 18014 Granada, Spain; deromero@ugr.es (D.R.-M.); beatriz.gonzalez.easp@juntadeandalucia.es (B.G.-A.); mariajoseases@hotmail.com (M.J.G.-A.); ajerez@ugr.es (A.F.H.); antonio.gm.gr@gmail.com (A.G.-M.)
[3] Statistics and Operations Research Department, Faculty of Sciences, University of Granada, 18071 Granada, Spain
[4] Andalusian School of Public Health (EASP), 18011 Granada, Spain
[5] CIBER of Epidemiology and Public Health (CIBERESP), Instituto de Salud Carlos III, 28029 Madrid, Spain
[6] Department of Legal Medicine and Toxicology, University of Granada, 18016 Granada, Spain
[7] Department of Pharmacology and Pediatrics, University of Málaga, 29010 Málaga, Spain; spburillo@ugr.es
* Correspondence: marina.lacasana.easp@juntadeandalucia.es (M.L.); jarufian@ugr.es (J.Á.R.-H.)
† These authors contributed equally to this work.
‡ These authors contributed equally to this work.

Abstract: During pregnancy, controlling nutrition is crucial for the health of both mother and foetus. While polyphenols have positive health effects, some studies show harmful outcomes during pregnancy. This study evaluated polyphenol intake in a cohort of mother–child pairs and examined its effects on foetal anthropometric parameters. Polyphenol intake was assessed using food frequency questionnaires (FFQs) and 24-h dietary recalls, and analysed with the Phenol-Explorer database. Gestational age and birth measurements were retrieved from medical records. Statistical analyses validated dietary records and assessed polyphenol impact using multivariate generalised linear models. The study found that mean gestational age was 39.6 weeks, with a mean birth weight of 3.33 kg. Mean total polyphenol intake by FFQ was 2231 mg/day, slightly higher than 24-h recall data. Flavonoids and phenolic acids constituted 52% and 37% of intake, respectively, with fruits and legumes as primary sources. This study highlights the use of FFQs to estimate polyphenol intake. Furthermore, the study found associations between polyphenol consumption and anthropometric parameters at birth, with the effects varying depending on the type of polyphenol. However, a more precise evaluation of individual polyphenol intake is necessary to determine whether the effects they produce during pregnancy may be harmful or beneficial for foetal growth.

Keywords: foetal anthropometry; polyphenols; pregnant women; 24-h dietary recalls; food frequency questionnaire

1. Introduction

Balanced maternal nutrition during pregnancy is a pivotal area of study, as it exerts a significant influence on foetal growth and the overall well-being of both mother and offspring [1,2]. Numerous epidemiological studies suggest that diets rich in plant-based foods have long-term beneficial effects on both the foetus and maternal health [3,4]. Among the compounds contributing to these effects are polyphenols, with over 8000 molecules so far [5]. These compounds are secondary metabolites derived from plants and play a crucial role in their survival and adaptation. Phenolic compounds can be classified into five broad categories: flavonoids, phenolic acids, lignans, stilbenes and other polyphenols [6–8]. The primary dietary sources of polyphenols include vegetables, fruits, cereals, nuts, legumes, chocolate and similar foods [9,10]. Due to their beneficial effects on health, dietary polyphenols have received considerable attention. They are primarily recognised for their antioxidant activity, which is associated with other beneficial properties such as modulation of inflammatory responses, anti-obesogenic activity and reduction of the risk of cardiovascular disease [3,10–14]. Additionally, polyphenols have been linked to neuroprotective functions [15–17] and the inhibition of tumour growth in various types of cancers, including those affecting the colon, prostate and breast [11–13]. Given their health benefits, there is considerable public interest in increasing polyphenol intake through diet, nutraceuticals, fortified foods, beverages and dietary supplements [18].

Although the beneficial effects of polyphenols are well documented, concerns have been raised about the potential health risk of these compounds [9,14,19–23]. At present, the toxicity of polyphenols remains uncertain, but the availability of polyphenol-rich foods and supplements is growing. Amid increasing concern, a database named ToxDP2 has been created [21], providing comprehensive data on 415 dietary polyphenols that may have toxicological effects. In addition, studies suggest that consumption of large amounts of polyphenols may have pro-oxidant effects. They have also been associated with hepatotoxicity or an increased risk of certain types of cancer [10,14,19,21,24,25]. One of the major risks associated with polyphenol consumption is the constriction of the foetal ductus arteriosus during the third trimester of pregnancy [9,19–21,23,26–35], which may lead to potentially serious consequences, including perinatal pulmonary hypertension, heart failure and foetal death [20,28]. Therefore, understanding the relationship between polyphenol consumption and its effects on maternal and foetal health is essential.

Commonly, methods used to evaluate dietary polyphenol consumption during pregnancy involve the use of dietary records such as food frequency questionnaires (FFQs) [30,36,37]. In addition, accurate quantification requires a database containing polyphenol concentrations in various foods. Phenol-Explorer is one of the most widely used databases for this purpose [8]. Considering the above, this study aimed to evaluate polyphenol consumption in a cohort of pregnant women from South-eastern Spain and its potential effects on foetal health, focusing on anthropometric measurements at birth.

2. Materials and Methods

2.1. Patient Selection and Study Design

This prospective, population-based, pregnant-women birth cohort study, known as the GENEIDA Project, "Genetics, early life environmental exposures and infant development in Andalusia" (https://www.easp.es/web/geneida/, accessed on 12 August 2024), started in 2014 in a well-defined geographic area of South-eastern Spain (Almería). Inclusion criteria for enrolment included pregnant women aged 17 years or older who intended to give birth at the referral hospital. Additionally, participants were required to have singleton pregnancies (not resulting from assisted reproductive technology) and no pre-existing chronic diseases. Furthermore, they could not currently be receiving medical treatment, and could not have any language barriers.

Women were enrolled in the study at their first antenatal visit at the hospital (around 12–13 weeks of gestation) and were followed throughout pregnancy, delivery and after birth at different children's development ages (1, 2, 4 and 7–8 years). A total of 800 women were recruited, and the final analysis was based on 680 women (85%). Pregnant women completed the same FFQ on two occasions, initially during the first trimester and subsequently during the third trimester. Simultaneously, 24-h dietary recalls were conducted in a subsample of 40 women for this specific study.

This study was approved by the Biomedical Research Ethics Committee of Andalusia, and all participants provided written and informed consent. The study objectives were clearly explained and participants had the right to withdraw from the study and request withdrawal of their data at any time. Throughout the study, we adhered to the ethical principles of the World Medical Association's Declaration of Helsinki, as well as the ethical and legal standards of Spanish legislation.

2.2. *Dietary Assessment*

A variety of dietary records were administered to study participants. A semi-quantitative FFQ previously validated for assessing total nutrient intake was used for dietary recording [38]. The FFQ covered 141 items, which were further classified into 28 food subgroups. These items included specific traditional dishes, spices and foods most frequently consumed in the study area. Respondents had nine options to choose from, ranging from "never" or "almost never" to "more than six times a day". The 24-h dietary recall method was selected as the reference system to validate the FFQ for the polyphenol intake [30]. This validation was performed in a subsample of the study population. The data from this subsample were collected from those participants who volunteered to take part. All foods and beverages consumed in the previous 24-h dietary recalls were compiled over three non-consecutive days, including two weekdays and one weekend day.

Both dietary records were completed twice during pregnancy: the first covered the time before the first trimester of pregnancy and the second during the third trimester. To enhance response rates and data accuracy, trained interviewers assisted participants in completing the questionnaires, thereby minimising bias.

2.3. *Quantitative Estimation of Total Polyphenol Intake*

The Phenol-Explorer 3.6 database was used to estimate polyphenol intake. This resource provided data on the total polyphenol content of foods using the Folin–Ciocalteu method. Additionally, we determined the concentrations of individual polyphenol families and subfamilies [8]. The mean total polyphenol intake (MTPI) of each participant was estimated from the mean of the Folin–Ciocalteu total polyphenol content and the sum of the concentrations of each polyphenol subfamily. The subfamilies of phenolic compounds were categorised into several main groups based on Phenol-Explorer criteria: (a) flavonoids (including anthocyanins, chalcones, dihydrochalcones, dihydroflavonols, flavanols, flavanones, flavones, flavonols and isoflavonoids); (b) phenolic acids (such as hydroxybenzoic acids, hydroxycinnamic acids, hydroxyphenylacetic acids and hydroxyphenyl propanoic acids); (c) lignans (lignans); (d) stilbenes (stilbenes); and (e) other polyphenols (alkylmethoxyphenols, alkylphenols, furanocoumarins, hydroxybenzaldehydes, hydroxybenzoketones, hydroxycinnamaldehydes, hydroxycoumarins, methoxyphenols, naphtoquinones, tyrosols and other polyphenols). Some subfamilies were transformed into dichotomous variables due to the large number of participants who did not consume foods containing these polyphenols. The foods were classified into eleven groups: cereals and derived products, vegetables, fruits, legumes, nuts, oils, fruit derivatives (e.g., fruit juices), chocolate and coffee, spices and infusions, alcoholic beverages and processed foods (such as pizzas, lasagnas, etc.). Processed foods were separated according to their main ingredients following typical commercial recipes and were adjusted using cooking yield factors to estimate the total phenols of that food in the diet [6–8]. Any food lacking polyphenols was excluded from the study. For the estimation of polyphenols in 24-h dietary recalls, a previously developed and validated tool was used [39].

2.4. *General Questionnaire, Medical Records and Anthropometric Measurements*

Information from participants was collected using a structured questionnaire administered by trained staff during their hospital appointment scheduled for the first and third trimesters of pregnancy. The questionnaire covered sociodemographic characteristics, working life and occupational exposure, exposure at home and living environment, obstetric history and prior illnesses. Pregnant women self-reported relevant data such as pre-pregnancy weight and height during the first trimester of pregnancy. Weight at 32 weeks' gestation was extracted from medical records. Body mass index (BMI) was calculated from height and weight using the function (kg/m^2). The gestational age of the pregnancy, defined as the time elapsed between the first day of the last menstrual cycle and the time of delivery, along with anthropometric measurements, including birth weight, height and head circumference, was obtained from hospital records in accordance with relevant guidelines and standardised protocols [40–42]. The ponderal index was calculated using the following formula: weight (g) $\times$ 100/(length, cm)^3. Specific z-scores for weight, length and head circumference at birth were calculated. These adjustments are described in more detail in previous studies [43].

2.5. Data Analysis

Statistical data were analysed using the SPSS statistical package version 26.0, R software version 4.3.2 and Python version 3.7. Bivariate and multivariate generalised linear models (GLMs) were used to evaluate the impact of polyphenol intake on height z-score, weight z-score, head circumference (HC) z-score and ponderal index. The mother's polyphenol intake during the first and third trimesters of pregnancy was used as the independent variable, and all models were adjusted for energy intake to ensure accurate estimation. The following confounders and covariates were identified based on previous studies and considered for adjustment in the multivariate models: energy intake, family's monthly income, gestational weight gain, gestational age at the first prenatal visit, infant sex, marital status, maternal education, maternal stress, mother's age, physical exercise, pre-pregnancy BMI, history of repeated abortions, rural/urban residence, supplement intake, type of delivery, alcohol consumption, ethnicity, parity, season and smoking. Variables were mapped and their relationships analysed using a directed acyclic diagram (DAG) generated by DAGitty version 3.0 software (Figure 1).

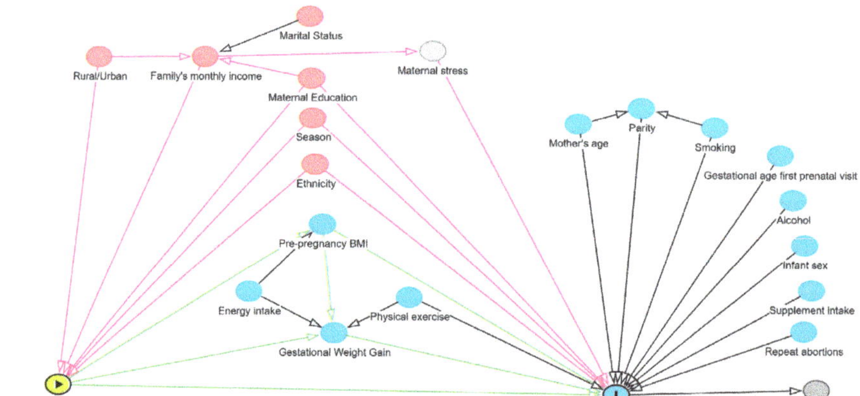

Figure 1. Direct acyclic graph (DAG) that displays the potential relationship between the variables and covariates considered for this study. "Triangle" indicates the exposure variable and "I" is the outcome. Red circles: confounding variables. Blue circles: covariates (causality associated with health outcomes). Light grey circle: variable not available in our study. Dark grey circle: descendant variable. Green arrows: causal path. Pink arrows: biasing path.

With this information, and using a stepwise method of variable selection, the following confounding factors were finally selected for inclusion in multivariate models: height z-score (smoking, alcohol intake and repeated abortions); weight z-score (smoking, repeated abortions, maternal education and parity); head circumference z-score (smoking, mother's age, maternal physical exercise, supplement intake, education and parity), and ponderal index (smoking, mother's age, maternal education and parity).

Means and standard deviations (SD) for all polyphenol intakes were obtained for the 24-h dietary recalls and the two FFQs. Previously, the validity and reproducibility of the polyphenol intake FFQ were assessed using statistical approaches, in line with the methodology previously used for nutrients [38]. Briefly, the methodologies commonly used for validation of nutritional parameters include the correlation coefficient, quintile ranking and limits of agreement (LOA). In particular, Spearman's correlation coefficient was determined for MTPI according to the distribution in the different food groups. In quintile ranking, polyphenol intake was divided into quintiles and the percentage of data correctly classified in the same or adjacent quintiles was calculated. The LOA technique, or Bland–Altman method, is a graphical technique where the limits of agreement are established as ±1.96 SD of the mean difference between the polyphenol intakes obtained from two questionnaires. In this technique, the percentage of data falling within these graphical limits was counted. The significance level was set at $p < 0.05$.

3. Results

3.1. Characteristics of the Study Population

The characteristics of 680 pregnant women and their newborns from the GENEIDA cohort are shown in Table 1.

Table 1. Demographic characteristic of the study population ($n = 680$).

Characteristics	No. (%), Mean ± SD
Maternal characteristics	
Maternal age	31.05 ± 4.86
Education:	
Primary education	335 (49.3%)
Secondary education	162 (23.8%)
Higher education	183 (26.9%)
Parity:	
0 (primiparous)	262 (38.5%)
≥1 (multiparous)	418 (61.5%)
Repeat abortions:	
Yes	54 (7.9%)
No	626 (92.1%)
Smoking:	
Never	569 (83.6%)
Only 1st trimester	29 (4.3%)
During all pregnancy	82 (12.1%)
Alcohol consumption:	
Never	133 (19.5%)
Only 1st trimester	282 (41.5%)
During all pregnancy	265 (39.0%)
Vitamin supplement intake:	
Never	538 (79.1%)
Sometime during pregnancy	129 (19.0%)
During all pregnancy	12 (1.8%)
Physical exercise:	
Never	14 (2.1%)
Sometime during pregnancy	138 (20.3%)
During all pregnancy	528 (77.6%)
Energy intake (Kcal):	
1st trimester	2404 ± 739
3rd trimester	2054 ± 670
Pre-pregnancy BMI (kg/m^2)	24.23 ± 4.68
Gestational weight gain (kg)	11.23 ± 5.42

Table 1. *Cont.*

Characteristics	No. (%), Mean ± SD
Infant characteristics	
Infant sex:	
Male	349 (51.3%)
Female	331 (48.7%)
Length of gestation (weeks)	39.87 ± 1.25
Ponderal index	2.55 ± 0.25
Birth weight (g)	3329.30 ± 427.05
Birth length (cm)	50.70 ± 2.09
Head circumference (cm)	33.75 ± 1.52

The mean maternal age was 31 years with a standard deviation of 4.8 years old. The mean height of the participants was 1.64 m and pre-pregnancy weight 64.7 kg. The pre-pregnancy BMI was 24.2 ± 4.5 kg/m^2. The mean gestational age was 39 weeks with a standard deviation of 1.3 weeks and 48.7% of the newborns were girls. Regarding the anthropometric characteristics of the newborns, the mean birth weight was 3.33 kg, the mean birth length 50.7 cm, the head circumference 33.8 cm and the ponderal index 2.55.

3.2. Validity and Reproducibility of FFQ

The validation study used dietary information provided by 40 out of the 680 pregnant women participating in the study. These women completed all the FFQ and 24-h dietary recalls. The correlation coefficients for MTPI according to distribution in the different food groups ranged from 0.42 (for fruit polyphenols) to 0.02 (for legume polyphenols). In the case of mean total polyphenol intake, a statistically significant (but low) correlation coefficient of 0.3 was found. According to quintile classification, polyphenol intakes for each food group in the same (or adjacent) quintile ranged from 76.7% to 53.5% for the groups "chocolate and coffee" and "oils", respectively (Table 2). The limits of the agreement varied from 95.4% to 90.7%.

Table 2. Validation of daily intake of total polyphenols based on food frequency questionnaire (FFQ) and 24-h dietary recalls (n = 40).

	FFQ 1	FFQ 2	Correlation Coefficient	Agreement by Quintiles (%) [a]	Agreement by LOA (%) [b]
	Mean ± SD	**Mean ± SD**			
Mean total polyphenol intake (mg)	2158 ± 1023	1875 ± 835	0.303 *	67.4	95.4
Vegetables (mg) †	476 ± 321	312 ± 296	0.369 *	62.8	93.1
Spices and infusions (mg) †	7.33 ± 5.02	139 ± 209	0.326 *	67.4	95.4
Cereals and derived products (mg)	230 ± 131	234 ± 126	0.314 *	69.8	90.7
Legumes (mg) †	676 ± 408	219 ± 395	0.015	60.5	93.1
Fruits (mg)	358 ± 185	407 ± 279	0.418 **	69.8	90.7
Fruit derivatives (mg)	68.5 ± 30.9	49.3 ± 81.5	0.224	62.8	90.7
Oils (mg) †	29.5 ± 15.8	12.3 ± 9.57	−0.086	53.5	95.4
Nuts (mg) †	45.9 ± 10.4	33.4 ± 68.8	0.261	67.4	95.4
Processed foods (mg) †	66.8 ± 49.3	65.1 ± 81.1	−0.056	67.4	90.7
Chocolate and coffee (mg)	418 ± 345	564 ± 527	0.347 *	76.7	93.1
Alcoholic beverages (mg)	5.07 ± 2.73	4.87 ± 9.01	0.260	65.1	90.7

[a] Correctly classified if classified into same or adjacent (±1) quintiles. [b] Overall proportion of agreement limits between both questionnaires, corresponding to Bland–Altman plots. * Correlation significant at $p < 0.05$ level; ** Correlation significant at $p < 0.01$ level. † Significant differences ($p < 0.05$), paired-sample sign test, observed between total polyphenol intakes obtained by FFQ and 24-h dietary recalls.

For reproducibility, FFQs during the first and third trimesters of pregnancy were compared. The correlations between the two FFQs regarding the contribution of MTPI and the polyphenol families are shown in Table 3. Comparisons were also made between the different food groups. Correlation coefficients ranged from 0.52 to 0.32 for the vegetable and cereal groups, respectively. In relation to the polyphenol intake, the ranges varied from 0.141 for stilbenes to 0.406 for phenolic acids. For MTPI, the polyphenol families and all food groups had significant correlations with $p < 0.01$. The percentage of food groups classified in the same quintile by the two FFQs ranged from 74.5% for the group of vegetables to 65% for the fruit group. In the case of polyphenol families, the mean values classified in the same quintile were 66.2%. The limits of agreement for all values were distributed over 94.7% (Table 3).

Table 3. Reproducibility analysis of polyphenol intakes (mg) based on two food frequency questionnaires (FFQ), during first and third trimesters of pregnancy (n = 680).

	FFQ 1	FFQ 2	Correlation Coefficient	Agreement by Quintiles (%) [a]	Agreement by LOA (%) [b]
	Mean ± SD	Mean ± SD			
Mean total polyphenol intakes	2388 ± 905	2075 ± 932	0.355 **	65.2	94.1
Flavonoids	624 ± 364	518 ± 353	0.336 **	69.8	93.5
Phenolic acids	461 ± 225	350 ± 200	0.406 **	65.6	95.7
Lignans	68.3 ± 45.4	57.8 ± 45.7	0.376 **	68.9	94.4
Stilbenes	0.47 ± 0.53	0.2 ± 0.24	0.141 **	60.1	96.6
Other polyphenols	60.5 ± 46.9	50.6 ± 40.9	0.321 **	67.5	94.1

[a] Correctly classified if placed into the same or adjacent (±1) quintiles. [b] Overall proportion of agreement limits between both questionnaires, corresponding to Bland–Altman plots. ** Correlation significant at $p < 0.01$ level.

3.3. Total Polyphenol Intake

The MTPI for the 680 women during pregnancy was 2231 ± 757 mg/day calculated on the basis of information provided by the FFQs, and 1875 ± 835 mg/day from the 24-h dietary recalls (40 pregnant women). The total polyphenol consumption estimated from the FFQs was slightly higher when compared with the average of the 24-h dietary recalls. Total polyphenol content of food calculated by the Folin–Ciocalteu method was 3367 ± 1167 mg/day, while 1069 ± 421 mg/day was obtained with the sum of the concentrations of the individual polyphenol subfamilies. The flavonoid group was the most abundant polyphenol family, accounting for about 52% of the total intake. Phenolic acids accounted for 37% of the total, making them the second-most abundant group. Lignans and other polyphenols each represented about 5%, while stilbenes were the minority group. If we focus on subfamilies, flavanols (33%), hydroxycinnamic acids (21%), flavanones and anthocyanins are the most representative, accounting for 73% of the total intake. The results by subfamily of phenolic compounds are shown in the Supplementary Material (Supplementary File S1).

Of the 11 food groups, legumes (28.5%), fruits (25.3%), vegetables (15.2%) and chocolate and coffee (14.1%) were the major dietary sources of total polyphenols in the diet of the GENEIDA cohort. Within each food group, the main contributors were identified and were consistent with the 24-h dietary recalls. Lentils, cocoa powder, apples, chocolate, oranges, tomatoes, gazpacho and capsicum were the foods with the highest contribution to dietary polyphenols in relation to total polyphenol intake and regular food consumption.

3.4. Relationship between Polyphenol Intake and Anthropometric Measures at Birth

Bivariate and multivariate GLMs were used to evaluate the potential effects of polyphenol intake (total, by families or subfamilies) on different birth anthropometric measures (height z-score, weight z-score, head circumference z-score and ponderal index) at different trimesters of pregnancy and the average of the two calculated (Supplementary File S2).

Figure 2 presents the resulting regression coefficients of polyphenols (total and families) in the multivariate models, including their confidence intervals. Beta coefficients indicate that polyphenols significantly increased birth anthropometric measures for some of the polyphenol families at some gestational periods. The intake of phenolic acids during the third trimester, which accounted for over 30% of the total intake, was significantly associated with increased head circumference at birth. Also, phenolic acids showed a near-significant positive relationship with weight during the first trimester and on average. Lastly, stilbenes exhibited a significant positive association with both height and weight at birth in the third trimester.

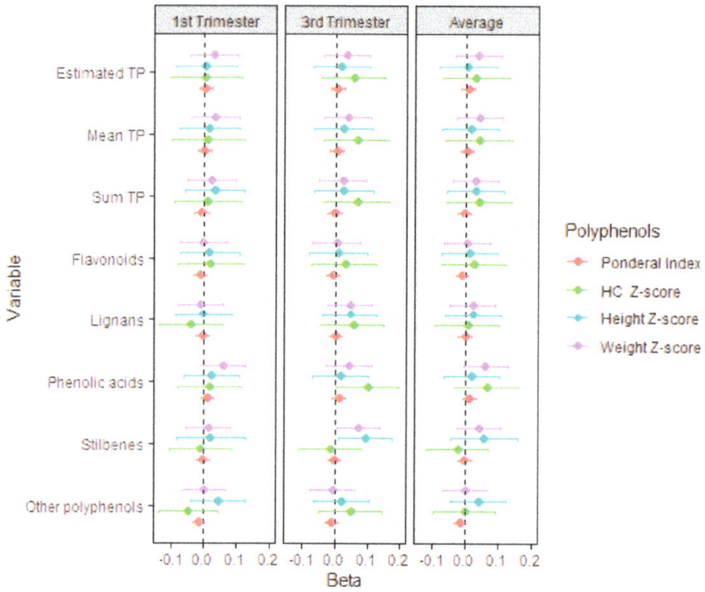

Figure 2. Associations between sum of total polyphenol intake and by family groups and anthropometric measures at birth. GLM adjusted for height z-score (smoking, alcohol and repeat abortions); weight z-score (smoking, repeat abortions, maternal education and parity); head circumference (HC) z-score (smoking, mother's age, maternal, physical exercise, supplement intake, education and parity); and ponderal index (smoking, mother's age, maternal education and parity). Regression coefficients and 95% confidence intervals are presented. TP: total polyphenols.

An in-depth analysis, taking into account the subfamilies of polyphenols, revealed significant associations (Figure 3). Statistically significant inverse associations were found, particularly during the first trimester of pregnancy, between the ponderal index and intake of hydroxyphenyl acetic acids, as well as between hydroxyphenyl propanoic acids and tyrosols. However, significant direct associations were observed between different subfamilies of polyphenols and anthropometry at birth measures, with the exception of dihydroflavonols. Only some of the positive direct associations remained when considering average pregnancy intake and anthropometric measures at birth.

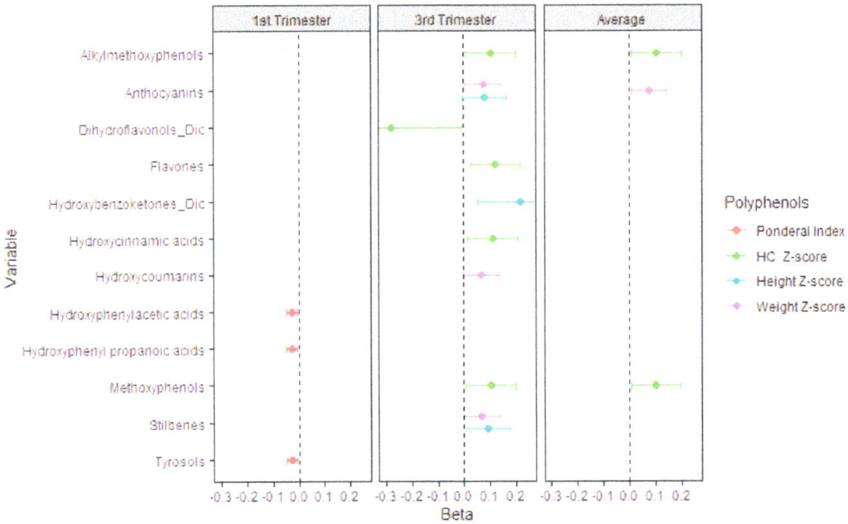

Figure 3. Associations between intake of polyphenols by subfamilies during pregnancy and anthropometric measures at birth (only statistically significant associations are shown). GLM adjusted for height z-score (smoking, alcohol and repeat abortions); weight z-score (smoking, repeat abortions, maternal education and parity); head circumference (HC) z-score (smoking, mother's age, maternal, physical exercise, supplement intake, education and parity); and ponderal index (smoking, mother's age, maternal education and parity). Regression coefficients and 95% confidence intervals are presented. Figure presents the results of the models that had statistically significant effects.

4. Discussion

4.1. Validation and Reproducibility

In the current study, carried out in a population of healthy pregnant women in the south of Spain, the intake of total polyphenols was evaluated using various dietary assessment tools. Although the FFQ used is a valid and reproducible tool for assessing nutrients [38], it is essential to demonstrate its validity and reproducibility specifically for polyphenol intake. Although FFQs are widely used to estimate total polyphenol intake, only a few have been adequately validated [36,44]. Furthermore, finding validated tools specifically for estimating polyphenol intake in pregnant women poses additional challenges [30]. Our study included correlation coefficients, percentages of LOA, and the percentage of agreement by quintiles (as shown in Tables 2 and 3). The results obtained were comparable to the values observed for the validation of other nutrients [38]. Similarly to the validation of different macro and micronutrients, the correlation coefficients for validation analysis of polyphenol intake were low, while the rest of the statistical tests yielded optimal results. These correlation coefficients were comparable to those reported by other studies that validated different FFQ in pregnant women [45]. Interestingly, the reproducibility analysis revealed higher correlation coefficients than those obtained from the validation (Tables 2 and 3). This is consistent with the findings of other FFQ validation and reproducibility studies. Overall, the results indicate an acceptable level of validity and high reproducibility for all food groups and polyphenol intakes during pregnancy. This was evidenced by a percentage of agreement by quintiles higher than 60% and LOA exceeding 90% in both cases that was consistent with other studies [17,29]. Therefore, the use of this FFQ represents a valuable tool for the estimation of polyphenol intake during pregnancy.

4.2. Polyphenol Intake

The total consumption of polyphenols, around 2 g/day, is consistent with findings from other studies [12,44,46,47]. In the present study, statistically significant differences were observed between total polyphenol intakes obtained by the FFQ and 24-h dietary recalls for vegetables, spices and infusions, legumes, nuts, processed foods and oils (Table 2). The FFQ revealed higher contributions from legumes, while the 24-h diet recall indicated greater contributions from spices and infusions. These discrepancies underscore the importance of detailed recording to accurately assess the true contribution of polyphenols from certain foods such as spices and infusions [48], which gives consistency to the results found. Given that FFQs often inadequately cover spice and infusion food groups, the current trend involves incorporating them into new FFQs that are undergoing validation [49].

Looking closely at the data from our study, foods with the highest dietary polyphenol content were also identified as sources of polyphenols in other studies [50,51]. Among populations with the highest polyphenol intake, legumes were the primary food group contributing to daily polyphenol intake. Recent studies have emphasised the significant role of legumes, accounting for up to 32% of total dietary polyphenol intake [52]. Cocoa and chocolate were additional sources of polyphenol intake in women of the GENEIDA cohort, aligning with findings from previous studies [53].

When comparing the average intake of food groups during the first and third trimesters of pregnancy, a general decrease in consumption across various foods was observed. Specifically, there was a lower intake of processed foods, chocolate, coffee and alcoholic beverages. Such a decrease may be attributed to heightened awareness of maintaining a healthy diet during pregnancy [54].

Flavonoids, phenolic acids and lignans were the families that contributed most to daily polyphenol intake, as also reported by previous studies [11,55]. Similar results were found for the subfamilies of phenolic compounds [11,56].

The limited data available on polyphenol consumption in pregnant women make comparisons difficult. In a comprehensive cohort study involving 120 pregnant Brazilian women, the average polyphenol intake was 1048 $\pm$ 362 mg/day [30]. This amount is similar to the sum of the concentrations of individual polyphenol subfamilies found in our study, although both exceeded the levels reported for pregnant women in China [57]. Additionally, a study validating an FFQ in the general population (aged 20–60 years) revealed polyphenol intake similar to that observed in the GENEIDA cohort (2111 mg/day) [58].

Polyphenol intakes among European women vary between 653 and 1552 mg per day [25]. For example, the cohort of women in the HAPIEE (Health, Alcohol and Psychosocial factors In Eastern Europe) had an average polyphenol intake of 1726 $\pm$ 662 mg/day [59]. In the GENEIDA cohort, fruits, vegetables and cocoa products were major contributors to daily polyphenol intake. There are notable differences in the consumption of polyphenols between different parts of the world. These variations may stem from differences in population characteristics, dietary behaviours, or the tools and databases employed to assess food intake [59].

Most academic sources evaluate polyphenol intake based on individual polyphenols or families, but few combine the results to estimate total intake, which may provide a less realistic estimate [56]. Furthermore, it is important to consider the databases used because although some researchers prefer to use their individual databases, Phenol-Explorer tends to be one of the most commonly used options [60,61]. Despite Phenol-Explorer being one of the most widely used approaches, polyphenol content databases have limitations and may underestimate intake. The MTPI was devised for this reason, aiming to supplement overall values rather than merely summing up individual polyphenols. A clear example of daily polyphenol intake in the Spanish population illustrates this variation. Records show values ranging from 671 mg/day [25] to as high as 2590–3016 mg/day [37]. The difference lies in whether the approximations include extractable or non-extractable polyphenols, which depends on the dietary records and databases used.

4.3. Relationship between Prenatal Polyphenol Intake and Birth Anthropometry and Foetal Development

Some studies suggest that a high intake of polyphenols may impair foetal development and contribute to different problems such as low birth weight [19–21,23,26–29,31–35]. These studies are based on the properties of polyphenols similar to anti-inflammatory drugs, which may be harmful during foetal development by interacting with the foetal ductus arteriosus [32].

The ductus arteriosus is an essential structure in foetal circulation, connecting the pulmonary artery with the aortic arch during foetal life. It begins to close within the first hours after birth, becoming part of the adult circulation pattern by 72 h [28]. Foetal ductus arteriosus constriction is a clinical disorder caused by inhibition of the prostaglandin synthesis pathway, and has long been associated with maternal intake of nonsteroidal anti-inflammatory drugs in late pregnancy [32]. Over the years, researchers have studied the potential association between polyphenol intake and constriction of the foetal ductus arteriosus, which, although rare, is a condition often considered idiopathic [32]. The effects of polyphenols on ductal dynamics have been well documented in animal studies [35], and include reduced litter size, foetal head circumference and foetal abdominal circumference in mice [27]. Evidence from several studies supports a cause–effect relationship between maternal consumption of polyphenol-rich substances (such as herbal teas, orange and grape juice, chocolate and cocoa) and constriction of the foetal ductus arteriosus [23,28,31,33–35]. Recommendations to prevent foetal ductal constriction during the third trimester of pregnancy have been subject to debate, and include possible dietary modifications to reduce tea, chocolate or cocoa consumption [28]. As part of these guidelines, a low-polyphenol diet has been proposed for women with foetal ductal constriction. Notably, the majority of foetuses receiving this dietary intervention showed reversal after a three-week period of low-polyphenol intake, suggesting the effectiveness of this intervention [23,31,33].

Similar ductal problems have been identified [19]. For example, cases of premature closure of the ductus arteriosus have been associated with maternal consumption of functional foods with high anthocyanin content [29], or excessive tea consumption [26]. After identifying possible causes, pregnant women were advised to reduce the consumption of these foods and, at the end of the dietary intervention, a progressive improvement of ductal constriction was observed [26]. Furthermore, other harmful consequences have been documented, including an increased likelihood of neural tube defects in a Chinese population that regularly consumed tea [62].

However, there is certain discordance, as other studies found no significant harmful effects after conducting similar research. Despite high levels of hydroxytyrosol supplementation in pigs, no effect on ductus arteriosus constriction was observed during pregnancy [15,63]. On the other hand, certain studies have shown beneficial effects for pregnant women, including improvements in blood pressure and reductions in gestational diabetes [3,57].

In this study, the intake of polyphenols in the GENEIDA cohort was estimated to evaluate whether the intake of these chemical species is associated with anthropometric measures at birth. Results indicate that foetal growth can be influenced by certain types of polyphenols in varying ways, and the observed trends underscore the importance of considering not only the total intake of polyphenols but also the specific types consumed. This approach is consistent with the fact that polyphenols can function as both antioxidants and pro-oxidants, depending on their structure and concentration [24].

The findings of our study indicate that the effect of polyphenols on pregnancy varies not only with the specific type of polyphenol, but also with the trimester of pregnancy during which exposure occurs (Supplementary File S2). This suggests that the physiological changes occurring in the mother throughout pregnancy may influence how different polyphenol structures affect the course of pregnancy and foetal development.

Despite the results obtained, further research is needed to explore the effect of polyphenols on foetal development, as suggested by other studies [22], especially by studying specific subfamilies [21,24]. In light of the results obtained, it is possible to see how families of polyphenols such as tyrosol or other polyphenols can have certain negative associations with anthropometric parameters at birth. Similarly, this phenomenon can be observed within certain subfamilies, such as certain phenolic acids. On the other hand, our study indicates that lignans can significantly affect anthropometric parameters in a positive manner. Our results are also consistent with previous studies that have found beneficial effects of lignans intake in pregnant women [64]. However, other studies have examined the oestrogenic effects of these compounds and their potential impact on pregnancy, highlighting the need for further studies to ensure their safety [65]. For these reasons, precaution should be taken during the latter stages of pregnancy, when it is advisable to limit the consumption of foods rich in polyphenols. For instance, in Brazil, guidelines for foetal cardiovascular health recommend limiting the intake of foods with a high polyphenol content during the last three months of pregnancy [28].

The significance of this issue lies in the fact that numerous dietary supplements and nutraceuticals currently consumed contain high levels of polyphenols. For instance, individuals who take supplements may consume up to 100 times more polyphenols daily [18]. While this heightened intake could be beneficial for health, some harmful effects may occur during specific life stages, such as pregnancy. Hence, careful control of polyphenol intake during gestation is necessary.

4.4. Strengths and Limitations of the Present Study

While the FFQ may overestimate dietary polyphenol intake, it is important to note that our results were estimated from a large population-based cohort of pregnant women. Additionally, the validity and reproducibility of the tools used for assessing polyphenol intake are important aspects to consider. Limitations of using databases should also be considered; although Phenol-Explorer is widely used at present, perhaps the inclusion of additional information could complete the results. Despite the remarkable results obtained, the associations found, although significant, remain somewhat inconclusive. This study is one of the few to date that highlight the importance of distinguishing between the various types of polyphenols when making recommendations of dietary restrictions during pregnancy, as some of them may be beneficial for foetal development while others may have adverse effects.

5. Conclusions

This study highlights the importance of comprehensively evaluating polyphenol intake during pregnancy, due to its impact on anthropometric measurements at birth. The results indicate that a validated FFQ can be an effective and reliable tool for estimating polyphenol consumption in pregnant women. In the GENEIDA cohort, legumes, fruits, vegetables, chocolate and coffee were the primary dietary sources of total polyphenols. The findings suggest that the intake of different polyphenol families and subfamilies may have diverse effects on foetal development. Some polyphenols may have beneficial effects, while others could be harmful. This underscores the importance of considering not only the overall quantity of polyphenols consumed, but also the specific classes of polyphenols ingested. Further research is required to elucidate the impact of individual polyphenol intake on maternal and foetal health during pregnancy.

These findings are crucial for the formulation of more precise dietary guidelines and recommendations during pregnancy to ensure optimal neonatal development.

Supplementary Materials: The following supporting information can be downloaded at https://www.mdpi.com/article/10.3390/nu16183096/s1: Supplementary File S1: Results by subfamily of phenolic compounds; Supplementary File S2: Bivariate and multivariate GLM.

Author Contributions: Conceptualisation, D.H.-N., D.R.-M., S.P.d.l.C., M.L. and J.Á.R.-H.; methodology, D.H.-N., D.R.-M., B.G.-A., A.F.H., S.P.d.l.C. and M.L.; software, D.H.-N. and D.R.-M.; data curation, D.R.-M., B.G.-A., M.J.G.-A., A.F.H., B.N.-P., A.D.-O., A.G.-M. and S.P.-B.; writing—original draft preparation, D.H.-N.; writing—review and editing, D.R.-M., M.L. and J.Á.R.-H.; visualisation, D.H.-N. and D.R.-M.; supervision, M.L. and J.Á.R.-H.; funding acquisition, M.L. All authors have read and agreed to the published version of the manuscript.

Funding: This research was funded by the Institute of Health Carlos III (PI13/01559), including The European Regional Development Fund (FEDER). Regional Health Council of Andalusia (Spain) (PI-045-2014). This manuscript was also supported by the Plan propio de Investigación y Transferencia of the University of Granada under the programme "Intensificación de la Investigación, modalidad B".

Institutional Review Board Statement: The study was conducted in accordance with the Declaration of Helsinki, and approved by the Biomedical Research Ethics Committee of Andalusia (25 November 2014).

Informed Consent Statement: Informed consent was obtained from all subjects involved in the study.

Data Availability Statement: The data presented in this study are available on request from the corresponding author. The data are not publicly available due to confidentiality concerns.

Acknowledgments: We gratefully acknowledge the contribution of health care staff of the Poniente University Hospital, and women participating in the GENEIDA project, without whom this study would not have been possible.

Conflicts of Interest: The authors declare no conflicts of interest.

References

1. Loy, S.-L.; Marhazlina, M.; Nor Azwany, Y.; Hamid Jan, J.M. Higher Intake of Fruits and Vegetables in Pregnancy Is Associated with Birth Size. *Southeast Asian J. Trop. Med. Public Health* **2011**, *42*, 1214. [PubMed]
2. Tovar, A.; Kaar, J.L.; McCurdy, K.; Field, A.E.; Dabelea, D.; Vadiveloo, M. Maternal Vegetable Intake during and after Pregnancy. *BMC Pregnancy Childbirth* **2019**, *19*, 267. [CrossRef] [PubMed]
3. Santangelo, C.; Varì, R.; Scazzocchio, B.; Filesi, C.; Masella, R. Management of Reproduction and Pregnancy Complications in Maternal Obesity: Which Role for Dietary Polyphenols? *Biofactors* **2014**, *40*, 79–102. [CrossRef] [PubMed]
4. Simmons, K.; Meloncelli, N.; Kearney, L.; Maher, J. Low Vegetable Intake in Pregnancy and Associated Maternal Factors: A Scoping Review. *Nutr. Res.* **2022**, *99*, 78–97. [CrossRef] [PubMed]
5. Manach, C.; Williamson, G.; Morand, C.; Scalbert, A.; Rémésy, C. Bioavailability and Bioefficacy of Polyphenols in Humans. I. Review of 97 Bioavailability Studies. *Am. J. Clin. Nutr.* **2005**, *81*, 230S–242S. [CrossRef]
6. Neveu, V.; Perez-Jiménez, J.; Vos, F.; Crespy, V.; du Chaffaut, L.; Mennen, L.; Knox, C.; Eisner, R.; Cruz, J.; Wishart, D. Phenol-Explorer: An Online Comprehensive Database on Polyphenol Contents in Foods. *Database* **2010**, *2010*, bap024. [CrossRef]
7. Rothwell, J.A.; Urpi-Sarda, M.; Boto-Ordonez, M.; Knox, C.; Llorach, R.; Eisner, R.; Cruz, J.; Neveu, V.; Wishart, D.; Manach, C. Phenol-Explorer 2.0: A Major Update of the Phenol-Explorer Database Integrating Data on Polyphenol Metabolism and Pharmacokinetics in Humans and Experimental Animals. *Database* **2012**, *2012*, bas031. [CrossRef]
8. Rothwell, J.A.; Perez-Jimenez, J.; Neveu, V.; Medina-Remon, A.; M'hiri, N.; García-Lobato, P.; Manach, C.; Knox, C.; Eisner, R.; Wishart, D.S. Phenol-Explorer 3.0: A Major Update of the Phenol-Explorer Database to Incorporate Data on the Effects of Food Processing on Polyphenol Content. *Database* **2013**, *2013*, bat070. [CrossRef]
9. Nacka-Aleksić, M.; Pirković, A.; Vilotić, A.; Bojić-Trbojević, Ž.; Jovanović Krivokuća, M.; Giampieri, F.; Battino, M.; Dekanski, D. The Role of Dietary Polyphenols in Pregnancy and Pregnancy-Related Disorders. *Nutrients* **2022**, *14*, 5246. [CrossRef]
10. Scalbert, A.; Manach, C.; Morand, C.; Rémésy, C.; Jiménez, L. Dietary Polyphenols and the Prevention of Diseases. *Crit. Rev. Food Sci. Nutr.* **2005**, *45*, 287–306. [CrossRef]
11. Coletro, H.N.; Bressan, J.; Diniz, A.P.; Hermsdorff, H.H.M.; Pimenta, A.M.; Meireles, A.L.; Mendonca, R.d.D.; Carraro, J.C.C. Total Polyphenol Intake, Polyphenol Subtypes, and Prevalence of Hypertension in the CUME Cohort. *J. Am. Coll. Nutr.* **2023**, *42*, 15–26. [CrossRef] [PubMed]
12. Condezo-Hoyos, L.; Gazi, C.; Pérez-Jiménez, J. Design of Polyphenol-Rich Diets in Clinical Trials: A Systematic Review. *Food Res. Int.* **2021**, *149*, 110655. [CrossRef] [PubMed]
13. Cory, H.; Passarelli, S.; Szeto, J.; Tamez, M.; Mattei, J. The Role of Polyphenols in Human Health and Food Systems: A Mini-Review. *Front. Nutr.* **2018**, *5*, 87. [CrossRef] [PubMed]
14. Delgado, A.M.; Issaoui, M.; Chammem, N. Analysis of Main and Healthy Phenolic Compounds in Foods. *J. AOAC Int.* **2019**, *102*, 1356–1364. [CrossRef] [PubMed]
15. Hahn, M.; Baierle, M.; Charão, M.F.; Bubols, G.B.; Gravina, F.S.; Zielinsky, P.; Arbo, M.D.; Cristina Garcia, S. Polyphenol-Rich Food General and on Pregnancy Effects: A Review. *Drug Chem. Toxicol.* **2017**, *40*, 368–374. [CrossRef]
16. Martín, M.A.; Goya, L.; de Pascual-Teresa, S. Effect of Cocoa and Cocoa Products on Cognitive Performance in Young Adults. *Nutrients* **2020**, *12*, 3691. [CrossRef]

17. Mori, N.; Sawada, N.; Ishihara, J.; Kotemori, A.; Takachi, R.; Murai, U.; Kobori, M.; Tsugane, S. Validity of a Food Frequency Questionnaire for the Estimation of Total Polyphenol Intake Estimates and Its Major Food Sources in the Japanese Population: The JPHC FFQ Validation Study. *J. Nutr. Sci.* **2021**, *10*, e35. [CrossRef]
18. Ly, C.; Yockell-Lelievre, J.; Ferraro, Z.M.; Arnason, J.T.; Ferrier, J.; Gruslin, A. The Effects of Dietary Polyphenols on Reproductive Health and Early Development. *Hum. Reprod. Update* **2014**, *21*, 228–248. [CrossRef]
19. Navarrete-Muñoz, E.M.; Valera-Gran, D.; Garcia-de-la-Hera, M.; Gonzalez-Palacios, S.; Riaño, I.; Murcia, M.; Lertxundi, A.; Guxens, M.; Tardón, A.; Amiano, P. High Doses of Folic Acid in the Periconceptional Period and Risk of Low Weight for Gestational Age at Birth in a Population Based Cohort Study. *Eur. J. Nutr.* **2019**, *58*, 241–251. [CrossRef]
20. Ono, K.; Nitta, A.; Tanaka, S.; Shiraishi, M.; Mizutani, A.; Matsubara, T. A Case of Premature Constriction of the Ductus Arteriosus in an Infant Caused by Intake of Rooibos Tea during Pregnancy. *Dokkyo Med. J.* **2022**, *1*, 72–75. [CrossRef]
21. Sinha, M.; Sachan, D.K.; Bhattacharya, R.; Singh, P.; Parthasarathi, R. ToxDP2 Database: Toxicity Prediction of Dietary Polyphenols. *Food Chem.* **2022**, *370*, 131350. [CrossRef] [PubMed]
22. Tresserra-Rimbau, A.; Lamuela-Raventos, R.M.; Moreno, J.J. Polyphenols, Food and Pharma. Current Knowledge and Directions for Future Research. *Biochem. Pharmacol.* **2018**, *156*, 186–195. [CrossRef] [PubMed]
23. Zielinsky, P.; Piccoli, A.L., Jr.; Vian, I.; Zílio, A.M.; Naujorks, A.A.; Nicoloso, L.H.; Barbisan, C.W.; Busato, S.; Lopes, M.; Klein, C. Maternal Restriction of Polyphenols and Fetal Ductal Dynamics in Normal Pregnancy: An Open Clinical Trial. *Arq. Bras. Cardiol.* **2013**, *101*, 217–225. [CrossRef] [PubMed]
24. Granato, D.; Mocan, A.; Câmara, J.S. Is a Higher Ingestion of Phenolic Compounds the Best Dietary Strategy? A Scientific Opinion on the Deleterious Effects of Polyphenols in Vivo. *Trends Food Sci. Technol.* **2020**, *98*, 162–166. [CrossRef]
25. Zamora-Ros, R.; Cayssials, V.; Jenab, M.; Rothwell, J.A.; Fedirko, V.; Aleksandrova, K.; Tjønneland, A.; Kyrø, C.; Overvad, K.; Boutron-Ruault, M.-C. Dietary Intake of Total Polyphenol and Polyphenol Classes and the Risk of Colorectal Cancer in the European Prospective Investigation into Cancer and Nutrition (EPIC) Cohort. *Eur. J. Epidemiol.* **2018**, *33*, 1063–1075. [CrossRef]
26. Costa, V.; Carriço, A.; Valente, F. Constricción Prematura Del Ductus Arterioso: Consecuencias Del Consumo Excesivo de Té Negro y de Hierbas. *Prog. Obstet. Ginecol.* **2013**, *56*, 144–146. [CrossRef]
27. Finn-Sell, S.L.; Cottrell, E.C.; Greenwood, S.L.; Dilworth, M.R.; Cowley, E.J.; Sibley, C.P.; Wareing, M. Pomegranate Juice Supplementation Alters Utero-Placental Vascular Function and Fetal Growth in the eNOS−/− Mouse Model of Fetal Growth Restriction. *Front. Physiol.* **2018**, *9*, 1145. [CrossRef]
28. Pedra, S.R.; Zielinsky, P.; Binotto, C.N.; Martins, C.N.; da Fonseca, E.S.V.B.; Guimarães, I.C.B.; Corrêa, I.V.d.S.; Pedrosa, K.L.M.; Lopes, L.M.; Nicoloso, L.H.S. Brazilian Fetal Cardiology Guidelines-2019. *Arq. Bras. Cardiol.* **2019**, *112*, 600–648. [CrossRef]
29. Tanaka, M.; Miyakoshi, K.; Yamada, M.; Kadohira, I.; Minegishi, K.; Yoshimura, Y. Functional Foods for the Fetus? *Acta Obstet. Gynecol. Scand.* **2011**, *90*, 1172–1173. [CrossRef]
30. Vian, I.; Zielinsky, P.; Zilio, A.M.; Mello, A.; Lazzeri, B.; Oliveira, A.; Lampert, K.V.; Piccoli, A.; Nicoloso, L.H.; Bubols, G.B. Development and Validation of a Food Frequency Questionnaire for Consumption of Polyphenol-Rich Foods in Pregnant Women. *Matern. Child. Nutr.* **2015**, *11*, 511–524. [CrossRef]
31. Zielinsky, P.; Manica, J.; Piccoli Jr, A.; Areias, J.; Nicoloso, L.; Menezes, H.; Frajndlich, R.; Busato, A.; Petracco, R.; Hagemann, L. OP18. 03: Experimental Study of the Role of Maternal Consumption of Green Tea, Mate Tea and Grape Juice on Fetal Ductal Constriction. *Ultrasound Obstet. Gynecol.* **2007**, *30*, 515. [CrossRef]
32. Zielinsky, P.; Piccoli, A.L.; Manica, J.L.L.; Nicoloso, L.H.S. New Insights on Fetal Ductal Constriction: Role of Maternal Ingestion of Polyphenol-Rich Foods. *Expert Rev. Cardiovasc. Ther.* **2010**, *8*, 291–298. [CrossRef]
33. Zielinsky, P.; Piccoli, A.; Manica, J.; Nicoloso, L.; Vian, I.; Bender, L.; Pizzato, P.; Pizzato, M.; Swarowsky, F.; Barbisan, C. Reversal of Fetal Ductal Constriction after Maternal Restriction of Polyphenol-Rich Foods: An Open Clinical Trial. *J. Perinatol.* **2012**, *32*, 574–579. [CrossRef] [PubMed]
34. Zielinsky, P.; Martignoni, F.V.; Vian, I. Deleterious Effects of Maternal Ingestion of Cocoa upon Fetal Ductus Arteriosus in Late Pregnancy. *Front. Pharmacol.* **2014**, *5*, 281. [CrossRef] [PubMed]
35. Zielinsky, P.; Busato, S. Prenatal Effects of Maternal Consumption of Polyphenol-rich Foods in Late Pregnancy upon Fetal Ductus Arteriosus. *Birth Defects Res. Part C Embryo Today Rev.* **2013**, *99*, 256–274. [CrossRef]
36. Burkholder-Cooley, N.M.; Rajaram, S.S.; Haddad, E.H.; Oda, K.; Fraser, G.E.; Jaceldo-Siegl, K. Validating Polyphenol Intake Estimates from a Food-Frequency Questionnaire by Using Repeated 24-h Dietary Recalls and a Unique Method-of-Triads Approach with 2 Biomarkers–3. *Am. J. Clin. Nutr.* **2017**, *105*, 685–694. [CrossRef]
37. Saura-Calixto, F.; Serrano, J.; Goni, I. Intake and Bioaccessibility of Total Polyphenols in a Whole Diet. *Food Chem.* **2007**, *101*, 492–501. [CrossRef]
38. Hinojosa-Nogueira, D.; Romero-Molina, D.; Giménez-Asensio, M.J.; Gonzalez-Alzaga, B.; Lopéz-Flores, I.; de la Cueva, S.P.; Rufián-Henares, J.Á.; Hernández, A.F.; Lacasaña, M. Validity and Reproducibility of a Food Frequency Questionnaire to Assess Nutrients Intake of Pregnant Women in the South-East of Spain. *Nutrients* **2021**, *13*, 3032. [CrossRef]
39. Hinojosa-Nogueira, D.; Pérez-Burillo, S.; García-Rincón, I.; Rufián-Henares, J.A.; Pastoriza, S. A Useful and Simple Tool to Evaluate and Compare the Intake of Total Dietary Polyphenols in Different Populations. *Public Health Nutr.* **2021**, *24*, 3818–3824. [CrossRef]
40. De Onis, M.; Habicht, J.-P. Anthropometric Reference Data for International Use: Recommendations from a World Health Organization Expert Committee. *Am. J. Clin. Nutr.* **1996**, *64*, 650–658. [CrossRef]

41. Lourenção, L.F.d.P.; de Paula, N.C.; Cardoso, M.A.; Santos, P.R.; de Oliveira, I.R.C.; Fonseca, F.L.A.; da Veiga, G.L.; Alves, B.d.C.A.; Graciano, M.M.d.C.; Pereira-Dourado, S.M. Biochemical Markers and Anthropometric Profile of Children Enrolled in Public Daycare Centers. *J. Pediatr.* **2022**, *98*, 390–398. [CrossRef] [PubMed]
42. World Health Organization. *Physical Status: The Use of and Interpretation of Anthropometry, Report of a WHO Expert Committee*; World Health Organization: Geneva, Switzerland, 1995; ISBN 92-4-120854-6.
43. Gimenez-Asensio, M.J.; Hernandez, A.F.; Romero-Molina, D.; Gonzalez-Alzaga, B.; Luzardo, O.P.; Henríquez-Hernández, L.A.; Boada, L.D.; García-Cortés, H.; Lopez-Flores, I.; Sanchez-Piedra, M.D.; et al. Effect of Prenatal Exposure to Organophosphates and Pyrethroid Pesticides on Neonatal Anthropometric Measures and Gestational Age. *Environ. Res.* **2023**, *232*, 116410. [CrossRef] [PubMed]
44. Hoge, A.; Guillaume, M.; Albert, A.; Tabart, J.; Dardenne, N.; Donneau, A.-F.; Kevers, C.; Defraigne, J.-O.; Pincemail, J. Validation of a Food Frequency Questionnaire Assessing Dietary Polyphenol Exposure Using the Method of Triads. *Free Radic. Biol. Med.* **2019**, *130*, 189–195. [CrossRef]
45. Ogawa, K.; Jwa, S.-C.; Kobayashi, M.; Morisaki, N.; Sago, H.; Fujiwara, T. Validation of a Food Frequency Questionnaire for Japanese Pregnant Women with and without Nausea and Vomiting in Early Pregnancy. *J. Epidemiol.* **2017**, *27*, 201–208. [CrossRef] [PubMed]
46. Aali, Y.; Ebrahimi, S.; Shiraseb, F.; Mirzaei, K. The Association between Dietary Polyphenol Intake and Cardiometabolic Factors in Overweight and Obese Women: A Cross-Sectional Study. *BMC Endocr. Disord.* **2022**, *22*, 120. [CrossRef]
47. Shahar, S.; Lin, C.H.; Haron, H. Development and Validation of Food Frequency Questionnaire (FFQ) for Estimation of the Dietary Polyphenol Intake among Elderly Individuals in Klang Valley. *Malays. J. Health Sci.* **2014**, *12*, 33–39.
48. Opara, E.I.; Chohan, M. Culinary Herbs and Spices: Their Bioactive Properties, the Contribution of Polyphenols and the Challenges in Deducing Their True Health Benefits. *Int. J. Mol. Sci.* **2014**, *15*, 19183–19202. [CrossRef]
49. Madani, Z.; Javardi, M.S.M.; Karandish, M.; Movahedi, A. Promoting and Updating Food Frequency Questionnaire Tool to Measure Food Consumption and Nutrient Intake Analysis. *Int. J. Prev. Med.* **2021**, *12*, 165.
50. Pinto, P.; Cardoso, S.; Pimpao, R.C.; Tavares, L.; Ferreira, R.B.; Santos, C.N. Daily Polyphenol Intake from Fresh Fruits in Portugal: Contribution from Berry Fruits. *Int. J. Food Sci. Nutr.* **2013**, *64*, 1022–1029. [CrossRef]
51. Perez-Jimenez, J.; Fezeu, L.; Touvier, M.; Arnault, N.; Manach, C.; Hercberg, S.; Galan, P.; Scalbert, A. Dietary Intake of 337 Polyphenols in French Adults. *Am. J. Clin. Nutr.* **2011**, *93*, 1220–1228. [CrossRef]
52. Nascimento-Souza, M.A.; de Paiva, P.G.; Pérez-Jiménez, J.; Franceschini, S.d.C.C.; Ribeiro, A.Q. Estimated Dietary Intake and Major Food Sources of Polyphenols in Elderly of Viçosa, Brazil: A Population-Based Study. *Eur. J. Nutr.* **2018**, *57*, 617–627. [CrossRef] [PubMed]
53. Wisnuwardani, R.W.; De Henauw, S.; Androutsos, O.; Forsner, M.; Gottrand, F.; Huybrechts, I.; Knaze, V.; Kersting, M.; Le Donne, C.; Marcos, A. Estimated Dietary Intake of Polyphenols in European Adolescents: The HELENA Study. *Eur. J. Nutr.* **2018**, *58*, 2345–2363. [CrossRef] [PubMed]
54. Alabduljabbar, S.; Zaidan, S.A.; Lakshmanan, A.P.; Terranegra, A. Personalized Nutrition Approach in Pregnancy and Early Life to Tackle Childhood and Adult Non-Communicable Diseases. *Life* **2021**, *11*, 467. [CrossRef]
55. Pounis, G.; Di Castelnuovo, A.; Bonaccio, M.; Costanzo, S.; Persichillo, M.; Krogh, V.; Donati, M.B.; De Gaetano, G.; Iacoviello, L. Flavonoid and Lignan Intake in a Mediterranean Population: Proposal for a Holistic Approach in Polyphenol Dietary Analysis, the Moli-Sani Study. *Eur. J. Clin. Nutr.* **2016**, *70*, 338–345. [CrossRef]
56. Yahya, H.M.; Day, A.; Lawton, C.; Myrissa, K.; Croden, F.; Dye, L.; Williamson, G. Dietary Intake of 20 Polyphenol Subclasses in a Cohort of UK Women. *Eur. J. Nutr.* **2016**, *55*, 1839–1847. [CrossRef] [PubMed]
57. Gao, Q.; Zhong, C.; Zhou, X.; Chen, R.; Xiong, T.; Hong, M.; Li, Q.; Kong, M.; Xiong, G.; Han, W. Inverse Association of Total Polyphenols and Flavonoids Intake and the Intake from Fruits with the Risk of Gestational Diabetes Mellitus: A Prospective Cohort Study. *Clin. Nutr.* **2021**, *40*, 550–559. [CrossRef]
58. Hoge, A.; Guillaume, M.; Donneau, A.-F.; Albert, A.; Cheramy-Bien, J.-P.; Tabart, J.; Kevers, C.; Dommes, J.; Defraigne, J.-O.; Pincemail, J. Validation Study of a Food Frequency Questionnaire for the Measurement of Food Consumption in Polyphenols: Use of a Urinary Bioamarker. Preliminary Results. *Free Radic. Biol. Med.* **2017**, *108*, S40. [CrossRef]
59. Grosso, G.; Stepaniak, U.; Topor-Mądry, R.; Szafraniec, K.; Pająk, A. Estimated Dietary Intake and Major Food Sources of Polyphenols in the Polish Arm of the HAPIEE Study. *Nutrition* **2014**, *30*, 1398–1403. [CrossRef]
60. Bondonno, N.P.; Murray, K.; Bondonno, C.P.; Lewis, J.R.; Croft, K.D.; Kyrø, C.; Gislason, G.; Tjønneland, A.; Scalbert, A.; Cassidy, A.; et al. Flavonoid Intake and Its Association with Atrial Fibrillation. *Clin. Nutr.* **2020**, *39*, 3821–3828. [CrossRef]
61. Mérida, D.M.; Vitelli-Storelli, F.; Moreno-Franco, B.; Rodríguez-Ayala, M.; López-García, E.; Banegas, J.R.; Rodríguez-Artalejo, F.; Guallar-Castillón, P. Polyphenol Intake and Mortality: A Nationwide Cohort Study in the Adult Population of Spain. *Clin. Nutr.* **2023**, *42*, 1076–1085. [CrossRef]
62. Sridharan, S.; Archer, N.; Manning, N. Premature Constriction of the Fetal Ductus Arteriosus Following the Maternal Consumption of Camomile Herbal Tea. *Ultrasound Obstet. Gynecol.* **2009**, *34*, 358–359. [CrossRef] [PubMed]
63. Garcia-Contreras, C.; Vazquez-Gomez, M.; Barbero, A.; Pesantez, J.L.; Zinellu, A.; Berlinguer, F.; Gonzalez-Añover, P.; Gonzalez, J.; Encinas, T.; Torres-Rovira, L. Polyphenols and IUGR Pregnancies: Effects of Maternal Hydroxytyrosol Supplementation on Placental Gene Expression and Fetal Antioxidant Status, DNA-Methylation and Phenotype. *Int. J. Mol. Sci.* **2019**, *20*, 1187. [CrossRef] [PubMed]

64. Tang, R.; Chen, M.; Zhou, K.; Chen, D.; Yu, J.; Hu, W.; Song, L.; Hang, B.; Wang, X.; Xia, Y. Prenatal Lignan Exposures, Pregnancy Urine Estrogen Profiles and Birth Outcomes. *Environ. Pollut.* **2015**, *205*, 261–268. [CrossRef]
65. Li, J.; Ma, X.; Luo, L.; Tang, D.; Zhang, L. The What and Who of Dietary Lignans in Human Health: Special Attention to Estrogen Effects and Safety Evaluation. *J. Agric. Food Chem.* **2023**, *71*, 16419–16434. [CrossRef] [PubMed]

nutrients

MDPI

Article

Body Composition Analysis of the Clinical Routine Using Air Displacement Plethysmography: Age-Group-Specific Feasibility Analysis among Preterm Infants

Lennart A. Lücke [1,2], Niels Rochow [3,4,5,*], Katja Knab [3], Stefan Schäfer [3], Jasper L. Zimmermann [3], Anastasia Meis [3], Stephanie Lohmüller-Weiß [3], Adel Szakacs-Fusch [3], Ursula Felderhoff-Müser [6] and Christoph Fusch [3,7]

1 Department of Anaesthesiology and Intensive Care Medicine, Campus Charité Mitte und Charité Campus Virchow-Klinikum, Charité-Universitätsmedizin, 13353 Berlin, Germany; lennart-alexander.luecke@charite.de
2 Research Department of Child Nutrition, University Hospital of Pediatrics and Adolescent Medicine, St. Josef-Hospital, Ruhr University Bochum, 44791 Bochum, Germany
3 Department of Pediatrics, Paracelsus Medical University, Breslauer Str. 201, 90471 Nürnberg, Germany; christoph.fusch@klinikum-nuernberg.de (C.F.)
4 DeuZWEG German Center for Growth, Development and Health Encouragement during Childhood and Youth, 10249 Berlin, Germany
5 Department of Pediatrics, University Medicine Rostock, 18057 Rostock, Germany
6 Department of Pediatrics I, Neonatology, Pediatric Intensive Care, and Pediatric Neurology, University Hospital Essen, University of Duisburg-Essen, Hufelandstr. 55, 45147 Essen, Germany
7 Department of Pediatrics, McMaster University, Hamilton, ON L8S 4L8, Canada
* Correspondence: niels.rochow@klinikum-nuernberg.de; Tel.: +49-(0)-911-398-2307

Abstract: Body composition assessments using air displacement plethysmography (ADP, PEAPOD®) have been introduced into clinical practice at a few neonatal units. To allow accurate body composition assessments in term and preterm infants, a workflow for routine testing is needed. The aim of this study was to analyze the feasibility of weekly routine ADP testing. We analyzed (1) postnatal ages at first ADP assessment, (2) the number of weekly routine in-hospital assessments, and (3) the workload of body composition measurements using ADP in clinical practice on the basis of an retrospective analysis of our own clinical operating procedures. The retrospective analysis of weekly routine ADP testing proved feasible at Nuremberg Children's Hospital. The analysis of postnatal age at the first ADP test revealed differences across groups, with extremely preterm infants starting at a mean postmenstrual age of 36.6 weeks, very preterm infants starting at 34.2 weeks, and moderate to late preterm infants starting at 35.3 weeks. The mean number of tests before discharge was significantly greater in the extremely preterm group ($n = 3.0$) than in the very preterm ($n = 2.4$) and moderate to late preterm groups ($n = 1.7$). The workload of the procedure is reasonable, at 8–13 min per test cycle. The study proved that weekly routine ADP assessments in preterm infants are feasible. However, the initiation of routine testing in extremely preterm infants starts at a significantly greater postnatal age than in the more mature population. ADP assessments can be safely and easily integrated into clinical practice and may be valuable tools for providing additional information on nutritional status and infant growth. A standardized routine protocol allowing identical measurement conditions across healthcare institutions and a standardized interpretation tool for age-adapted body composition data, however, would improve comparability and usability.

Keywords: neonate; air–displacement plethysmography; body composition; lean mass; method analysis; clinical routine; standardization

1. Introduction

Preterm infants rely on optimum external nutritional management and feeding, whereas a healthy fetus in a healthy pregnancy stays in utero until term and receives adequate placental nutrition for the growth of body mass, organs, and particularly the brain. High survival rates and low neonatal morbidity have led to a focus on improving the quality of survival [1,2]. In preterm infants, an optimum body composition (fat and fat-free mass) is key to lowering the risk for chronic diseases later in life and negative neurodevelopmental outcomes. Both decreased and excessive fat mass increase the risk for metabolic and cardiovascular diseases [3–5]. A greater fat-free mass has been related to improved neurodevelopmental outcomes [6–8].

Establishing a framework for routine body composition analysis, interpretation, and nutritional intervention is a common goal in neonatal research to further improve the quality of survival [9]. Various methods, such as anthropometric measurements, bioelectrical impedance analysis, dual-energy X-ray absorptiometry, and air displacement plethysmography (ADP), have been used to evaluate body composition [10–12].

ADP is a promising, noninvasive, and radiation-free method for body composition analysis in clinical practice. This method has been validated by various studies [13–17] and has been suggested as the gold standard for routine body composition assessments in preterm and term-born infants [12]. An increasing number of centers have introduced regular ADP measurements and shared experiences for routine assessments in neonatal intensive care units (NICUs) [18,19].

These studies, however, have neither reported the feasibility of testing in clinical practice for differing age groups of preterm infants nor established standardized protocols for ADP testing in clinical practice. At the Children's University Hospital, Nuremberg, body composition measurements were introduced in 2019 into the clinical routine using ADP. To the best of our knowledge, this study is the first to analyze the feasibility of routine ADP assessments in preterm infants.

This study aimed to analyzed the following

- The feasibility of weekly routine ADP assessments for preterm infants;
- Preterm infants' readiness for first ADP testing across different gestational ages at birth and number of repeated tests during in-hospital routine;
- The workload of body composition measurements using ADP in clinical practice.

2. Materials and Methods

2.1. Study Design

This quality improvement study was performed from March to September 2021 at the neonatal Level III intensive care unit of the Children's Hospital at Nuremberg General Hospital, South Campus of Paracelsus Medical School of Nuremberg. The infants were evaluated for testing on the basis of the inclusion criteria (see Section 4.2) and selected from our REDCap NICU database for retrospective analysis [20,21]. Anonymized data were exported and accessed from October 2021 to December 2021.

Prior to the study, the standard operating procedure for ADP measurements was approved by our institutional review board (#SZ_D_028.21-IX-1). In accordance with German professional regulations for physicians, the present retrospective study did not require additional Ethics Committee approval because it was a quality improvement study, with all prior data being available on a routine basis and analyzed anonymously. In our NICU, parents and legal guardians of all our patients are, orally and in writing, informed about our standards of care and routine procedures, their indications, their nature, risks, and benefits. This information is documented by the physician and approved by the parents' signatures. The use of extended anthropometry by the ADP is included herein.

2.1.1. Nutrition

All infants were fed according to our local clinical guidelines [22]. In general, infants with a birth weight < 1000 g or born at a gestational age < 28 + 0/7 weeks were fed an exclusively human milk diet including a human milk-based fortifier and ready-to-feed milk (Humavant, Prolacta Bioscience Inc., Groot-Bijgaarden, Belgium) for the first 4 weeks after reaching full enteral feeding (150 mL/kg/d). Preterm infants with a gestational age of

28 + 1/7 to 33 + 6/7 weeks received their mother's own milk (MOM), which was targeted and bovine-fortified (Aptamil FMS, Danone GmbH, Frankfurt, Germany), or preterm formula at 80 kcal/100 mL (Aptamil Prematil, Danone GmbH, Frankfurt, Germany). Breastmilk analysis for target fortification was performed twice per week, and the macronutrient content was adjusted using modules to reach the ESPGHAN recommendations [12,17,18]. Infants born at a gestational age of 34 + 0/7 to 36 + 6/7 weeks received standard fortified MOM (Aptamil FMS, Danone GmbH, Frankfurt, Germany) or preterm formula at 73 kcal/100 mL (Aptamil PDF, Danone GmbH, Frankfurt, Germany). Term-born infants ($\geq$37 + 0/7) were fed MOM or term formula (Aptamil Pronutra Pre, Danone GmbH, Frankfurt, Germany).

2.1.2. Body Composition and Anthropometric Measurements

Body composition assessments were performed via ADP (PEAPOD, COSMED, Inc., Concord, CA, USA), and the details have been previously described [23,24]. ADP relies on a two-compartment model dividing the body into fat mass and fat-free mass on the basis of measured body density data. Body density was calculated from body volume and weight. Body weight was measured via an inbuilt PEAPOD scale. Body volume was calculated as the difference in the compressible air volume of the measuring chamber before and after the subject was placed in the chamber. The estimation of body volume relies on the main assumption that the density of fat mass is constant (0.9007 kg/L) and that the density of fat-free mass is dependent on gestational age. Reference data for fat mass and fat-free mass were obtained by Fomon et al. and Butte et al. [25,26]. Detailed information about the measurement procedure, technical information, and physical conditions of the device has been described elsewhere [23,27].

2.2. The Clinical Procedure at the Children's University Hospital Nuremberg

2.2.1. Inclusion Criteria and Testing Procedure

Weekly body composition measurements were conducted at a predefined time window between 8.30 a.m. and 11.00 a.m. ADP measurements were only performed in clinically stable infants, preferably on Tuesdays. The following inclusion criteria had to be met for eligibility: FiO_2 of 21%, no respiratory support, and no episodes of significant desaturation (SaO_2 < 85%) and/or bradycardia (<80/min) requiring stimulation within the last 48 h.

The measurements were performed in the following sequence: (i) body length via a length board, (ii) head circumference via nonstretchable tape, and (iii) body weight and body volume via PEAPOD. The PEAPOD is located in a designated room away from open windows, fans, or heating/cooling ducts to meet the criteria for test location presented in the PEAPOD operator manual (room temperature: 20–28 °C, humidity: 20–70%, pressure: 562–795 mmHg) [27]. The PEAPOD was not moved throughout the study period. The measurements were performed by trained research staff in the PEAPOD room, which was heated to a constant temperature of 26 °C. Body weight was measured to a resolution of 0.1 g via a digital scale integrated within the PEAPOD. The resolution of the length board (Infantometer Seca 416, Hamburg, Germany) and nonstretchable tape was 1 mm. The time required for a single PEAPOD measurement (time within the test chamber) is less than 3 min.

2.2.2. Testing Workflow

The ADP testing routine was developed on the basis of the operator's manual provided by the manufacturer of the PEAPOD and the previous experience of the research group with the PEAPOD at McMaster University, Hamilton, ON, Canada [28]. PEAPOD measurements were performed by at least two operators: one assigned to operate the PEAPOD (PEAPOD operating nurse) and one assigned to childcare (PEAPOD nurse). The following testing workflow was implemented:

1. Screening: One day prior to the test day, the study nurse screened all neonates in the units. On the test day, eligibility for testing was evaluated using inclusion and exclusion criteria (see Testing Procedure). The attending physician confirmed clinical

stability. A list of all infants to be tested on that day was provided to the unit to inform the bedside nurses which infants were being measured.

2. Preparation: The PEAPOD operating nurse was switched on the PEAPOD at least two hours before the first body composition assessment on the day to allow for system warm-up and equilibration. When tests started early in the day, the PEAPOD system was switched on the night before the test day. Automated volume calibration was started before each volume measurement. Manual system calibration was performed at the beginning of each test day. The results from the quality control tests were reviewed once a month.
3. Testing: The PEAPOD nurse transferred infants from the unit to the PEAPOD room after a final infant stability check-up was requested from the nurse at the unit. The infants were undressed prior to testing. Head circumference and length measurements were performed together by the PEAPOD operating nurse and the PEAPOD nurse. The PEAPOD measurements were coordinated and performed by the PEAPOD operating nurse. The detailed instructions for operating the PEAPOD device are described in the manual of the PEAPOD operator [27].
4. Body composition data: The PEAPOD operating nurse was responsible for obtaining and printing the body composition data. The results were visualized on individual body composition graphs and added to the patient's folder, which was accessible to the physicians, thus allowing interpretation of body composition data.
5. Responsible physicians evaluated body composition tests: However, no standardized recommendations for individual interventions based on body composition results have been published.

2.3. *Data Analysis*

Descriptive statistical analysis was performed. The subjects were grouped by GA at birth into "extremely preterm" (<28 weeks), "very preterm" (28–31 + 6/7 weeks), "moderate- and late preterm" (32–36 + 6/7 weeks), and "term" infants (≥37 weeks) [29]. Time stamps from the PEAPOD database were used to assess the duration per test. For statistical analysis, Microsoft Excel Professional Plus 2016, Microsoft Excel® Office 365 (Redmond, DC, USA) and IBM SPSS Statistics for Windows, Version 26.0 (Armonk, NY, USA) were used. Violin and boxplots were generated via GraphPad Prism version 6 for Windows (GraphPad Software, San Diego, CA, USA; www.graphpad).

3. Results

3.1. *Feasility and Infants' Readiness*

A total of n = 429 tests were performed for 260 subjects (n = 185 preterm and n = 85 term infants; Table 1). Over the course of the study period, a total of 206 preterm infants were born or admitted to our NICU, resulting in 89.8% of the infants being tested following routine clinical protocols. No adverse effects, such as infection, episodes of apnea or desaturation, were observed during the study period.

Table 1. Frequency of routine clinical PEAPOD assessments per gestational age (GA) group. Wk. – weeks, m – male, f – female, PMA – postmenstrual age in weeks, * = statistically significant difference between the GA groups ($p < 0.05$).

Groups per GA	Extremely Preterm; <28 wk.	Very Preterm; 28 to 31 + 6/7 wk.	Moderate and Late Preterm; 32 to 36 + 6/7 wk.	Term Infants; ≥37 wk.	All Subjects
Number of subjects (m/f)	14 (11/3)	28 (19/9)	143 (81/62)	75 (48/27)	260 (159/101)
Total number of tests	42	65	244	78	429
Mean GA (weeks)	26.3	30	34.4	39	33.6

Table 1. *Cont.*

Groups per GA	Extremely Preterm; <28 wk.	Very Preterm; 28 to 31 + 6/7 wk.	Moderate and Late Preterm; 32 to 36 + 6/7 wk.	Term Infants; ≥37 wk.	All Subjects
Week of life at first PEAPOD test	10.5 ± 3.2 *	4.4 ± 2.4 *	1 ± 0.7 *	0.7 ± 0.6 *	2.5
PMA at first PEAPOD test	36.6	34.2	35.3	39.9	35.5
Number of tests before discharge	3.1 ± 1.4 *	2.4 ± 1.4	1.7 ± 1.1	1.1 ± 0.2 *	1.65 ± 0.9

3.2. Weekly Routine Testing

Postnatal age at first ADP testing significantly differed between the groups. Measurements in the extremely preterm group could be initiated at 10.5 ± 3.2 weeks of life. This chronological age was significantly greater than that of the other three groups (very preterm: 4.4 ± 2.4 weeks, moderate and late preterm: 1 ± 0.7 weeks, and term infants: 0.7 ± 0.6 weeks, $p < 0.01$). The mean PMA at the first ADP test was highest in the extremely preterm group (36.6 ± 2.7 weeks). The mean PMAs of the very preterm and moderate-to-late preterm infants were 34.2 ± 1.9 and 35.3 ± 1.1 weeks, respectively (Table 1). The median PMA at the first test in the extremely preterm group was comparable to the median of the moderate–late preterm group (36 weeks). The median PMA at the first test in the very preterm group was comparable to that in the 1st quartile in the moderate–late preterm group (34 weeks, Figure 1). The mean number of tests before discharge was greater in the extremely preterm group (n = 3.1 ± 1.4) than in the very preterm (n = 2.4 ± 1.4), moderate-to-late preterm (n = 1.7 ± 1.1), and term groups (n = 1.1 ± 0.2; sig. $p < 0.01$; Table 1).

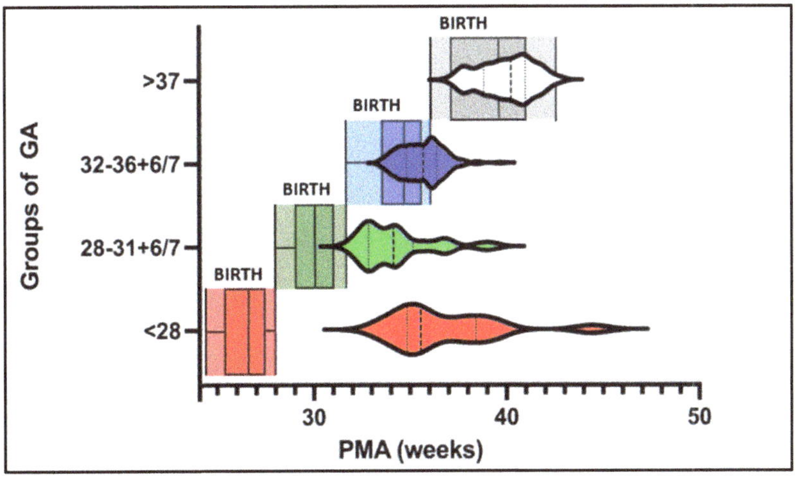

Figure 1. Distribution of gestational age at birth (GA, boxplot) and postmenstrual age (PMA; weeks, Violin plot) at first body composition measurement.

3.3. Personnel Requirements

The time per test was dependent on the number of staff available. When tests were performed by two operators (one PEAPOD nurse and one PEAPOD operating nurse), the time per full testing cycle was 13 ± 3 min. When body composition testing was performed by three operators (two PEAPOD nurses and one PEAPOD operating nurse), the required time per full testing cycle significantly decreased to 8 ± 0.6 min. The test frequency significantly increased due to the greater efficiency of transport between the neonatal unit and the PEAPOD room, as did the undressing and measuring of the subsequent child, with the actual ADP measurement still running.

Throughout the study period, a mean of twelve body composition assessments were performed on the weekly testing day. This corresponds to a weekly mean cumulative work time of 312 min with two operators (12.8 min × 12 tests × 2 operators) and 288 min with three operators (8 min × 12 tests × 3 operators).

4. Discussion

The retrospective analysis of the feasibility of routine ADP testing in preterm infants revealed positive results, with almost 90% of infants born at the Nuremberg NICU being tested during the study period. No adverse effects from routine testing were observed. The data revealed a later start of testing in extremely premature infants than in older infants. Longer hospitalizations of premature extremely premature infants resulted in a significantly greater number of repeated body composition tests. The required workload per routine ADP test was reasonable at 8–13 min, depending on the number of nurses available.

4.1. Feasibility of ADP Testing in Routine Clinical Practice

Our retrospective analysis demonstrated the potential of ADP to be successfully transferred from a research-only method to a standard clinical method and proposed that almost all clinically stable infants in the NICU can be successfully tested without adverse effects. While Bell et al. recommended using body composition assessment as a tool for routine clinical practice, Aljanini et al., similar to us, demonstrated the feasibility of introducing ADP into routine clinical practice [19].

The data indicate that during the study period, 89.8% of preterm infants admitted or born at our NICU underwent routine ADP assessments. A small fraction of the remaining 10.2% of infants who could not be assessed in a clinical setting were affected for three main reasons: (1) clinical instability, (2) nursing during scheduled assessment, and (3) early discharge or transfer to a different hospital.

4.2. Routine Testing

4.2.1. Postnatal Age at the First Test

Different institutions have recently implemented ADP assessments in clinical practice [18,19,24]. Although the clinical settings and assessment procedures were methodically described, they were neither retrospectively analyzed nor formulated as standardized protocols for routine assessment.

In our cohort, body composition measurements were initiated significantly later at a higher postmenstrual age in infants with a lower GA. This phenomenon is most likely due to the periods of clinical instability and prolonged respiratory support in the groups born extremely or very prematurely. Bruckner et al. reported similar findings. The first PEAPOD test was initiated at significantly greater postnatal ages in extremely preterm infants (days of life: 89 ± 28) than in very preterm infants (days of life: 39 ± 15) [30].

Our sample size (n = 429) is large enough to describe the feasibility of ADP assessments for different groups of premature infants. However, improved outcomes and earlier weaning of extremely preterm infants might allow earlier body composition assessment.

4.2.2. Repeated Testing

We demonstrated that the highest number of weekly body composition tests (n = 3) before discharge were performed in the extremely preterm group (Figure 1). This observation can be explained by the length of hospital stay of infants born at a younger gestational age [31].

We demonstrated that the applicability and usability of ADP measurements during hospital stays significantly vary among different groups of GA at birth (Figure 1):

Extremely and very preterm infants: Although the first measurements were possible starting at 31 weeks PMA, when infants were not receiving respiratory support, the median time was 36 weeks PMA. Despite this relatively late PMA, the prolonged hospital stay allows repeated body composition tests (mean number of measurements = 3) before discharge in this group. This hints at a large enough window for repeated weekly body composition analysis before discharge, opening the option to plot body composition growth trends and introduce nutritional intervention on the basis of body composition data during the hospital stay.

Moderate and late preterm infants: Body composition measurements can be initiated soon after birth (1 ± 0.7 weeks of life). A mean of two ADP measurements before discharge limits longitudinal assessment during the NICU stay. However, it allows individual adjustment of nutritional management. We suggest initiating nutritional adjustments if necessary and performing follow-up measurements after discharge.

Term infants: Due to the short hospitalization period, repeated ADP testing is limited during normal hospital stays. This does not allow continuous plotting of body composition reference charts during hospital stays. Hence, the value of routine body composition assessments in this GA group regarding nutritional monitoring and intervention during hospital stays is limited. Body composition assessments for the adjustment of discharge nutritional regimens, however, could provide value.

4.2.3. Frequency

A recent study by Lücke et al. revealed that at weekly intervals, the reproducibility of the ADP method is sufficient for monitoring body composition along trajectories [24].

At MetroHealth Medical Center, infants are tested once during their hospital stay (either at term or prior to discharge) [19]. In contrast, both the NICU Nuremberg and Cincinnati Children's Medical Center perform weekly ADP testing.

The decision between repeated or single body composition assessments depends on institutional focus. While single body composition assessments may reduce the workload, continuous body composition assessments provide options for continuous monitoring of nutritional status and for creating body composition growth trajectories. The lack of established recommendations for nutritional or therapeutic consequences from repeated body composition assessments limits the indication for high-frequency testing on a routine basis.

4.2.4. Time and Personnel Requirements

For safety reasons, each ADP test requires at least one PEAPOD operating nurse and one PEAPOD nurse. In our study, the time per ADP test decreased significantly when three, not two, nurses were available (from 13 min to 8 min). This significant reduction in the total time requirement per test was due to an improved, more efficient workflow. Staffing with two PEAPOD nurses will allow the preceding infant to be prepared for the assessment while another infant is still inside the PEAPOD. The time required per test at NICU Nuremberg was slightly greater (8 ± 0.6 min with two PEAPOD nurses) than the 5–7 min testing time estimated by Alja'nini et al. [19]. In his publication, however, it is unclear whether testing cycles included dressing, undressing, and logistics between the unit and the PEAPOD room. Additionally, it remains unclear how much personnel were involved in the presented testing routine, making a comparison of the cumulative work time impossible. For an average of 12 body composition assessments per week, the required cumulative work time at NICU Nuremberg was up to 5 h for all three operators. Overall, the workload is reasonable, and the time-per-test efficiency is optimal for all three operators.

4.2.5. Clinical Significance

Overall, routine body composition measurements provide valuable information for monitoring growth and nutritional status. In particular, high fat mass and reduced fat-free mass are related to suboptimal neurodevelopment and risk for metabolic and cardiovascular diseases later in life [6,32,33]. An optimum body composition is associated with improved neurological outcomes [6,7].

We aim to use body composition data for growth interpretation and to adjust nutritional management by plotting body composition data in reference graphs. These practices, however, are not yet standardized, leaving space for both different interpretations and different interventions (e.g., nutritional management) between medical practitioners and healthcare institutions. Salas et al. reported that simply providing body composition data have little effect on physician decisions or nutritional management [18].

This indicates the need for standardization of (1) the testing routine, (2) visualization and interpretation of body composition data, and (3) nutritional intervention regimens to efficiently use valuable body composition data.

In our NICU, we have taken first steps toward this process by defining an easily reproducible clinical procedure and standardizing the visualization of body composition data via reference charts by Norris et al., Hamatschek et al., and Demerath et al. [34–36]. At our hospital, the data from weekly body composition assessments are graphed into reference charts and provided to physicians to allow individual nutritional management. The evaluation and interpretation of individual body composition growth trajectories are performed weekly on the basis of alignment or deviation from percentiles.

This information is obtained by individually adjusting the nutritional supply during hospital stays and modifying postdischarge nutritional regimens on the basis of individual requirements (personalized or precision medicine).

4.3. *Future Clinical Utility of Body Composition Data*

A standardized protocol for routine testing would lower the threshold for implementing measurements in clinical practice while enhancing the comparability of body composition data across different childcare institutions.

Further investigations should address a model on how body composition data can help to further standardize individualized nutritional management by providing different quantities of macronutrients on the basis of infants' needs (e.g., different protein–energy ratios or carbohydrate–nonprotein ratios).

Therefore, as an important next step, research should aim to determine the optimum body composition that leads to optimum neurocognitive development while preventing vascular and metabolic diseases. Therefore, exact nutritional intervention guidelines must be formulated to guide the interpretation of body composition results in routine clinical practice.

Furthermore, individual nutritional intervention could allow earlier discharge from the hospital.

4.4. *Limitations of the ADP Method*

Noninvasive procedures can be implemented in clinical practice with a reasonable workload. Like all indirect body composition assessments, the PEAPOD device relies on assumptions. The FM density is constant, and the FFM density is only modified by sex and age [26]. Individual changes in body compartment density may lead to errors in estimation. A detailed description of the methodical limitations can be found in a recent article by our group [24]. Nevertheless, the PEAPOD has been validated by various comparability studies [13,14,16,17]. Furthermore, the ADP method was identified as the single "most accurate and reliable method for assessing body composition in preterm infants" in a review analyzing body composition methods in premature infants by Nagel et al. [12].

Another limitation of this method is that infants must be clinically stable before tests can be performed. Hence, body composition tests were initiated at significantly later postnatal and postmenstrual ages in infants with lower GA. Further noninvasive body composition methods, such as new BIA devices, should be reassessed for accuracy and reliability, as they could complement early body composition measurements with the PEAPOD.

4.5. Limitations and Strengths of the Study

This manuscript does not address data from body composition testing. Hence, individual fat and fat-free masses were not analyzed. This has been performed in a previous paper [24]. This manuscript solely analyses the applicability of this method in clinical practice and the presented testing protocol in clinical practice for different groups of premature infants.

A limitation of our protocol is that it does not provide a standardized guide for the interpretation and clinical utility of body composition data. This should be the aim of further investigations to improve outcomes.

A key strength of our study is that the PEAPOD tests were integrated into the clinical routine, and the study was performed under "real-life" conditions. During the entire study period, one single PEAPOD operating nurse was responsible for testing, thereby reducing measurement bias. In addition, only clinically stable infants without respiratory support were tested in routine clinical practice, providing a large, homogeneous cohort of both preterm (n = 185) and term infants (n = 75) with a total of n = 429 measurements.

5. Conclusions

The retrospective analysis of our data proved the feasibility of weekly routine ADP assessments in preterm infants. However, the initiation of routine testing in extremely preterm infants starts at a significantly greater postnatal age than in more mature groups. ADP assessments can be safely, easily and reasonably integrated into routine clinical practice. Body composition data may be a valuable tool for providing additional information on nutritional status and infant growth. A standardized routine protocol allowing identical measurement conditions across healthcare institutions and a standardized interpretation tool for age-adapted body composition data, however, will improve the comparability and usability of the method.

Author Contributions: Conceptualization, L.A.L., N.R. and C.F.; methodology, L.A.L., N.R. and C.F.; software, L.A.L. and N.R.; validation, L.A.L., N.R. and C.F.; formal analysis, L.A.L., N.R. and C.F.; investigation, L.A.L., A.S.-F., K.K., S.S., J.L.Z., U.F.-M., A.M. and S.L.-W.; data curation, L.A.L. and N.R.; writing—original draft preparation, L.A.L. and N.R.; writing—review and editing, L.A.L., N.R. and C.F.; visualization, L.A.L.; supervision, C.F.; project administration, N.R.; funding acquisition, C.F. All authors have read and agreed to the published version of the manuscript.

Funding: This research received no external funding.

Institutional Review Board Statement: The study was conducted in accordance with the Declaration of Helsinki and approved by the Institutional Review Board of Paracelsus Medical University (protocol code SZ_D_028.21-IX-1, file number: IRB-2023-17 and initial date of approval 3 March 2021 (Document translation to English on 12 October 2023)).

Informed Consent Statement: Written informed consent was obtained from the parents or legal guardians of the parents for all infants being tested during the routine assessments.

Data Availability Statement: The original contributions presented in the study are included in the article, and further inquiries can be directed to the corresponding author.

Conflicts of Interest: The authors declare that they have no conflicts of interest.

References

1. Costeloe, K.L.; Hennessy, E.M.; Haider, S.; Stacey, F.; Marlow, N.; Draper, E.S. Short Term Outcomes after Extreme Preterm Birth in England: Comparison of Two Birth Cohorts in 1995 and 2006 (the EPICure Studies). *BMJ* **2012**, *345*, e7976. [CrossRef]

2. Stoll, B.J.; Hansen, N.I.; Bell, E.F.; Walsh, M.C.; Carlo, W.A.; Shankaran, S.; Laptook, A.R.; Sánchez, P.J.; Van Meurs, K.P.; Wyckoff, M.; et al. Trends in Care Practices, Morbidity, and Mortality of Extremely Preterm Neonates, 1993–2012. *JAMA* **2015**, *314*, 1039–1051. [CrossRef] [PubMed]
3. Hofman, P.L.; Regan, F.; Jackson, W.E.; Jefferies, C.; Knight, D.B.; Robinson, E.M.; Cutfield, W.S. Premature Birth and Later Insulin Resistance. *N. Engl. J. Med.* **2004**, *351*, 2179–2186. [CrossRef] [PubMed]
4. Ong, K.K.; Ahmed, M.L.; Emmett, P.M.; Preece, M.A.; Dunger, D.B. Association between Postnatal Catch-up Growth and Obesity in Childhood: Prospective Cohort Study. *BMJ* **2000**, *320*, 967–971. [CrossRef] [PubMed]
5. Carr, H.; Cnattingius, S.; Granath, F.; Ludvigsson, J.F.; Edstedt Bonamy, A.-K. Preterm Birth and Risk of Heart Failure up to Early Adulthood. *J. Am. Coll. Cardiol.* **2017**, *69*, 2634–2642. [CrossRef] [PubMed]
6. Ramel, S.E.; Gray, H.L.; Christiansen, E.; Boys, C.; Georgieff, M.K.; Demerath, E.W. Greater Early Gains in Fat-Free Mass, but Not Fat Mass, Are Associated with Improved Neurodevelopment at 1 Year Corrected Age for Prematurity in Very Low Birth Weight Preterm Infants. *J. Pediatr.* **2016**, *173*, 108–115. [CrossRef] [PubMed]
7. Pfister, K.M.; Zhang, L.; Miller, N.C.; Ingolfsland, E.C.; Demerath, E.W.; Ramel, S.E. Early Body Composition Changes Are Associated with Neurodevelopmental and Metabolic Outcomes at 4 Years of Age in Very Preterm Infants. *Pediatr. Res.* **2018**, *84*, 713–718. [CrossRef] [PubMed]
8. Bua, J.; Risso, F.M.; Bin, M.; Vallon, F.; Travan, L.; Paviotti, G. Association between Body Composition at Term Equivalent Age and Bayley Scores at 2 Years in Preterm Infants. *J. Perinatol. Off. J. Calif. Perinat. Assoc.* **2021**, *41*, 1852–1858. [CrossRef] [PubMed]
9. Bell, K.A.; Ramel, S.E.; Robinson, D.T.; Wagner, C.L.; Scottoline, B.; Belfort, M.B. Body Composition Measurement for the Preterm Neonate: Using a Clinical Utility Framework to Translate Research Tools into Clinical Care. *J. Perinatol. Off. J. Calif. Perinat. Assoc.* **2022**, *42*, 1550–1555. [CrossRef] [PubMed]
10. Dung, N.Q.; Fusch, G.; Armbrust, S.; Jochum, F.; Fusch, C. Body Composition of Preterm Infants Measured during the First Months of Life: Bioelectrical Impedance Provides Insignificant Additional Information Compared to Anthropometry Alone. *Eur. J. Pediatr.* **2007**, *166*, 215–222. [CrossRef] [PubMed]
11. Koo, W.W.K.; Walters, J.C.; Hockman, E.M. Body Composition in Neonates: Relationship Between Measured and Derived Anthropometry with Dual-Energy X-ray Absorptiometry Measurements. *Pediatr. Res.* **2004**, *56*, 694–700. [CrossRef] [PubMed]
12. Nagel, E.; Hickey, M.; Teigen, L.; Kuchnia, A.; Curran, K.; Soumekh, L.; Earthman, C.; Demerath, E.; Ramel, S. Clinical Application of Body Composition Methods in Premature Infants. *J. Parenter. Enter. Nutr.* **2020**, *44*, 785–795. [CrossRef]
13. Roggero, P.; Giannì, M.L.; Amato, O.; Piemontese, P.; Morniroli, D.; Wong, W.W.; Mosca, F. Evaluation of Air-Displacement Plethysmography for Body Composition Assessment in Preterm Infants. *Pediatr. Res.* **2012**, *72*, 316–320. [CrossRef]
14. Ma, G.S.; Yao, M.J.; Liu, Y.; Lin, A.W.; Zou, H.; Urlando, A.; Wong, W.W.; Nommsen-Rivers, L.; Dewey, K.G. Validation of a New Pediatric Air-Displacement Plethysmograph for Assessing Body Composition in Infants. *Am. J. Clin. Nutr.* **2004**, *79*, 653–660. [CrossRef] [PubMed]
15. Mazahery, H.; von Hurst, P.R.; McKinlay, C.J.D.; Cormack, B.E.; Conlon, C.A. Air Displacement Plethysmography (Pea Pod) in Full-Term and Pre-Term Infants: A Comprehensive Review of Accuracy, Reproducibility, and Practical Challenges. *Matern. Health Neonatol. Perinatol.* **2018**, *4*, 12. [CrossRef] [PubMed]
16. Ellis, K.J.; Yao, M.; Shypailo, R.J.; Urlando, A.; Wong, W.W.; Heird, W.C. Body-Composition Assessment in Infancy: Air-Displacement Plethysmography Compared with a Reference 4-Compartment Model. *Am. J. Clin. Nutr.* **2007**, *85*, 90–95. [CrossRef]
17. Frondas-Chauty, A.; Louveau, I.; Le Huërou-Luron, I.; Rozé, J.-C.; Darmaun, D. Air-Displacement Plethysmography for Determining Body Composition in Neonates: Validation Using Live Piglets. *Pediatr. Res.* **2012**, *72*, 26–31. [CrossRef] [PubMed]
18. Salas, A.A.; Jerome, M.L.; Chandler-Laney, P.; Ambalavanan, N.; Carlo, W.A. Serial Assessment of Fat and Fat-Free Mass Accretion in Very Preterm Infants: A Randomized Trial. *Pediatr. Res.* **2020**, *88*, 733–738. [CrossRef]
19. Alja'nini, Z.; McNelis, K.M.; Viswanathan, S.; Goddard, G.R.; Merlino-Barr, S.; Collin, M.; Groh-Wargo, S. Infant Body Composition Assessment in the Neonatal Intensive Care Unit (NICU) Using Air Displacement Plethysmography: Strategies for Implementation into Clinical Workflow. *Clin. Nutr. ESPEN* **2021**, *43*, 212–222. [CrossRef] [PubMed]
20. Harris, P.A.; Taylor, R.; Minor, B.L.; Elliott, V.; Fernandez, M.; O'Neal, L.; McLeod, L.; Delacqua, G.; Delacqua, F.; Kirby, J.; et al. The REDCap Consortium: Building an International Community of Software Platform Partners. *J. Biomed. Inform.* **2019**, *95*, 103208. [CrossRef] [PubMed]
21. Harris, P.A.; Taylor, R.; Thielke, R.; Payne, J.; Gonzalez, N.; Conde, J.G. Research Electronic Data Capture (REDCap)—A Metadata-Driven Methodology and Workflow Process for Providing Translational Research Informatics Support. *J. Biomed. Inform.* **2009**, *42*, 377–381. [CrossRef] [PubMed]
22. Agostoni, C.; Buonocore, G.; Carnielli, V.P.; De Curtis, M.; Darmaun, D.; Decsi, T.; Domellöf, M.; Embleton, N.D.; Fusch, C.; Genzel-Boroviczeny, O.; et al. Enteral Nutrient Supply for Preterm Infants: Commentary from the European Society of Paediatric Gastroenterology, Hepatology and Nutrition Committee on Nutrition. *J. Pediatr. Gastroenterol. Nutr.* **2010**, *50*, 85–91. [CrossRef]
23. Urlando, A.; Dempster, P.; Aitkens, S. A New Air Displacement Plethysmograph for the Measurement of Body Composition in Infants. *Pediatr. Res.* **2003**, *53*, 486–492. [CrossRef] [PubMed]
24. Lücke, L.; Fusch, C.; Knab, K.; Schäfer, S.; Zimmermann, J.L.; Felderhoff-Müser, U.; Meis, A.; Lohmüller-Weiß, S.; Szakacs-Fusch, A.; Rochow, N. Reproducibility of Air Displacement Plethysmography in Term and Preterm Infants—A Study to Enhance Body Composition Analysis in Clinical Routine. *Nutrients* **2024**, *16*, 1810. [CrossRef] [PubMed]

25. Fomon, S.J.; Haschke, F.; Ziegler, E.E.; Nelson, S.E. Body Composition of Reference Children from Birth to Age 10 Years. *Am. J. Clin. Nutr.* **1982**, *35*, 1169–1175. [CrossRef] [PubMed]
26. Butte, N.F.; Hopkinson, J.M.; Wong, W.W.; Smith, E.O.; Ellis, K.J. Body Composition during the First 2 Years of Life: An Updated Reference. *Pediatr. Res.* **2000**, *47*, 578–585. [CrossRef] [PubMed]
27. COSMED PEA POD® Infant Body Composition System Operator's Manual 2019. Available online: https://www.bioclinicalservices.com.au/cosmed-srl/clinical/pea-pod-operators-manual-rev-n (accessed on 1 May 2024).
28. Rochow, N.; Fusch, G.; Ali, A.; Bhatia, A.; Therefore, H.Y.; Iskander, R.; Chessell, L.; El Helou, S.; Fusch, C. Individualized Target Fortification of Breast Milk with Protein, Carbohydrates, and Fat for Preterm Infants: A Double-Blind Randomized Controlled Trial. *Clin. Nutr.* **2021**, *40*, 54–63. [CrossRef] [PubMed]
29. Moutquin, J.-M. Classification and Heterogeneity of Preterm Birth. *BJOG Int. J. Obstet. Gynaecol.* **2003**, *110* (Suppl. 20), 30–33. [CrossRef]
30. Bruckner, M.; Khan, Z.; Binder, C.; Morris, N.; Windisch, B.; Holasek, S.; Urlesberger, B. Extremely Preterm Infants Have a Higher Fat Mass Percentage in Comparison to Very Preterm Infants at Term-Equivalent Age. *Front. Pediatr.* **2020**, *8*, 61. [CrossRef]
31. Murki, S.; Vardhelli, V.; Deshabhotla, S.; Sharma, D.; Pawale, D.; Kulkarni, D.; Kumar, P.; Kabra, N.S.; Sundaram, M.; Plakkal, N.; et al. Predictors of Length of Hospital Stay among Preterm Infants Admitted to Neonatal Intensive Care Unit: Data from a Multicentre Collaborative Network from India (INNC: Indian National Neonatal Collaborative). *J. Paediatr. Child Health* **2020**, *56*, 1584–1589. [CrossRef] [PubMed]
32. Crane, J.D.; Yellin, S.A.; Ong, F.J.; Singh, N.P.; Konyer, N.; Noseworthy, M.D.; Schmidt, L.A.; Saigal, S.; Morrison, K.M. ELBW Survivors in Early Adulthood Have Higher Hepatic, Pancreatic and Subcutaneous Fat. *Sci. Rep.* **2016**, *6*, 31560. [CrossRef] [PubMed]
33. Parlapani, E.; Agakidis, C.; Karagiozoglou-Lampoudi, T. Anthropometry and Body Composition of Preterm Neonates in the Light of Metabolic Programming. *J. Am. Coll. Nutr.* **2018**, *37*, 350–359. [CrossRef] [PubMed]
34. Hamatschek, C.; Yousuf, E.I.; Möllers, L.S.; Therefore, H.Y.; Morrison, K.M.; Fusch, C.; Rochow, N. Fat and Fat-Free Mass of Preterm and Term Infants from Birth to Six Months: A Review of Current Evidence. *Nutrients* **2020**, *12*, 288. [CrossRef] [PubMed]
35. Norris, T.; Ramel, S.E.; Catalano, P.; Caoimh, C.N.; Roggero, P.; Murray, D.; Fields, D.A.; Demerath, E.W.; Johnson, W. New Charts for the Assessment of Body Composition, According to Air-Displacement Plethysmography, at Birth and across the First 6 Month of Life. *Am. J. Clin. Nutr.* **2019**, *109*, 1353–1360. [CrossRef] [PubMed]
36. Demerath, E.W.; Johnson, W.; Davern, B.A.; Anderson, C.G.; Shenberger, J.S.; Misra, S.; Ramel, S.E. New Body Composition Reference Charts for Preterm Infants. *Am. J. Clin. Nutr.* **2017**, *105*, 70–77. [CrossRef]

nutrients

Article

Total Gestational Weight Gain Is Explained by Leptin and Body Fat, Regardless of Pre-Pregnancy Body Mass Index and Other Adipokines, in Mexican Adolescents

Gabriela Chico-Barba [1,2], Reyna Sámano [2,*], Hugo Martínez-Rojano [3], Rosa María Morales-Hernández [2], Edgar Barrientos-Galeana [2], Andrea Luna-Hidalgo [2], Martha Kaufer-Horwitz [4], Gregorio T. Obrador [5] and Antonio Rafael Villa-Romero [6,*]

1 Programa de Maestría y Doctorado en Ciencias Médicas, Odontológicas y de la Salud, Facultad de Medicina, Universidad Nacional Autónoma de México, Mexico City 04510, Mexico; gabyc3@gmail.com
2 Coordinación de Nutrición y Bioprogramación, Instituto Nacional de Perinatología, Mexico City 11000, Mexico
3 Sección de Posgrado e Investigación, Escuela Superior de Medicina, Instituto Politécnico Nacional, Mexico City 11340, Mexico; hmartinez_59@yahoo.com.mx
4 Dirección de Nutrición, Instituto Nacional de Ciencias Médicas y Nutrición Salvador Zubirán, Mexico City 14080, Mexico
5 School of Medicine, Universidad Panamericana, Mexico City 03920, Mexico
6 División de Investigación, Facultad de Medicina, Universidad Nacional Autónoma de México, Mexico City 04510, Mexico
* Correspondence: ssmr0119@yahoo.com.mx (R.S.); avilla@unam.mx (A.R.V.-R.)

Abstract: Pre-pregnancy body mass index (pBMI) is a predictor of gestational weight gain (GWG). However, other factors, such as adipokines and inflammation markers, may also be associated with GWG. The aim of the study was to determine the association of leptin, adiponectin, irisin, and C-reactive protein, with GWG in adolescents. A longitudinal study was conducted from 2018 to 2023 in adolescents with a clinically healthy pregnancy. The assessments included sociodemographic and clinical data, pBMI, percent of body fat, serum concentrations of leptin, adiponectin, irisin, and high-sensitivity C-reactive protein (hsCRP), and total GWG adequacy. Cox regression models were performed, the outcome variables were inadequate and excessive GWG. In 198 participants, being overweight/obesity was marginally associated with a protective effect against inadequate GWG (HR = 0.44, 95%CI = 0.18–1.06), regardless of maternal characteristics and adipokines. Leptin (HR = 1.014, 95%CI = 1.008–1.021), and body fat percent (HR = 1.11, 95%CI = 1.05–1.17) were associated with a higher risk of excessive GWG, independent of other maternal variables such as pBMI, while adiponectin was associated with a lower risk. These findings suggest that, in Mexican adolescents, adipose tissue and its adipokines during pregnancy may play a more significant role in the final GWG than body weight.

Keywords: leptin; adiponectin; irisin; C-reactive protein; teenage pregnancy; inflammation; gestational weight gain

1. Introduction

Adolescent pregnancy is a public health problem in low- and middle-income countries [1]. Mexico ranks among the highest in Latin America [2], with approximately 15.3% of total births attributed to women under 20 years old [3]. Teenage mothers face increased risk of adverse perinatal outcomes, including preeclampsia, infections, postpartum hemorrhage, and maternal mortality [4–6]. Additionally, infants born to adolescent mothers are more likely to experience low birth weight, be small for gestational age, and experience intrauterine growth restriction [4–6].

Gestational weight gain (GWG) may play a role in the aforementioned perinatal outcomes [7–9]. GWG is predominantly explained by the increase in fat mass [10] and is regulated by diet, exercise, and maternal characteristics such as age, pre-pregnancy body mass index (BMI), and metabolic factors [10]. Among these metabolic factors, adipokines such as leptin [11–13], adiponectin [12,14], and the adipomyokine irisin [15], may be associated with both inadequate and excessive GWG. Leptin and adiponectin are the most studied adipokines in pregnancy outcomes and GWG, but there are others, such as chemerin, resistin, and visfatin with scarce evidence [16].

Leptin, secreted by white adipose tissue, regulates metabolic and endocrine functions [17]. During pregnancy, the placenta also secretes leptin, leading to hyperleptinemia and leptin resistance, thus contributing to changes in energy balance [18,19]. Evidence suggests that higher leptin serum concentrations are associated with excessive weight gain in adolescents [20,21]. However, studies describing the mechanisms by which leptin may regulate GWG are limited [22]. For instance, one proposal is that central regulation of appetite in the hypothalamus is altered in leptin resistance, favoring increased food intake and more weight gain [23].

In contrast, adiponectin, another hormone derived from white adipose tissue with actions opposite to leptin, decreases during pregnancy and exhibits anti-inflammatory properties on microglia cells [14,22,24,25].

Irisin, a novel hormone primarily secreted by skeletal muscle during exercise but also by fat tissue, is considered an adipomyokine [26]. Its levels increase during pregnancy and it regulates maternal and fetal glucose levels, with most studies focusing on its relation to gestational diabetes [27–29]. Although there is no evidence for the association of irisin and GWG, its role in the conversion of white to brown adipose tissue, stimulated by exercise [26], makes irisin a promising adipomyokine to be studied in the context of gestational weight outcomes.

Limited evidence exists regarding the role or association of adiponectin and irisin in GWG in both adults and adolescents [12,30].

Furthermore, leptin and irisin act as pro-inflammatory hormones [17,31], while adiponectin exhibits anti-inflammatory properties [24]. Pregnancy itself induces inflammation [32], as does obesity in non-pregnant individuals due to the secretion of pro-inflammatory proteins by adipose tissue [31]. High-sensitivity C-reactive protein (hsCRP), the principal and most studied inflammatory marker, increases in both scenarios [33,34], with reported increments of 3% in hsCRP for every 1 kg increase in gestational weight [35].

Moreover, the prevalence of overweight and obesity among Mexican female adolescents is approximately 41% [36], predisposing them to begin pregnancy with higher body fat levels. Pre-pregnancy overweight and obesity are associated with excessive weight gain during pregnancy [37,38].

Adipokines, such as leptin, adiponectin and irisin, are mediators of the inflammatory response and metabolic regulation. Although the mechanisms are not fully described, leptin and other adipokines could be prognostic factors for metabolic diseases and for events such as insufficient or excessive weight gain during pregnancy. Studies on the association between adipokines and GWG focused on adult women in high-income countries or in nutritional and health contexts different from those of Mexican adolescents [11–13,20,25,39]. It is necessary to identify these biomarkers in adolescents since their levels of adipokines and inflammation markers could vary due to the stage of fat mass accretion they are in, in addition to the changes caused by pregnancy. Increased fat tissue before or during pregnancy predisposes women to retain weight, and it predisposes offspring to metabolic diseases, as the maternal pregnancy metabolic and inflammatory environment plays a crucial role in the early origins of disease [40–43]. Identifying metabolic and inflammatory factors related to GWG is essential for understanding the mechanisms predisposing young girls to gain more or less weight than recommended during pregnancy. Therefore, this study aimed to determine the association of leptin, adiponectin, irisin, and hsCRP with total gestational weight gain in adolescents, evaluating their potential as prognostic factors.

2. Materials and Methods

2.1. Study Design and Sample Collection

We conducted a follow-up study at the Instituto Nacional de Perinatología (INPer) in Mexico City from 2018 to 2023. Participants were selected through convenient sampling based on consecutive cases meeting the following inclusion criteria: pregnant adolescents aged 10–19 years (as defined by the World Health Organization [44]), receiving medical antenatal care at INPer, primigravida, and with a healthy singleton pregnancy. All participants were recruited during their outpatient consultation at INPer. Exclusion criteria were having pre-pregnancy chronic or inflammatory diseases such as type I or II diabetes, cardiac, kidney, autoimmune, or psychiatric diseases, as well as the consumption of alcohol, tobacco, or drugs during pregnancy. The sample size was calculated with a 95% confidence level, based on a correlation coefficient of 0.26 between leptin and gestational weight gain in adolescents [20], as leptin is the most studied adipokine. The calculated sample size was 114 participants. However, accounting for an expected 15% loss rate, a total of 131 participants was required.

2.2. Sociodemographic and Clinical Variables

During the initial assessment, with one legal guardian present, information on age, occupation, marital status, education, and socioeconomic status was collected through a questionnaire. Menarche age and gestational age, determined by last menstrual period to determine the trimester of initiation of prenatal care, were obtained from medical records. Physical activity was asked as a direct question, with a yes or no response. Dietary intake was assessed using a single 24-h recall; total energy intake (kcal/d) was determined in the Nutrickal® software https://www.nutrikcal.mx/NutriKcalVO.html (Mexico City, Mexico). The sociodemographic, anthropometric, clinical, and dietetic measurements were performed by six trained nutritionist.

2.3. Anthropometric Evaluation

In the first visit, weight before pregnancy was self-reported, which is an accurate measurement of real pre-pregnancy weight [45,46]. In addition, height was measured with a manual stadiometer (SECA 222, Hamburg, Germany 0.1 cm accuracy).

Pre-pregnancy body mass index (pBMI) was calculated using pre-pregnancy weight and height; then, pBMI classification was obtained with AnthroPlus® https://www.who.int/tools/growth-reference-data-for-5to19-years/application-tools (World Health Organization, Geneva, Switzerland) according to z-scores: underweight ≤ -2, normal weight -2 to +1, overweight 1 to 1.99, and obesity >+2 [47].

Body fat percent was obtained using an InBody 770® Body Composition Analyzer (InBody Co., Ltd, Seoul, Korea). This assessment was performed during morning hours (from 8:00 to 10:00 h) in fasting conditions, with an empty bladder and light clothes.

Maternal weight was measured using a digital scale (TANITA, Tokyo, Japan, model BWB-800; 0.010 kg accuracy). Final weight was assessed one or two weeks before delivery. We calculated total GWG by the difference between the last measured weight and the pre-pregnancy weight.

Then, to assess the GWG as a continuous variable, we calculated the percentage adequacy of GWG by dividing the total GWG by the expected GWG and multiplying the result by 100 [48]. The expected GWG was obtained with the following formula: expected weight gain = recommended weight gain for the first trimester + ((gestational age final − 13.86 weeks) × (recommended weight gain rate in second and third trimesters)). According to IOM recommendations, the recommended GWG rates were based on pBMI as follows: low and normal weight 2 kg, overweight 1 kg, and obesity 0.5 kg for the first trimester, and low weight 0.51 kg, normal weight 0.42 kg, overweight 0.28 kg, and obesity 0.22 kg/week for second and third trimesters [10].

To assess the GWG as a categorical variable, the percentage adequacy of GWG was categorized into inadequate (<90%), adequate (90 to <125%), and excessive ($\geq$125%) [49].

2.4. Biochemical Determinations

A nurse collected blood sample between 7 and 8 a.m., after fasting 8 to 10 h. Then, serum was obtained after centrifugation for 10 min at 3500 rpm; samples were frozen at −70 °C until processing. Leptin, adiponectin and irisin were determined by ELISA technique.

For leptin and adiponectin, we used an absorbance microplate reader (ELISA Bio-Rad, model 680 Bench-mark Plus, Bio-Rad, Hercules, CA, USA) and ELISA Human Immunoassay kit (Quantikine® ELISA Human Immunoassay, R&D Systems Inc., Minneapolis, MN, USA), respectively, following manufacturer's instructions.

Irisin was determined using the Human irisin ELISA kit (My BioSource.com, MBS 706887, San Diego, CA, USA).

High-sensitivity C-reactive protein (hsCRP) was measured by colorimetric method (Respons 910, DiaSys Diagnostic Systems, Holzheim, Germany) with a detection range of 0.1 mg/L.

The biochemical determinations were performed by three clinical chemist.

2.5. Statistical Analyses

Frequencies, measures of central tendency and dispersion were obtained to describe the sample characteristics. Kruskal–Wallis and Mann–Whitney U tests were used to compare serum adipokines concentrations according to pBMI and GWG category. Additionally, Spearman's Rho was calculated to correlate the biochemical variables.

To determine the association of the serum concentrations of the adipokines with GWG, we performed Cox regression models, where time was determined in days (gestational age minus weeks of gestation at the moment of blood sample); the outcome variables were inadequate and excessive GWG. Both models were adjusted by pBMI, maternal age, physical activity, and energy intake. Hazard ratios with 95%CI were obtained.

A sensitivity analysis was performed in participants that started the study between 18 and 30 weeks of gestation, as the metabolic and inflammatory status are similar during these weeks. In this way, we excluded the effect of gestational age in the adipokines status.

All the analyses we performed using IBM SPSS Statistics for Windows, version 23.0 (IBM Corp., Armonk, NY, USA).

2.6. Ethical Aspects

The study was approved by the Institutional Ethics, Biosafety, and Research Committees (INPer registration number 2017-2-101). Written informed assent was obtained from the adolescents and written informed consent was obtained from their legal guardians. Confidentiality was guaranteed by assigning an ID number for each participant during data collection and analysis. All participants were informed that their medical care would not be affected by their participation in the study.

3. Results

A total of 198 adolescents were included in the analysis. Figure 1 shows the flow chart of participant selection. Table 1 shows the participants characteristics at the first visit. Mean age was 15.9 ± 1.4 years, most of them were single, homemakers and had a pBMI of normal weight.

Figure 2 shows the total GWG by pBMI. Inadequate GWG was most common in participants with pre-pregnancy normal weight, while excessive GWG was more frequent in those living with pre-pregnancy overweight/obesity.

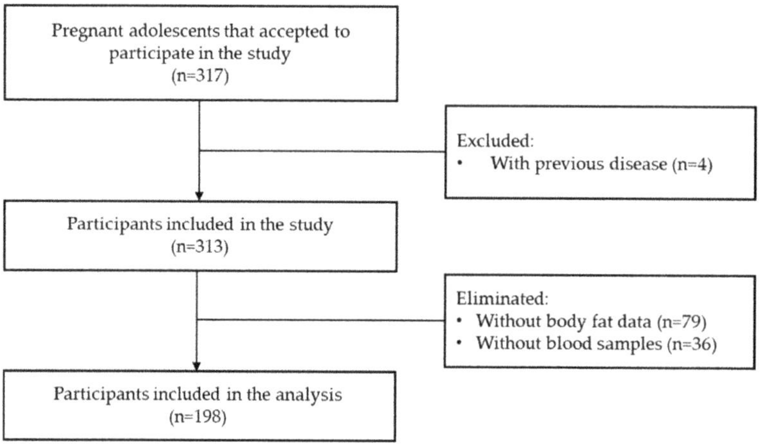

Figure 1. Flowchart of the participants' selection.

Table 1. General characteristics of pregnant adolescents at first visit (*n* = 198).

Characteristics	Variable		*n* (%)
Sociodemographic	Age, years *		15.9 ± 1.4
	Age, group		
		≤15 years	64 (32.3)
		≥16 years	134 (67.7)
	Occupation		
		Homemaker	165 (83.3)
		Student	29 (14.6)
		Employee	4 (2.0)
	Marital status		
		Single	147 (74.2)
		With partner	51 (25.8)
	Socioeconomic level		
		Low	96 (48.5)
		Middle	88 (44.4)
		High	14 (7.1)
	Education, years **		9.0 (8.0–10.0)
Clinical	Menarche, years **		11.6 ± 1.4
	Trimester		
		First	12 (6.1)
		Second	106 (53.5)
		Third	80 (40.4)
Anthropometrical	Pre-pregnancy weight, kg **		52.0 (46.0–57.25)
	Height, cm **		155.0 (151.0–158.3)
	Pre-pregnancy BMI, kg/m^2 **		21.6 (15.0–33.9)
	Pre-pregnancy BMI		
		Underweight	2 (1.0)
		Normal weight	151 (76.3)
		Overweight	32 (16.2)
		Obesity	13 (6.6)
	GWG, kg **		11.5 (8.8–14.5)
	GWG adequacy, % **		99.1 (78.5–140.6)
	GWG category		
		Inadequate	77 (38.9)
		Adequate	56 (28.3)
		Excessive	65 (32.8)
	Body fat, % *		35.7 ± 5.9

Table 1. *Cont.*

Characteristics	Variable		*n* (%)
Biochemical	Leptin (ng/mL) **		35.3 (20.6–49.5)
	Adiponectin (ng/mL) **		8627.9 (6065.8–13,275.1)
	Irisin (ng/mL) **		669.1 (380.6–1043.8)
	C-reactive protein (mg/L) **		3.4 (2.0–5.3)
Lifestyle	Physical activity		
		Yes	54 (27.3)
	Energy intake, kcal/d **		1944 (1564–2315)
	Protein adequacy, % **		15.8 (13.0–19.1)
	Lipid adequacy, % **		33.9 (28.0–39.3)
	Carbohydrate adequacy, % **		51.0 (45.0–57.4)

* Mean ± standard deviation, ** Median (percentile 25–percentile 75). BMI: body mass index, GWG: gestational weight gain.

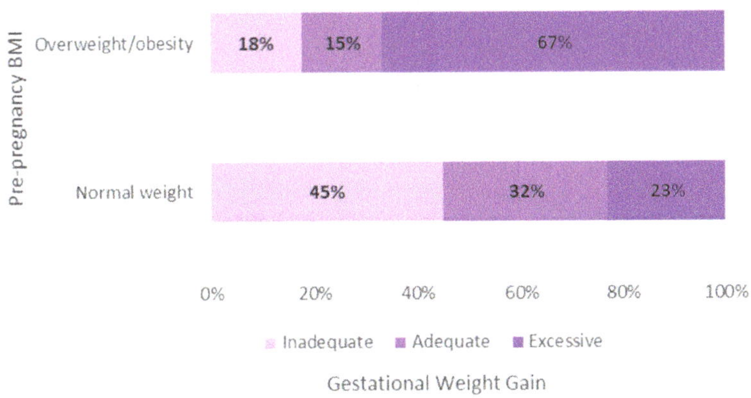

Figure 2. Total gestational weight gain according to pre-pregnancy body mass index.

Leptin, Adiponectin, Irisin, hsCRP, and Total Gestational Weight Gain

The median concentrations of leptin, adiponectin, irisin, and hsCPR were 35.3 ng/mL, 8627.9 ng/mL, 669.1 ng/mL, and 3.4 mg/L, respectively (Table 1).

Among adolescents with normal pBMI, differences in median concentrations were observed for leptin and adiponectin, between GWG categories (Kruskal–Wallis test, $p = 0.023$ and $p = 0.001$). Irisin showed almost statistical significance ($p = 0.076$).

For participants with overweight/obesity pBMI, only leptin median concentrations differed significantly between GWG categories (Kruskal–Wallis test, $p = 0.038$).

The correlations among the anthropometric and biochemical variables can be seen in the Supplementary file (Table S1).

Figure 3 shows the serum concentrations of each adipokine based on pBMI and GWG categories. In individuals with a normal pBMI, leptin concentrations differed significantly between the inadequate and excessive GWG groups, as well as between the adequate and excessive GWG groups. Among those living with pre-pregnancy overweight or obesity, significant differences in median leptin concentrations were observed only between the adequate and excessive GWG groups. For adiponectin, differences were found only among the GWG categories in women with a normal pBMI. Lastly, in adolescents with a normal pBMI, irisin levels differed between the inadequate an excessive GWG groups. No differences in hsCRP levels were found between the GWG categories.

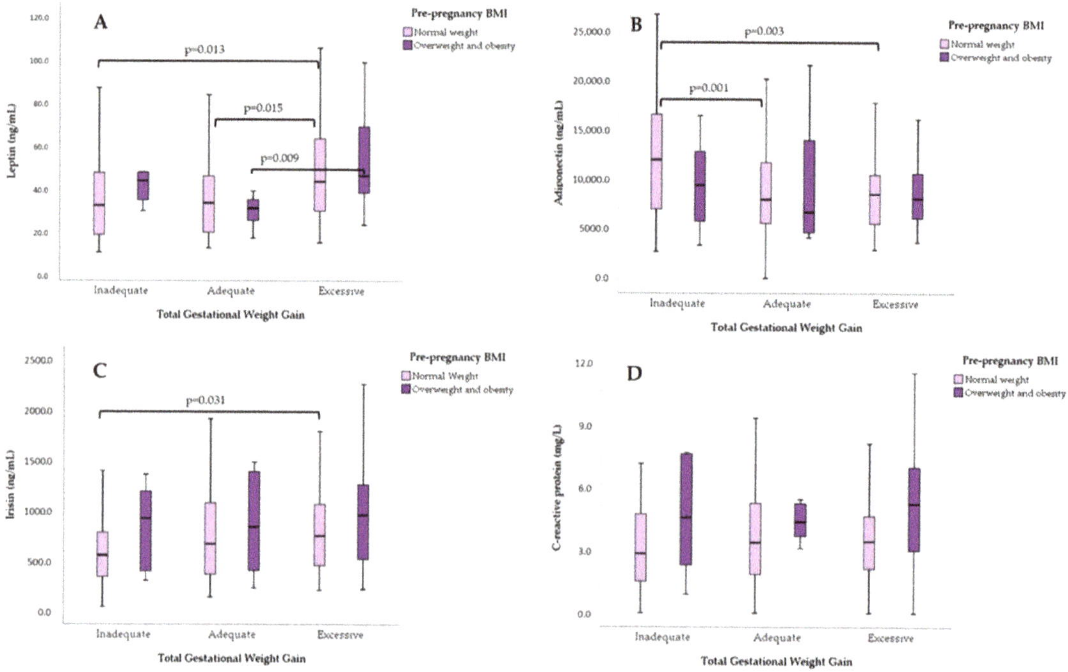

Figure 3. Serum concentrations of (**A**) leptin, (**B**) adiponectin, (**C**) irisin, and (**D**) hs-CRP, according to pre-pregnancy BMI and total gestational weight gain. U-Mann–Whitney test for pair comparisons.

According to the Cox regression models, pre-pregnancy overweight/obesity showed a nearly statistically significant association as a protective factor (HR = 0.44, 95%CI = 0.18–1.06) for inadequate GWG, regardless of maternal characteristics and the other adipokine concentrations, (see Table 2). On the other hand, leptin (HR = 1.014, 95%CI = 1.008–1.021), adiponectin (HR = 0.99994, 95%CI = 0.99988–0.99999), and body fat (HR = 1.11, 95%CI = 1.05–1.17) were associated with higher risk of having excessive GWG, as shown in Table 3.

Table 2. Cox regression model for inadequate gestational weight gain according to maternal clinical and biochemical characteristics.

Variable	Inadequate Gestational Weight Gain HR	95%CI	*p*-Value
Age (years)	0.87	0.72–1.04	0.129
Leptin (ng/mL)	1.005	0.99–1.01	0.130
Adiponectin (ng/mL)	1.00001	0.99997–1.00005	0.568
Irisin (ng/mL)	1.0004	0.9998–1.001	0.117
hsCRP (mg/L)	1.01	0.98–1.02	0.589
Pre-pregnancy BMI			
Normal weight	Ref.	Ref.	Ref.
Overweight/obesity	0.44	0.18–1.06	0.066
Body fat (%)	0.96	0.91–1.01	0.140
Physical activity			
Yes	Ref.	Ref.	Ref.
No	0.73	0.44–1.19	0.210
Energy intake (kcal/d)	1.0001	0.9998–1.0004	0.415

HR: Hazard Ratio, 95%CI: 95% Confidence Interval, Ref.: category of reference.

Table 3. Cox regression model for excessive gestational weight gain according to maternal clinical and biochemical characteristics.

	Excessive Gestational Weight Gain		
Variable	**HR**	**95%CI**	***p*-Value**
Age (years)	0.89	0.75–1.07	0.223
Leptin (ng/mL)	1.014	1.008–1.021	<0.001
Adiponectin (ng/mL)	0.99994	0.99988–0.99999	0.038
Irisin (ng/mL)	1.0003	0.9997–1.0009	0.279
hsCRP (mg/L)	0.99	0.93–1.05	0.766
Pre-pregnancy BMI			
Normal weight	Ref.	Ref.	Ref.
Overweight/obesity	0.74	0.39–1.40	0.359
Body fat (%)	1.11	1.05–1.17	<0.001
Physical activity			
Yes	Ref.	Ref.	Ref.
No	0.78	0.44–1.31	0.369
Energy intake (kcal/d)	1.0001	0.9997–1.0005	0.408

HR: Hazard Ratio, 95%CI: 95% Confidence Interval, Ref.: category of reference.

The sensitivity analysis was performed in 126 participants who initiated the study from 18 to 30 weeks of gestation. The calculated hazard ratios showed similar associations for both outcomes, inadequate and excessive total GWG.

4. Discussion

In this observational study conducted on adolescents attending INPer in Mexico City, serum leptin concentrations were associated with a higher risk of excessive GWG along with body fat, while adiponectin was associated with a lower risk. Increases in leptin concentrations were particularly observed in adolescents living with pre-pregnancy overweight or obesity. None of the adipokines were associated with inadequate GWG, except for pre-pregnancy overweight and obesity, which were associated with a lower risk. Irisin and hsCRP showed no association with either inadequate or excessive GWG.

We found that 38.9% of the participants had inadequate GWG and 32.8% had excessive GWG. These results are very similar to the various frequencies of gestational weight gain in pregnant adolescents reported in different parts of the world, with fluctuations between 56% and 84% of adolescents typically experiencing inadequate gestational weight gain [50–52]. Therefore, inadequate gestational weight gain in pregnant adolescents is a health issue, as adolescents are a vulnerable group whose longitudinal growth is compromised [53–55] and they generally consume diets that are either excessive or deficient in quantity and/or quality [56], in addition to being exposed to adverse psychosocial risk factors that can influence gestational weight gain [57].

When GWG categories are divided by pBMI, we observed that excessive GWG was significantly higher in those living with overweight and obesity before pregnancy (67%), compared to those with normal weight (23%). These results are in accordance with previous findings from our study group [58], where we demonstrated that, in a group of adolescent mothers compared to adult mothers, adolescents had a higher gestational weight gain in kilograms compared to adults. These observations align with the United States Institute of Medicine's assumption that adolescents, especially the younger ones, are more likely to be categorized in a "lighter group" and therefore advised to gain more weight [10,59]. Regarding the evidence of the effects of pre-pregnancy body mass index and gestational weight gain on maternal and neonatal outcomes, it was reported that being underweight before pregnancy increases the risk of preterm birth and delivering a small-for-gestational-age newborn. On the other hand, overweight and obesity are high-risk factors for gestational diabetes, hypertensive syndrome, and fetal growth disorders. In terms of weight gain, women with insufficient gestational weight gain may experience anemia. Conversely, those with excessive weight gain have an increased risk of cesarean delivery, preeclampsia, gestational diabetes, blood transfusions, postpartum weight retention, and long-term obesity [60].

Since pre-pregnancy BMI determine GWG, we stratified serum concentrations of adipokines by these variables. We found that leptin concentrations were different across GWG categories among adolescents with normal weight pBMI, but among adolescents living with overweight/obesity before pregnancy, the only difference was found when comparing adequate vs. excessive GWG. Similar results were reported in several studies in adults [11,61–63], but few studies were performed in adolescents. For instance, Baratto, et al. [25], reported higher serum leptin concentration in Brazilian adolescents who started their pregnancy overweight or obese compared to adolescents who began their pregnancy with a normal body mass index. Therefore, we believe that leptin secreted by adipose tissue and the placenta is involved in the regulation of food intake, energy homeostasis, insulin secretion, and nutrient transport to the fetus, correlating with pre-pregnancy body mass index and adiposity [64]. In our study, adolescents with excessive gestational weight gain showed higher serum leptin concentrations, which is probably related to an abnormal accumulation of body fat, mainly visceral adipose tissue, leading to adipocyte dysfunction [65] and an alteration in adipokine profiles, where adiponectin decreases and leptin concentration increases [66]. Consequently, several studies reported that high leptin concentrations in the second and third trimesters of pregnancy correlate with excessive gestational weight gain [67].

Regarding the association of leptin with higher risk of excessive GWG, studies found a stronger association of leptin in the second trimester with excessive GWG in women living with overweight or obesity [11,13]. Our results are consistent with those reported by Fernandes MD et al. [20], who demonstrated a positive correlation between weight gain during pregnancy and serum leptin concentration in all trimesters of pregnancy. The higher leptin concentrations produced during pregnancy are related to weight gain as well as changes in hormone levels, which can stimulate leptin secretion [68]. Fernandes MD et al. [20] also observed a slight decrease in serum leptin concentrations in the second trimester, which was attributed to the development of insulin resistance during this period, as observed in other studies [25,68]. Therefore, it is crucial to demonstrate in future studies whether the slight decrease in leptin concentration in the second trimester is associated with normal gestational weight gain.

In addition to the association of leptin with excessive GWG, we found that percent body fat is also associated, regardless of pBMI. The majority of studies did not assess body fat, which is important since adipokines are secreted by adipose tissue. Only Lacroix et al. [11] included percent body fat in their analysis, finding that leptin is associated with GWG, adjusted by pBMI and body fat. All studies show a greater association between leptin and excessive GWG in individuals living with overweight and obesity compared to those with normal weight. However, when analyzing the percent body fat, we find that the association with pBMI is lost, as the amount of adipose tissue is more important than body weight. It is likely that the reason is leptin is produced and released mainly by adipose tissue into the bloodstream. Blood leptin levels reflect the size of adipose tissue and vary according to nutritional status [69]. Thus, leptin can function as a metabolic regulator linking the body's nutritional status with processes that require a lot of energy. During pregnancy, energy requirements are essential for adequate maternal weight gain to ensure the development of the fetus, placenta, and other maternal tissues [70]. Another important point related to leptin and reproduction is its secretion by the human placenta, further reinforcing its connection with pregnancy [71]. The formation of the placenta during human gestation is crucial for embryonic development and the success of pregnancy, as it facilitates metabolic exchange and the production of steroids, hormones, growth factors, and cytokines, all critical for maintaining pregnancy [72].

The increase in maternal leptin concentrations is also due to its secretion by the placenta. The mechanisms underlying the role of leptin in weight regulation during pregnancy are not yet well established. Leptin is involved in energy balance, but during gestation, adaptations occur in the central regulation of energy balance, including reduced transport into the brain and leptin resistance. However, these adaptations may not be as well established in individuals with obesity [73].

We found that adiponectin was associated with a lower risk of excessive GWG. This finding is consistent with results observed in adult Mexican women [63]. However, adiponectin showed no association with pre-pregnancy BMI or GWG in Brazilian pregnant adolescents [25]. It is important to note that the Brazilian study included only normal-weight adolescents, suggesting that the association may be present when higher body fat is involved. Adiponectin is secreted by adipocytes and participates in multiple functions such as insulin sensitization, stimulation of lipid metabolism, and glucose absorption, exhibiting anti-inflammatory properties and inversely correlating with body weight and fat mass [20,25]. During pregnancy, adiponectin concentration decreases due to an increase in fat mass.

We did not find any association between irisin and GWG. We hypothesized that since irisin is secreted by both adipose and muscle tissue [26] and is associated with gestational diabetes [27], it might also be associated with GWG. We included physical activity in our analysis, as irisin is stimulated by exercise. However, we found no associations, consistent with findings from another study [15]. This lack of association might be attributed to the generally low levels of physical activity among Mexican adolescents.

Regarding hsCRP, no associations were found with GWG. This result aligns with a study that assessed a panel of inflammatory markers in relation to GWG [13], as well as with the study by Logan et al. [12], who did not observe an association between hsCRP concentrations and gestational weight gain. However, Hrolfsdottir, et al. [35] found a positive association of hsCRP with greater GWG. It is important to note that the samples used in their study were stored for 20 years, suggesting potential differences in nutritional, health, and social environments compared to present-day conditions. While pregnancy is an inflammatory state [32], it appears that adipose tissue functions more in metabolic regulation than in inflammation, suggesting that the association of gestational weight gain with serum leptin concentrations is probably not related to the inflammatory response. Nonetheless, further studies are warranted.

This study has some limitations. Firstly, the participants were recruited at various stages of gestation, resulting in a heterogeneous sample. However, considering that maternal leptin concentrations typically peak in the late second and early third trimester [74], we conducted a sensitivity analysis on a subgroup of participants within a specific range of gestational weeks and found no significant differences in associations. Additionally, only 62.5% of the total sample were included in the analysis due to complete biochemical data availability, potentially affecting the results. Furthermore, body fat was assessed using bioimpedance, which can be influenced by hydration status, particularly at a more advanced gestational age when the volume of amniotic fluid is greater. Nonetheless, comparison with a subsample undergoing skin fold measurements revealed no statistical differences.

Despite these limitations, the study has notable strengths. We evaluated GWG according to IOM recommendations and as a percentage of adequacy, accounting for gestational age, thus providing specific total recommended gestational weight gain calculations. Additionally, we assessed pre-pregnancy BMI accordingly for adolescents, using the WHO growth chart for girls and age. Further, we included factors important for adipokine secretion in our analysis, such as body fat, energy intake, and physical activity.

5. Conclusions

In pregnant Mexican adolescents, both leptin and body fat percentage were associated with excessive GWG, independent of pBMI. This suggests that adipose tissue and its adipokines appear to play a more significant role in GWG than pre-pregnancy body weight. Future research should explore the interactions and physiological mechanisms of various adipokines beyond leptin, as well as other inflammatory markers, taking into account body composition and lifestyle factors.

It is essential to promote lifestyles that help adolescents start their pregnancy at an adequate and healthy weight, while providing necessary counseling and support to promote appropriate gestational weight gain.

According to recommendations from the Institute of Medicine of the United States, future research should focus on mechanisms underlying the effects of gestational weight gain on the mother–baby dyad, which may have adverse metabolic consequences later in their lives.

Supplementary Materials: The following supporting information can be downloaded at: https://www.mdpi.com/article/10.3390/nu16132147/s1, Table S1: Correlations between anthropometric, biochemical, and dietetic variables in Mexican pregnant adolescents, INPer 2018–2023.

Author Contributions: Conceptualization, G.C.-B., R.S., H.M.-R., M.K.-H., G.T.O. and A.R.V.-R.; methodology, G.C.-B., R.S., H.M.-R., M.K.-H., G.T.O. and A.R.V.-R.; validation, G.C.-B., R.S., R.M.M.-H., E.B.-G. and A.L.-H.; formal analysis, G.C.-B., E.B.-G., M.K.-H., G.T.O. and A.R.V.-R.; investigation, G.C.-B., R.S., H.M.-R., R.M.M.-H., E.B.-G. and A.L.-H.; resources, R.S., R.M.M.-H. and E.B.-G.; data curation, G.C.-B.; writing—original draft preparation, G.C.-B.; writing—review and editing, G.C.-B., R.S., H.M.-R., M.K.-H., G.T.O. and A.R.V.-R.; visualization, G.C.-B. and R.M.M.-H.; supervision, G.C.-B., R.S. and A.R.V.-R.; project administration, G.C.-B., R.S., A.L.-H. and A.R.V.-R.; funding acquisition, R.S. All authors have read and agreed to the published version of the manuscript.

Funding: This study was funded by the Instituto Nacional de Perinatología (registration numbers 2017-2-101 and 212250-494811) and by CONAHCyT (grants A3-S-40575 and CVU 288316 for Gabriela Chico-Barba's doctoral studies).

Institutional Review Board Statement: The study was approved by the Institute National of Perinatology Ethics Committee (registration number 2017-2-101, date of approval 29 September 2017).

Informed Consent Statement: Informed consent was obtained from all subjects involved in the study.

Data Availability Statement: The data presented in this study are available from the corresponding author upon reasonable request. The data are not publicly available due to privacy and ethical reasons.

Acknowledgments: We want to thank Cinthya Muñoz-Manrique for her insight in the data analysis. Additionally, we appreciate the assistance of Mari Cruz Tolentino-Dolores in the Nutrition Laboratory.

Conflicts of Interest: The authors declare no conflict of interest.

References

1. Adolescent Pregnancy. Available online: https://www.who.int/news-room/fact-sheets/detail/adolescent-pregnancy (accessed on 15 May 2024).
2. UNFPA Socioeconomic Consequences of Adolescent Pregnancy in Six Latin American Countries. Implementation of the MILENA methodology in Argentina, Colombia, Ecuador, Guatemala, Mexico and Paraguay. 2020. Available online: https://lac.unfpa.org/sites/default/files/pub-pdf/eng_-_informe_consecuencias_socioeconomicas_del_embarazo_en_la_adolescencia_en_seis_paises_de_america_latina_y_el_caribe._vf.pdf (accessed on 8 May 2024).
3. Natalidad y Fecundidad. Porcentaje de Nacimientos Registrados de Madres Adolescentes (Menores de 20 Años). Available online: https://www.inegi.org.mx/temas/natalidad/ (accessed on 8 May 2024).
4. Conde-Agudelo, A.; Belizán, J.M.; Lammers, C. Maternal-Perinatal Morbidity and Mortality Associated with Adolescent Pregnancy in Latin America: Cross-Sectional Study. *Am. J. Obstet. Gynecol.* **2005**, *192*, 342–349. [CrossRef] [PubMed]
5. Ganchimeg, T.; Ota, E.; Morisaki, N.; Laopaiboon, M.; Lumbiganon, P.; Zhang, J.; Yamdamsuren, B.; Temmerman, M.; Say, L.; Tunçalp, Ö.; et al. Pregnancy and Childbirth Outcomes among Adolescent Mothers: A World Health Organization Multicountry Study. *BJOG* **2014**, *121*, 40–48. [CrossRef] [PubMed]
6. Kawakita, T.; Wilson, K.; Grantz, K.L.; Landy, H.J.; Huang, C.C.; Gomez-Lobo, V. Adverse Maternal and Neonatal Outcomes in Adolescent Pregnancy. *J. Pediatr. Adolesc. Gynecol.* **2016**, *29*, 130–136. [CrossRef] [PubMed]
7. Dude, A.M.; Grobman, W.; Haas, D.; Mercer, B.M.; Parry, S.; Silver, R.M.; Wapner, R.; Wing, D.; Saade, G.; Reddy, U.; et al. Gestational Weight Gain and Pregnancy Outcomes among Nulliparous Women. *Am. J. Perinatol.* **2021**, *38*, 182–190. [CrossRef] [PubMed]

8. Mosquera, P.S.; Malta, M.B.; de Araújo Damasceno, A.A.; Neves, P.A.R.; Matijasevich, A.; Cardoso, M.A. MINA-Brazil Study Group Associations of Gestational Weight Gain with Perinatal Outcomes in Western Brazilian Amazon. *Matern. Child. Health J.* **2022**, *26*, 2030–2039. [CrossRef] [PubMed]
9. Yang, J.; Wang, M.; Tobias, D.K.; Rich-Edwards, J.W.; Darling, A.M.; Abioye, A.I.; Pembe, A.B.; Madzorera, I.; Fawzi, W.W. Gestational Weight Gain during the Second and Third Trimesters and Adverse Pregnancy Outcomes, Results from a Prospective Pregnancy Cohort in Urban Tanzania. *Reprod. Health* **2022**, *19*, 140. [CrossRef] [PubMed]
10. Rasmussen, K.M.; Yaktine, A.L.; Committee to Reexamine IOM Pregnancy Weight Guidelines; Food and Nutrition Board; Board on Children Youth and Families; Institute of Medicine; National Research Council. *Weight Gain During Pregnancy: Reexamining the Guidelines*; Institute fo Medicine: Washington, DC, USA; National Academy Press: Washington, DC, USA, 2009; ISBN 978-0-309-13113-1.
11. Lacroix, M.; Battista, M.-C.; Doyon, M.; Moreau, J.; Patenaude, J.; Guillemette, L.; Ménard, J.; Ardilouze, J.-L.; Perron, P.; Hivert, M.-F. Higher Maternal Leptin Levels at Second Trimester Are Associated with Subsequent Greater Gestational Weight Gain in Late Pregnancy. *BMC Pregnancy Childbirth* **2016**, *16*, 62. [CrossRef] [PubMed]
12. Logan, C.A.; Bornemann, R.; Koenig, W.; Reister, F.; Walter, V.; Fantuzzi, G.; Weyermann, M.; Brenner, H.; Genuneit, J.; Rothenbacher, D. Gestational Weight Gain and Fetal-Maternal Adiponectin, Leptin, and CRP: Results of Two Birth Cohorts Studies. *Sci. Rep.* **2017**, *7*, 41847. [CrossRef] [PubMed]
13. Wang, D.; Darling, A.M.; McDonald, C.R.; Perumal, N.; Liu, E.; Wang, M.; Aboud, S.; Urassa, W.; Conroy, A.L.; Hayford, K.T.; et al. Plasma Concentrations of Leptin at Mid-Pregnancy Are Associated with Gestational Weight Gain among Pregnant Women in Tanzania: A Prospective Cohort Study. *BMC Pregnancy Childbirth* **2021**, *21*, 675. [CrossRef]
14. Mazaki-Tovi, S.; Kanety, H.; Pariente, C.; Hemi, R.; Wiser, A.; Schiff, E.; Sivan, E. Maternal Serum Adiponectin Levels during Human Pregnancy. *J. Perinatol.* **2007**, *27*, 77–81. [CrossRef]
15. Hernández-Trejo, M.; Montoya-Estrada, A.; Torres-Ramos, Y.; Espejel-Núñez, A.; Guzmán-Grenfell, A.; Morales-Hernández, R.; Tolentino-Dolores, M.; Laresgoiti-Servitje, E. Oxidative Stress Biomarkers and Their Relationship with Cytokine Concentrations in Overweight/Obese Pregnant Women and Their Neonates. *BMC Immunol.* **2017**, *18*, 3. [CrossRef] [PubMed]
16. Gutaj, P.; Sibiak, R.; Jankowski, M.; Awdi, K.; Bryl, R.; Mozdziak, P.; Kempisty, B.; Wender-Ozegowska, E. The Role of the Adipokines in the Most Common Gestational Complications. *Int. J. Mol. Sci.* **2020**, *21*, 9408. [CrossRef] [PubMed]
17. Zhang, Y.; Chua, S. Leptin Function and Regulation. *Compr. Physiol.* **2017**, *8*, 351–369. [CrossRef] [PubMed]
18. Hauguel-de Mouzon, S.; Lepercq, J.; Catalano, P. The Known and Unknown of Leptin in Pregnancy. *Am. J. Obstet. Gynecol.* **2006**, *194*, 1537–1545. [CrossRef] [PubMed]
19. Hoggard, N.; Haggarty, P.; Thomas, L.; Lea, R.G. Leptin Expression in Placental and Fetal Tissues: Does Leptin Have a Functional Role? *Biochem. Soc. Trans.* **2001**, *29*, 57–63. [CrossRef] [PubMed]
20. Fernandes, M.D.; Daher, S.; de Sousa, L.M.; Baratto, I.; Lobo, T.F.; Júnior, E.A.; Guazzelli, C.A.F. Blood Level of Adipokines and Nutritional Status Variables in Adolescent Pregnancy. *Obstet. Gynecol. Sci.* **2020**, *63*, 683–689. [CrossRef] [PubMed]
21. Sámano, R.; Martínez-Rojano, H.; Chico-Barba, G.; Godínez-Martínez, E.; Sánchez-Jiménez, B.; Montiel-Ojeda, D.; Tolentino, M. Serum Concentration of Leptin in Pregnant Adolescents Correlated with Gestational Weight Gain, Postpartum Weight Retention and Newborn Weight/Length. *Nutrients* **2017**, *9*, 1067. [CrossRef] [PubMed]
22. Valencia-Ortega, J.; Solis-Paredes, J.M.; Saucedo, R.; Estrada-Gutierrez, G.; Camacho-Arroyo, I. Excessive Pregestational Weight and Maternal Obstetric Complications: The Role of Adipokines. *IJMS* **2023**, *24*, 14678. [CrossRef] [PubMed]
23. Trujillo, M.L.; Spuch, C.; Carro, E.; Señarís, R. Hyperphagia and Central Mechanisms for Leptin Resistance during Pregnancy. *Endocrinology* **2011**, *152*, 1355–1365. [CrossRef]
24. Fang, H.; Judd, R.L. Adiponectin Regulation and Function. *Compr. Physiol.* **2018**, *8*, 1031–1063. [CrossRef]
25. Baratto, I.; Daher, S.; Lobo, T.F.; Araujo Júnior, E.; Guazzelli, C.A.F. Adiponectin and Leptin Serum Levels in Normal Adolescent Pregnancies. *J. Matern.-Fetal Neonatal Med.* **2021**, *34*, 2019–2024. [CrossRef] [PubMed]
26. Boström, P.; Wu, J.; Jedrychowski, M.P.; Korde, A.; Ye, L.; Lo, J.C.; Rasbach, K.a.; Boström, E.A.; Choi, J.H.; Long, J.Z.; et al. A PGC1a Dependent Myokine that derives Browning of White Fat and Thermogenesis. *Nature* **2012**, *481*, 463–468. [CrossRef] [PubMed]
27. Du, X.L.; Jiang, W.X.; Lv, Z.T. Lower Circulating Irisin Level in Patients with Diabetes Mellitus: A Systematic Review and Meta-Analysis. *Horm. Metab. Res.* **2016**, *48*, 644–652. [CrossRef] [PubMed]
28. Wang, P.; Ma, H.; Hou, X.; Song, L.; Song, X.; Zhang, J. Reduced Plasma Level of Irisin in First Trimester as a Risk Factor for the Development of Gestational Diabetes Mellitus. *Diabetes Res. Clin. Pract.* **2018**, *142*, 130–138. [CrossRef] [PubMed]
29. Seven, A.; Yalinbas, E.; Kucur, S.K.; Kocak, E.; Isiklar, O.; Yuksel, B.; Timur, H.; Erbakirci, M.; Keskin, N. Comprehensive Evaluation of Irisin Levels in Fetomaternal Circulation of Pregnant Women with Obesity or Gestational Diabetes Mellitus. *Ir. J. Med. Sci.* **2019**, *188*, 1213–1219. [CrossRef] [PubMed]
30. Perichart-Perera, O.; Muñoz-Manrique, C.; Reyes-López, A.; Tolentino-Dolores, M.; Espino Y Sosa, S.; Ramírez-González, M.C. Metabolic Markers during Pregnancy and Their Association with Maternal and Newborn Weight Status. *PLoS ONE* **2017**, *12*, e0180874. [CrossRef] [PubMed]
31. Ren, Y.; Zhao, H.; Yin, C.; Lan, X.; Wu, L.; Du, X.; Griffiths, H.R.; Gao, D. Adipokines, Hepatokines and Myokines: Focus on Their Role and Molecular Mechanisms in Adipose Tissue Inflammation. *Front. Endocrinol.* **2022**, *13*, 873699. [CrossRef]

32. Palm, M.; Axelsson, O.; Wernroth, L.; Larsson, A.; Basu, S. Involvement of Inflammation in Normal Pregnancy. *Acta Obs. Gynecol. Scand.* **2013**, *92*, 601–605. [CrossRef]
33. Mor, G.; Cardenas, I.; Abrahams, V.; Guller, S. Inflammation and pregnancy: The Role of the Immune System at the Implantation Site. *Ann. N. Y. Acad. Sci.* **2012**, *1221*, 80–87. [CrossRef]
34. Unamuno, X.; Gómez-Ambrosi, J.; Rodríguez, A.; Becerril, S.; Frühbeck, G.; Catalán, V. Adipokine Dysregulation and Adipose Tissue Inflammation in Human Obesity. *Eur. J. Clin. Investig.* **2018**, *48*, e12997. [CrossRef]
35. Hrolfsdottir, L.; Schalkwijk, C.G.; Birgisdottir, B.E.; Gunnarsdottir, I.; Maslova, E.; Granström, C.; Strøm, M.; Olsen, S.F.; Halldorsson, T.I. Maternal Diet, Gestational Weight Gain, and Inflammatory Markers during Pregnancy. *Obesity* **2016**, *24*, 2133–2139. [CrossRef]
36. Shamah-Levy, T.; Gaona-Pineda, E.B.; Cuevas-Nasu, L.; Morales-Ruan, C.; Valenzuela-Bravo, D.G.; Méndez-Gómez Humaran, I.; Ávila-Arcos, M.A. Prevalence of Overweight and Obesity in Mexican School-Aged Children and Adolescents. Ensanut 2020-2022. *Salud Publica Mex* **2023**, *65*, s218–s224. [CrossRef]
37. Santos, S.; Voerman, E.; Amiano, P.; Barros, H.; Beilin, L.; Bergström, A.; Charles, M.; Chatzi, L.; Chevrier, C.; Chrousos, G.; et al. Impact of Maternal Body Mass Index and Gestational Weight Gain on Pregnancy Complications: An Individual Participant Data Meta-Analysis of European, North American and Australian cohorts. *BJOG* **2019**, *126*, 984–995. [CrossRef] [PubMed]
38. Sámano, R.; Chico-Barba, G.; Flores-Quijano, M.E.; Godínez-Martínez, E.; Martínez-Rojano, H.; Ortiz-Hernandez, L.; Nájera-Medina, O.; Hernández-Trejo, M.; Hurtado-Solache, C. Association of Pregestational BMI and Gestational Weight Gain with Maternal and Neonatal Outcomes in Adolescents and Adults from Mexico City. *Int. J. Environ. Res. Public Health* **2022**, *19*, 280. [CrossRef]
39. Enebe, J.T.; Enebe, N.O.; Nwagha, T.U.; Meka, I.A.; Nwankwo, M.E.; Izuka, E.O.; Egede, J.O.; Ugwu, I.A.; Okoro, N.I.; Okoye, H.C.; et al. Serum Leptin Levels and Relationship with Maternal Weight Gain at Term among Obese and Non-Obese Pregnant Women in Enugu, Nigeria: A Comparative Cross-Sectional Study. *J. Int. Med. Res.* **2023**, *51*, 03000605231213265. [CrossRef] [PubMed]
40. Itoh, H.; Ueda, M.; Suzuki, M.; Kohmura-Kobayashi, Y. Developmental Origins of Metaflammation; A Bridge to the Future between the DOHaD Theory and Evolutionary Biology. *Front. Endocrinol.* **2022**, *13*, 839436. [CrossRef] [PubMed]
41. Hotamisligil, G.S. Inflammation, Metaflammation and Immunometabolic disorders. *Nature* **2017**, *542*, 177–185. [CrossRef]
42. Ingvorsen, C.; Brix, S.; Ozanne, S.E.; Hellgren, L.I. The Effect of Maternal Inflammation on Foetal Programming of Metabolic Disease. *Acta Physiol.* **2015**, *214*, 440–449. [CrossRef]
43. Parisi, F.; Milazzo, R.; Savasi, V.M.; Cetin, I. Maternal Low-Grade Chronic Inflammation and Intrauterine Programming of Health and Disease. *IJMS* **2021**, *22*, 1732. [CrossRef]
44. Adolescent Health. Available online: https://www.who.int/health-topics/adolescent-health (accessed on 24 June 2024).
45. Headen, I.; Cohen, A.K.; Mujahid, M.; Abrams, B. The Accuracy of Self-Reported Pregnancy-Related Weight: A Systematic Review. *Obes. Rev.* **2017**, *18*, 350–369. [CrossRef]
46. Araújo, R.; Gama, S.; Barros, D.; Saunders, C.; Mattos, I. Validity of Self-Reported Weight, Height, and BMI in Mothers of the Research Birth in Brazil. *Rev. Saude Publica* **2017**, *51*, 115. [CrossRef] [PubMed]
47. de Onis, M.; Onyango, A.W.; Borghi, E.; Siyam, A.; Nishida, C.; Siekmann, J. Development of a WHO Growth Reference for School-Aged Children and Adolescents. *Bull. World Health Organ.* **2007**, *85*, 660–667. [CrossRef] [PubMed]
48. Widen, E.M.; Whyatt, R.M.; Hoepner, L.A.; Ramirez-Carvey, J.; Oberfield, S.E.; Hassoun, A.; Perera, F.P.; Gallagher, D.; Rundle, A.G. Excessive Gestational Weight Gain Is Associated with Long-Term Body Fat and Weight Retention at 7 y Postpartum in African American and Dominican Mothers with Underweight, Normal, and Overweight Prepregnancy BMI. *Am. J. Clin. Nutr.* **2015**, *102*, 1460–1467. [CrossRef]
49. Adu-Afarwuah, S.; Lartey, A.; Okronipa, H.; Ashorn, P.; Ashorn, U.; Zeilani, M.; Arimond, M.; Vosti, S.A.; Dewey, K.G. Maternal Supplementation with Small-Quantity Lipid-Based Nutrient Supplements Compared with Multiple Micronutrients, but Not with Iron and Folic Acid, Reduces the Prevalence of Low Gestational Weight Gain in Semi-Urban Ghana: A Randomized Controlled Trial. *J. Nutr.* **2017**, *147*, 697–705. [CrossRef] [PubMed]
50. Chavira-Suárez, E.; Ramírez-Mendieta, A.J.; Martínez-Gutiérrez, S.; Zárate-Segura, P.; Beltrán-Montoya, J.; Espinosa-Maldonado, N.C.; de la Cerda-Ángeles, J.C.; Vadillo-Ortega, F. Influence of Pre-Pregnancy Body Mass Index (p-BMI) and Gestational Weight Gain (GWG) on DNA Methylation and Protein Expression of Obesogenic Genes in Umbilical Vein. *PLoS ONE* **2019**, *14*, e0226010. [CrossRef] [PubMed]
51. Houghton, L.C.; Ester, W.A.; Lumey, L.H.; Michels, K.B.; Wei, Y.; Cohn, B.A.; Susser, E.; Terry, M.B. Maternal Weight Gain in Excess of Pregnancy Guidelines Is Related to Daughters Being Overweight 40 years later. *Am. J. Obs. Gynecol.* **2016**, *215*, 246.e1–246.e8. [CrossRef]
52. Groth, S.W.; Holland, M.L.; Smith, J.A.; Meng, Y.; Kitzman, H. Effect of Gestational Weight Gain and Prepregnancy Body Mass Index in Adolescent Mothers on Weight and Body Mass Index of Adolescent Offspring. *J. Adolesc. Health* **2017**, *61*, 626–633. [CrossRef]
53. Sámano, R.; Martínez-Rojano, H.; Chico-Barba, G.; Hernández-Trejo, M.; Guzmán, R.; Arteaga-Troncoso, G.; Figueroa-Pérez, M.A.; Morales, R.M.; Martínez, G. Associations between Prenatal Serum Levels of Leptin, IGF-I, and Estradiol and Adolescent Mothers' Height Gain during and after Pregnancy. *PLoS ONE* **2020**, *15*, e0228706. [CrossRef] [PubMed]

54. Lundeen, E.A.; Norris, S.A.; Martorell, R.; Suchdev, P.S.; Mehta, N.K.; Richter, L.M.; Stein, A.D. Adolescent Pregnancy and Attained Height among Black South African Girls: Matched-Pair Prospective Study. *PLoS ONE* **2016**, *11*, e0147861. [CrossRef] [PubMed]
55. Whelan, E.; Armson, B.A.; Ashley-Martin, J.; MacSween, K.; Woolcott, C. Gestational Weight Gain and Interpregnancy Weight Change in Adolescent Mothers. *J. Pediatr. Adolesc. Gynecol.* **2017**, *30*, 356–361. [CrossRef]
56. Marvin-Dowle, K.; Burley, V.J.; Soltani, H. Nutrient Intakes and Nutritional Biomarkers in Pregnant Adolescents: A Systematic review of STUDIES in Developed Countries. *BMC Pregnancy Childbirth* **2016**, *16*, 268. [CrossRef]
57. Singh, A.; Trumpff, C.; Genkinger, J.; Davis, A.; Spann, M.; Werner, E.; Monk, C. Micronutrient Dietary Intake in Latina Pregnant Adolescents and Its Association with Level of Depression, Stress, and Social Support. *Nutrients* **2017**, *9*, 1212. [CrossRef] [PubMed]
58. Sámano, R.; Chico-Barba, G.; Martínez-Rojano, H.; Godínez, E.; Rodríguez-Ventura, A.L.; Ávila-Koury, G.; Aguilar-Sánchez, K. Pre-Pregnancy Body Mass Index Classification and Gestational Weight Gain on Neonatal Outcomes in Adolescent Mothers: A Follow-Up Study. *PLoS ONE* **2018**, *13*, e0200361. [CrossRef]
59. Zheng, Z.; Bennett, W.L.; Mueller, N.T.; Appel, L.J.; Wang, X. Gestational Weight Gain and Pregnancy Complications in a High-Risk, Racially and Ethnically Diverse Population. *J. Women's Health* **2019**, *28*, 375–383. [CrossRef]
60. Sun, Y.; Shen, Z.; Zhan, Y.; Wang, Y.; Ma, S.; Zhang, S.; Liu, J.; Wu, S.; Feng, Y.; Chen, Y.; et al. Effects of Pre-Pregnancy Body Mass Index and Gestational Weight Gain on Maternal and Infant Complications. *BMC Pregnancy Childbirth* **2020**, *20*, 390. [CrossRef] [PubMed]
61. Suto, M.; Maeda, K.; Sato, M.; Kaji, T.; Irahara, M. Plasma Adipokine Concentrations in Overweight/Obese Pregnant Women: A Longitudinal Study. *Gynecol. Endocrinol.* **2019**, *35*, 242–246. [CrossRef]
62. Hinkle, S.N.; Rawal, S.; Liu, D.; Chen, J.; Tsai, M.Y.; Zhang, C. Maternal Adipokines Longitudinally Measured across Pregnancy and Their Associations with Neonatal Size, Length, and Adiposity. *Int. J. Obes.* **2019**, *43*, 1422–1434. [CrossRef]
63. Solis Paredes, J.M.; Perichart Perera, O.; Montoya Estrada, A.; Reyes Muñoz, E.; Espino Y Sosa, S.; Ortega Castillo, V.; Medina Bastidas, D.; Tolentino Dolores, M.; Sanchez Martinez, M.; Nava Salazar, S.; et al. Gestational Weight Gain Influences the Adipokine-Oxidative Stress Association during Pregnancy. *Obes. Facts* **2021**, *14*, 604–612. [CrossRef] [PubMed]
64. Andersson-Hall, U.; Svedin, P.; Svensson, H.; Lönn, M.; Mallard, C.; Holmäng, A. Longitudinal Changes in Adipokines and Free Leptin Index during and after Pregnancy in Women with Obesity. *Int. J. Obes.* **2020**, *44*, 675–683. [CrossRef]
65. Howell, K.R.; Powell, T.L. Effects of Maternal Obesity on Placental Function and Fetal Development. *Reproduction* **2017**, *153*, R97–R108. [CrossRef]
66. Kelly, A.C.; Powell, T.L.; Jansson, T. Placental Function in Maternal Obesity. *Clin. Sci.* **2020**, *134*, 961–984. [CrossRef] [PubMed]
67. Lappas, M.; Lim, R.; Price, S.; Prendergast, L.A.; Proietto, J.; Ekinci, E.I.; Sumithran, P. Exploring the Relationship between Maternal Circulating Hormones and Gestational Weight Gain in Women without Obesity: A Cross-Sectional study. *Int. J. Women's Health* **2020**, *12*, 455–462. [CrossRef] [PubMed]
68. Childs, G.V.; Odle, A.K.; MacNicol, M.C.; MacNicol, A.M. The Importance of Leptin to Reproduction. *Endocrinology* **2021**, *162*, bqaa204. [CrossRef] [PubMed]
69. Münzberg, H.; Morrison, C.D. Structure, Production and Signaling of Leptin. *Metabolism* **2015**, *64*, 13–23. [CrossRef]
70. Wauman, J.; Zabeau, L.; Tavernier, J. The Leptin Receptor Complex: Heavier Than Expected? *Front. Endocrinol.* **2017**, *8*, 30. [CrossRef] [PubMed]
71. Chehab, F.F. 20 years of leptin: Leptin and Reproduction: Past Milestones, Present Undertakings, and Future Endeavors. *J. Endocrinol.* **2014**, *223*, T37–T48. [CrossRef] [PubMed]
72. Pollheimer, J.; Knöfler, M. Signalling Pathways Regulating the Invasive Differentiation of Human Trophoblasts: A Review. *Placenta* **2005**, *26* (Suppl. A), S21–S30. [CrossRef] [PubMed]
73. Andrikopoulou, M.; Panigrahi, S.K.; Jaconia, G.D.; Gyamfi-Bannerman, C.; Smiley, R.M.; Page-Wilson, G. Pregnancy-specific Adaptations in Leptin and Melanocortin Neuropeptides in Early Human Gestation. *J. Clin. Endocrinol. Metab.* **2021**, *106*, dgab510. [CrossRef]
74. Tessier, D.R.; Ferraro, Z.M.; Gruslin, A. Role of Leptin in Pregnancy: Consequences of Maternal Obesity. *Placenta* **2013**, *34*, 205–211. [CrossRef]

nutrients

MDPI

Article

Prenatal Iodine Intake and Maternal Pregnancy and Postpartum Depressive and Anhedonia Symptoms: Findings from a Multiethnic US Cohort

Aderonke A. Akinkugbe [1,2,*], Yueh-Hsiu Mathilda Chiu [1,2], Srimathi Kannan [3], Veerle Bergink [4] and Rosalind J. Wright [1,2,5]

1 Department of Environmental Medicine and Climate Science, Icahn School of Medicine at Mount Sinai, New York, NY 10029, USA
2 Institute for Climate Change, Environmental Health and Exposomics, Icahn School of Medicine at Mount Sinai, New York, NY 10029, USA
3 Division of Metabolism, Endocrinology, and Diabetes, Department of Internal Medicine, University of Michigan, Ann Arbor, MI 48109, USA
4 Department of Psychiatry, Icahn School of Medicine at Mount Sinai, New York, NY 10029, USA
5 Department of Public Health, Icahn School of Medicine at Mount Sinai, New York, NY 10029, USA
* Correspondence: aderonke.akinkugbe@mssm.edu; Tel.: +1-(212)-824-7030

Abstract: Objective: Emerging evidence suggests that essential trace elements, including iodine, play a vital role in depressive disorders. This study investigated whether prenatal dietary iodine intake alone and in combination with supplemental iodine intake during pregnancy were associated with antepartum and postpartum depressive and anhedonia symptoms. **Methods**: The study population included 837 mothers in the PRogramming of Intergenerational Stress Mechanisms (PRISM) study. The modified BLOCK food frequency questionnaire was used to estimate prenatal dietary and supplemental iodine intake, while the 10-item Edinburg Postpartum Depression Scale (EPDS) ascertained depressive symptoms. Analyses considered the global EPDS score and the anhedonia and depressive symptom subscale scores using dichotomized cutoffs. Logistic regression estimating odds ratios and 95% confidence intervals (CIs) assessed associations of iodine intake in the second trimester of pregnancy and 6-month postpartum depressive and anhedonia symptoms considering dietary intake alone and combined dietary and supplementary intake in separate models. **Results**: Most women were Black/Hispanic Black (43%) and non-Black Hispanics (35%), with 39% reporting a high school education or less. The median (interquartile range, IQR) dietary and supplemental iodine intake among Black/Hispanic Black (198 (115, 337) μg/day) and non-Black Hispanic women (195 (126, 323) μg/day) was higher than the overall median intake level of 187 (116, 315) μg/day. Relative to the Institute of Medicine recommended iodine intake level of 160–220 μg/day, women with intake levels < 100 μg/day, 100–<160 μg/day, >220–<400 μg/day and ≥400 μg/day had increased adjusted odds of 6-month postpartum anhedonia symptoms (aOR = 1.74 (95% CI: 1.08, 2.79), 1.25 (95% CI: 0.80, 1.99), 1.31 (95% CI: 0.82, 2.10), and 1.47 (95% CI: 0.86, 2.51), respectively). The corresponding estimates for postpartum global depressive symptoms were similar but of smaller magnitude. **Conclusions:** Prenatal iodine intake, whether below or above the recommended levels for pregnant women, was most strongly associated with greater anhedonia symptoms, particularly in the 6-month postpartum period. Further studies are warranted to corroborate these findings, as dietary and supplemental iodine intake are amenable to intervention.

Keywords: iodine intake; pregnancy; postpartum; depressive symptoms; anhedonia; pregnancy cohort

1. Introduction

Mood disorders are common in the perinatal period. Perinatal maternal depression includes major and minor episodes during pregnancy (i.e., antenatal) and/or within the first 12 months after delivery (i.e., postpartum). The prevalence of antenatal depression is approximately 20%, while the prevalence of postpartum depression (PPD) ranges from 12 to 18% [1]. A recent report showed that the pooled global prevalence of PPD was 17.7%. PPD subtypes include an estimated 12-month prevalence of 9% for unipolar major depressive disorder and 3% for bipolar disorder [2].

Recent evidence underscores the need to consider the anhedonia depressive subtype, indexed as reduced interest or pleasure to stimuli previously perceived as rewarding consequent to impairment of the effort-based reward system [3]. Anhedonia has been reported in approximately 30% and 50% of individuals with unipolar and bipolar depressive disorder, respectively [4]. Mechanisms underlying anhedonia are distinct from depression. Anhedonia, which may be a surrogate indicator of future depressive illness, has been associated with increased depressive symptom severity and is a negative predictor of treatment response [2]. Studies on anhedonia in the postpartum period remain sparse, but it is estimated to occur in 23% of mothers [5,6]. In addition, women with symptoms suggestive of an anhedonia subtype in pregnancy are more likely to report depression during the postpartum period [2].

Mood disorders in the peripartum period are associated with a significant impact on maternal morbidity and mortality [7,8]. Psychological dysfunction also has implications for the offspring of affected women, being associated with suboptimal interactions between mothers and infants with consequent adverse effects on child cognitive, social, and emotional development, including high levels of child internalizing behaviors [9]. Thus, identifying contributing factors that are amendable to intervention is a critical public health focus.

Depletion of essential micronutrient reserves throughout pregnancy can increase a woman's risk for maternal depression [10,11]. Iodine is an essential micronutrient and the main element required for the synthesis of thyroid hormones, thyroxine (T4) and triiodothyronine (T3), which regulate multiple processes, including growth, metabolism, and reproduction. Thyroid hormones play important roles in modulating metabolic activity in the brain [12]. Thyroid dysfunction has also been linked to perinatal [13] and postpartum depression [13–15]. Iodine deficiency is common during pregnancy due not only to increased renal clearance [15] but also because increased maternal levels are needed to sustain maternal and fetal needs such that iodine requirements are 50% higher during pregnancy and lactation than any other period in the life course [16]. Thus, women of childbearing age are especially vulnerable to the adverse consequences of insufficient iodine intake, and an adequate supply of iodine nutrition before and during pregnancy is essential to adjust thyroid function to meet the increasing demands of pregnancy. Because of successful programs of universal salt iodization in formerly severely iodine-deficient regions, public health concerns have shifted from severe to mild-to-moderate iodine deficiency, which remains prevalent in many regions, especially among pregnant women [17]. Dietary guidelines set by the Institute of Medicine (IOM) recommends an estimated average requirement (EAR) of 160 μg/day, with 220 μg/day [18] being the recommended dietary allowance (RDA) during pregnancy, while the World Health Organization recommends a nutrient intake of iodine of 220 μg/day. Women of reproductive age, especially during pregnancy, fall short of these optimal dietary iodine guidelines.

Elucidating the link between habitual iodine intake during pregnancy and postpartum mood disorders remains understudied, and results have been mixed. One study in a population of pregnant women with mild-to-moderate iodine deficiency found that low dietary iodine levels in the second trimester were associated with higher perinatal and 6-month postpartum depression scores, while supplemental iodine intake was linked to higher postpartum depression [19]. Although it has been suggested that an abrupt increase in iodine from supplements, particularly in women with low intake from food, could cause a "stunning effect" on the thyroid gland and a temporary imbalance in thyroid hormones [20] that might affect mood, Wang et al., 2020 [21] found no differences in depression score 1-month postpartum and no difference in thyroid stimulating hormone (TSH). However, they reported a difference in free thyroxine (FT4) between groups that received iodine supplements (150 μg/day—the recommended supplemental intake level by the American Thyroid Association), as compared to those who received supplements without iodine and those who did not receive supplements. Depression scores were higher in the iodine supplement group, but the difference was not statistically significant [21]. Furthermore, no prior study has considered anhedonia symptoms separate from depressive symptom scores in the peripartum period with respect to mild-to-moderate iodine deficiency in pregnant women.

This study conducted in an ethnically diverse pregnancy cohort in the Northeastern United States (U.S.) examined associations between prenatal habitual dietary iodine intake alone and in combination with its supplemental counterpart and maternal depressive and anhedonia symptoms assessed in pregnancy and 6 months postpartum.

2. Materials and Methods

2.1. Study Population

Participants were mothers enrolled in the PRogramming of Intergenerational Stress Mechanisms (PRISM) study, an ongoing prospective pregnancy cohort originally designed to examine the influence of perinatal stress, maternal nutrition, and other environmental exposures on child development and health. Pregnant women were recruited between March 2011 and April 2020 from prenatal clinics in Boston and New York City hospitals. Eligibility included English or Spanish speaking, ≥18 years at enrollment, and carrying a singleton pregnancy. Women were excluded if they reported drinking ≥7 alcoholic beverages/week before pregnancy recognition or any alcohol consumption after becoming pregnant and having an infant born with congenital anomalies or neurological dysfunction that would impede their ability to participate in longitudinal follow-up. PRISM was conducted in accordance with prevailing ethical principles, and all procedures were approved by the human subject committees at the Brigham and Women's Hospital and Icahn School of Medicine at Mount Sinai; written informed consent was obtained in the participants' primary language. From a total of 1731 eligible mothers, after excluding mothers with more than one child from this study, 837 mothers with non-missing prenatal dietary iodine information were included in these analyses.

2.2. Exposures

Maternal Iodine: Prenatal dietary intake in the past 3 months was assessed in the second trimester of pregnancy with an interviewer-administered modified BLOCK98 FFQ (Block 2006_Bodnar FFQ, version 98.2, NutritionQuest, Berkeley, CA, USA) consisting of 120 food and beverage items [22,23]. The BLOCK98 FFQ incorporates dietary and questionnaire changes suggested by American national consumption data collected from the third National Health and Nutrition Examination Survey (NHANES III) [24,25] and has been validated in multi-cultural populations, including pregnant women [23,26]. The FFQ was administered in English or Spanish by bilingual research staff, reviewed for completion, and processed through the online BLOCK Dietary Data Systems (Berkeley, CA, USA) for micronutrient analysis using software developed at the National Cancer Institute (NCI). For each item on the FFQ, an average daily nutrient intake was calculated based on the nutrient content of the item and the frequency and portion size consumed. Nutrient values were calculated by multiplying the nutrient content of the food or beverage by the gram weight and frequency and summing across all food items. To compute iodine micronutrient values in foods, beverages, and dietary supplements, we used the most recent USDA, FDA, and ODS-NIH Database for the Iodine Content of Common Foods [27–29] and other scientific resources [30–32]. Supplementary data were linked to the NHANES dietary supplement files. For specific iodine-containing supplement use analysis, we identified supplements by their inclusion of iodine based on their ingredient identification codes on the dietary supplement database file. Estimates of iodine intake from dietary sources were generated through linkage to dietary intake tools and to the data generated by the

NHANES. To estimate updated iodine data from reported foods, the database developed by USDA version 3.0 [27], the Food and Drug Administration (FDA) Center for Food Safety and Applied Nutrition in College Park, MD, and the Office of Dietary Supplements, NIH, were utilized, along with the Office of Dietary Supplements, National Institutes of Health. After matching the consumed dietary supplement product with the ingredient information from the NHANES database, we categorized study participants as users or nonusers of dietary supplements with iodine. For these analyses, iodine intake from food and from food and supplements combined were categorized as <100 μg/day, 100–<160 μg/day, 160–220 μg/day (reference), 221–<400 μg/day, and ≥400 μg/day (due to the few mothers at or exceeding this intake level (12% and 15%, respectively, for dietary iodine and combined dietary and supplemental iodine). The reference group was chosen to reflect the IOM EAR of 160 μg/day and the RDA of 220 μg/day during pregnancy [18].

2.3. *Outcomes*

Global EPDS Score: The 10-item Edinburgh Postnatal Depression Scale (EPDS) can be used to assess depressive symptoms in the past 7 days as a unidimensional scale and as multidimensional subscales, including depressive and anhedonia symptoms in pregnant, postnatal, and non-pregnant women and it is validated in both English and Spanish populations [33–35]. The 10-item EPDS [8] was used to assess global antepartum depression in the second trimester, and postpartum depression was assessed 6 months after delivery. We focused on 6-month PPD in this study because it represents stable depression episodes unrelated to pregnancy. Women completed the EPDS 6-month postpartum either by telephone or during an in-person laboratory visit, and some completed IT at both visits (n = 455 (54%)). We used as the postpartum score non-missing values from either the telephone or the laboratory visits, and when both were available, we chose the higher total score of the two. Items included: "1: able to laugh", "2: looking forward", "3: self-blaming", "4: worrying", "5: scared", "6: things get on top of me (overwhelmed)", "7: difficult to sleep", "8: feeling sad", "9: crying", and "10: the thought of self-harming". Items were scored on a Likert scale from 0, indicating the most favorable condition, to 3, indicating the least favorable condition for each item. The range of the global EPDS score in this sample was 0–29 in the antepartum and postpartum periods.

The global EPDS score (antepartum and 6 months postpartum) was categorized into ≥10 vs. <10, a threshold that has been used as a consensus cutoff for screening for a concern of clinical depression [36]. A score of ≥10 on the EPDS scale has a reported sensitivity and specificity of 0.85 (95% CI: 0.79 to 0.90) and 0.84 (95% CI: 0.79 to 0.88), respectively [36]. We also considered a cutoff score of ≥13 vs. <13 (which is also commonly used) in a sensitivity analysis. Existing literature suggests that the EPDS can be used to assess multidimensional perinatal psychological functioning, although originally developed as a unidimensional scale. An exploratory and confirmatory factor analysis in the PRISM cohort identified 2-factor subconstructs (anhedonia and depressive symptoms) from the global EPDS [35]. The anhedonia subconstruct loaded on items 1 and 2, while the depression subconstruct loaded on items 3–9. Item 10 was not considered in the subconstruct analysis due to a very rare positive endorsement rate (only 0.8%).

Subscale Scores: We considered a depressive symptom subscale score using 7 items (questions 3–9) scored on the same 0 to 3 Likert scale; the range in our sample was 0–21. For data analysis, we used a median split of the total sub-score value (≥4 vs. <4) to indicate higher depressive vs. lower depressive subscale symptoms, respectively, for both the prenatal and 6-month postpartum periods.

Item 1: "In the past 7 days, I have been able to laugh and see the funny side of things", and item 2: "In the past 7 days, I have looked forward with enjoyment to things" assessed anhedonia subscale symptoms. Responses were scored on the same 0 to 3 Likert scale; the range in our sample was 0 to 6. We categorized those with a total score of 0 as having no anhedonia symptoms and those with a total score ≥ 1 as having symptoms of anhedonia, both during pregnancy and 6 months postpartum.

Covariates: We considered as adjustment covariates child sex (male, female); maternal age at birth (in years), parity (nulliparous, primiparous, or multiparous); self-reported pre-pregnancy depression diagnosis (yes or no); educational attainment (high school or less, and more than high school); race/ethnicity (Black/Hispanic Black, non-Black Hispanic, non-Hispanic white, other) and previous treatment for a thyroid disorder based on response to the self-reported question on treatment for thyroid disease in the past and abstraction from medical records.

2.4. Data Analysis

Descriptive statistics of frequencies and percentages summarized demographic variables, while the median (IQR) summarized dietary and supplemental iodine intake levels for the different demographic variables. Differences in iodine intake levels were assessed using the Wilcoxon rank-sum test. Missing data were as low as 2.4% for maternal race/ethnicity and as high as 31.5% for postpartum depression. Missing data were imputed using chained equations [37], with a total of 40 datasets imputed using 500 between imputation iterations. Regression analyses were conducted on both the imputed and unimputed datasets, and the results were qualitatively similar; therefore, imputed regression results are presented, and unimputed results are available for review in the supplemental material. Logistic regression estimating odds ratios and 95% confidence intervals (CIs) estimated associations separately between dietary and combined dietary and supplementary iodine intake levels in the 2nd trimester of pregnancy separately with antepartum and 6-month postpartum depressive and anhedonia symptoms. We evaluated effect measure modification by child sex and maternal race/ethnicity, setting a p-value for significant modification to $p < 0.1$, and the results indicated that both factors were not significant effect modifiers and were thus adjusted for as confounders in the main analyses. Due to running multiple models on correlated scales, we adjusted for multiple comparisons at a Bonferroni correction p-value < 0.025, considered statistically significant.

3. Results

3.1. Characteristics of Study Participants and Prenatal Iodine Intake

Most women were Black/Hispanic Black (43%) and non-Black Hispanics (35%). More than one-third reported having a high school education or less, and 25% reported a diagnosis of depression pre-pregnancy. The overall median (IQR) dietary and supplemental iodine intake level was 187 (116, 315) µg/day. We observed significant differences in dietary and supplemental iodine intake levels according to maternal race/ethnicity ($p = 0.05$), pre-pregnancy depression ($p = 0.02$), and prenatal global EPDS ≥ 10 ($p = 0.05$). The median (interquartile range, IQR) dietary and supplemental iodine intake among Black/Hispanic Black (198 (115, 337) µg/day) and non-Black Hispanic women (195 (126, 323) µg/day) was higher than the overall median intake level of 187 (116, 315) µg/day and was also higher than the median intake of dietary and supplemental iodine than the other racial/ethnic groups. Those reporting a diagnosis of depression pre-pregnancy had statistically significant ($p = 0.02$) higher median intake levels of dietary and supplemental iodine at 204 (131, 378) µg/day than those without pre-pregnancy depression whose median intake level was 181 (112, 304) µg/day. Similarly, those with a global EPDS ≥ 10 during pregnancy had a statistically significant ($p = 0.05$) higher median intake of 203 (127, 345) µg/day than those with a prenatal EPDS < 10 with a median intake of 177 (112, 312) µg/day. On the contrary, women with a 6-month postpartum global depressive symptom score EPDS ≥ 10 had lower but non-significant ($p = 0.6$) median dietary and supplemental iodine intake levels when compared to women with a postnatal global EPDS < 10 (168 (116, 324) vs. 191 (117, 319) µg/day, respectively). Likewise, women with postpartum anhedonia symptoms had significantly ($p = 0.04$) lower dietary/supplemental iodine intake levels 158 (108, 321) µg/day than those without postpartum anhedonia symptoms, 198 (126, 319) µg/day. There were no differences in iodine intake during pregnancy and the postpartum period for the depressive symptom subscale score (Table 1).

Table 1. Distribution of socio-demographic characteristics according to dietary and supplemental iodine intake, PRISM (Programming of Intergenerational Stress Mechanisms) pregnancy cohort.

	N	Percent	Food and Supplement Iodine (μg/Day), Median (IQR) #	*p*-Value
Overall	837	100	187 (116, 315)	
Maternal factors				
Age at birth, years, mean (SD) *	29.8 (5.92)			
Age at birth, years				0.4
18–<25	194	23.2	175 (111, 324)	
25–<35	473	56.5	188 (114, 310)	
≥35	170	20.3	198 (127, 320)	
Race/ethnicity				0.05
Non-Hispanic White	142	17.3	151 (110, 269)	
Black/Hispanic Black	352	43	198 (115, 337)	
Non-Black Hispanic	288	35.1	195 (126, 323)	
Other	37	4.52	153 (107, 281)	
Missing	18			
Education				0.6
High school or less	321	39.2	185 (111, 331)	
More than high school	496	60.7	191 (118, 311)	
Missing	20			
Depression pre-pregnancy				0.02
Yes	208	25.3	204 (131, 378)	
No	614	74.7	181 (112, 304)	
Missing	15			
Pregnancy depressive symptoms (Global EPDS)				0.05
<10	538	71.5	177 (112, 312)	
≥10	214	28.5	203 (127, 345)	
Missing	85			
Postpartum depressive symptoms (Global EPDS)				0.6
<10	454	79.2	191 (117, 319)	
≥10	119	20.8	168 (116, 324)	
Missing	264			
Pregnancy anhedonia symptoms				0.6
0	552	73.5	185 (115, 324)	
1–6	199	26.5	193 (120, 317)	
Missing	86			
Postpartum anhedonia symptoms				0.04
0	391	68.2	198 (126, 319)	
1–6	182	31.8	158 (108, 321)	
Missing	264			
Pregnancy depressive subscale symptoms				0.5
<4	339	45.1	180 (111, 318)	
≥4	413	54.9	193 (118, 322)	
Missing	85			
Postpartum depressive subscale symptoms				0.8
<4	292	51.0	188 (117, 323)	
≥4	281	49.0	187 (118, 315)	
Missing	264			
Thyroid disease §				0.4
Yes	52	6.33	170 (113, 278)	
No	769	93.7	190 (116, 320)	
Missing	16			
Child sex				0.8
Female	422	50.5	181 (116, 323)	
Male	413	49.5	192 (115, 305)	
Missing	2			

* SD—standard deviation; # IQR—interquartile range. § Treatment for a thyroid disease was based on self-report and medical record extraction. *p*-value for Wilcoxon–Mann–Whitney rank-sum test.

3.2. Regression Results

Figure 1 shows univariate dose–response curves for iodine intake (dietary alone (panel 1) and dietary/supplemental iodine (panel 2)) with antepartum and postpartum depressive (10-item global and 7-item subscale scores) and anhedonia symptoms. The shape of the dose–response for antepartum mood disorder symptoms was different from the shape of the dose–response observed in the postpartum period. Based on these plots, iodine intake, whether below or above recommended levels in pregnant women, was associated with greater global depressive and anhedonia symptoms, particularly in the postpartum period.

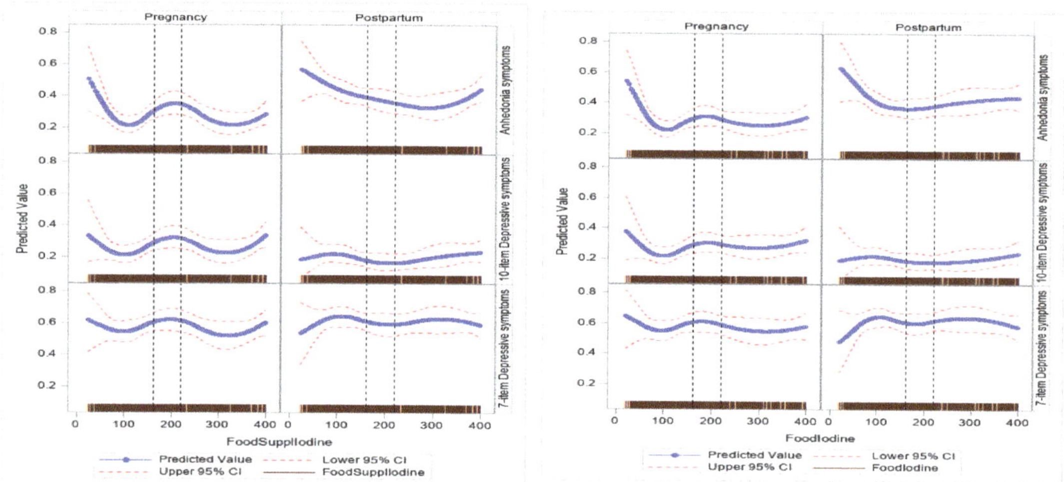

Dietary iodine   Dietary and Supplemental Iodine

Figure 1. Univariate dose–response curves for prenatal iodine intake with pregnancy and postpartum mental health outcomes.

3.2.1. Iodine Intake and Global EPDS Score—Antepartum

There was a suggested association between dietary iodine intake and greater odds of antepartum depression (EPDS $\geq$ 10) for intake levels greater than the recommended thresholds in the unadjusted and adjusted models. When compared to the reference (IOM recommended) of 160–220 µg/day, those in the 201–<400 µg/day and $\geq$400 µg/day had higher adjusted odds of having a global EPDS $\geq$ 10, OR = 1.09 (95% CI: 0.65, 1.83) and OR = 1.16 (95% CI: 0.65, 2.08), respectively. The estimates were similar for the combined dietary and supplemental iodine (Table 2).

3.2.2. Postpartum

There was a suggested association between low and high levels (relative to the reference of 160–220 µg/day) of the combined dietary and supplemental iodine intake and greater unadjusted and adjusted odds of the global 6-month postpartum EPDS score $\geq$ 10. Specifically, women with intake levels classified as <100 µg/day, 100–<160 µg/day, >220–<400 µg/day and $\geq$400 µg/day had greater adjusted odds of global postpartum depressive symptoms score $\geq$ 10 than the reference intake group (aOR = 1.39 (95% CI: 0.74, 2.63), 1.44 (95% CI: 0.80, 2.59), 1.31 (95% CI: 0.73, 2.35), and 1.12 (95% CI: 0.58, 2.17), respectively). We found a similar trend for dietary iodine alone but with smaller magnitudes (Table 3).

Table 2. Prenatal Iodine intake and maternal pregnancy mental health symptoms scores.

	Prenatal Anhedonia Symptoms		Prenatal Global EPDS Score	
	Odds Ratio (95% CI)		Odds Ratio (95% CI)	
Dietary Iodine Intake	Crude	Adjusted	Crude	Adjusted
<100 μg/day	1.03 (0.61, 1.73)	0.99 (0.58, 1.67)	0.87 (0.52, 1.47)	0.82 (0.48, 1.40)
100–<160 μg/day	1.14 (0.71, 1.84)	1.17 (0.72, 1.90)	0.97 (0.60, 1.57)	0.96 (0.59, 1.57)
160–220 μg/day	Ref.	Ref.	Ref.	Ref.
>220–<400 μg/day	1.05 (0.63, 1.75)	1.04 (0.62, 1.74)	1.13 (0.68, 1.86)	1.09 (0.65, 1.83)
≥400 μg/day	1.40 (0.80, 2.47)	1.29 (0.72, 2.30)	1.35 (0.77, 2.36)	1.16 (0.65, 2.08)
Dietary and supplemental iodine				
<100 μg/day	0.98 (0.58, 1.67)	0.96 (0.56, 1.65)	0.89 (0.52, 1.53)	0.86 (0.49, 1.50)
100–<160 μg/day	1.00 (0.62, 1.65)	1.04 (0.63, 1.71)	0.93 (0.56, 1.53)	0.93 (0.56, 1.56)
160–220 μg/day	Ref.	Ref.	Ref.	Ref.
>220–<400 μg/day	0.97 (0.60, 1.58)	0.97 (0.59, 1.60)	1.08 (0.66, 1.76)	1.07 (0.65, 1.77)
≥400 μg/day	1.19 (0.69, 2.05)	1.12 (0.64, 1.94)	1.33 (0.78, 2.29)	1.18 (0.68, 2.06)

Models were adjusted for child sex, maternal age at birth, maternal race/ethnicity, education, pre-pregnancy depression, parity, and previous treatment for a thyroid disease. Anhedonia was based on items 1 and 2 of the 10-item EPDS (Edinburg depression scale), and those with a score of ≥1 were categorized with anhedonia symptoms and 0 with no anhedonia symptoms. Global depressive symptoms were based on a score ≥ 10 on the 10-item EPDS depression scale. Reference for iodine intake was based on the IOM, EAR (160 μg/day), and RDA (220 μg/day) for pregnant women in the US.

Table 3. Prenatal iodine intake and maternal 6-month postpartum mental health outcomes symptoms scores.

	Postpartum Anhedonia Symptoms		Postpartum Global EPDS Score	
	Odds Ratio (95% CI)		Odds Ratio (95% CI)	
Dietary Iodine Intake	Crude	Adjusted	Crude	Adjusted
<100 μg/day	1.74 (1.09, 2.78)	1.74 (1.08, 2.79)	1.20 (0.68, 2.13)	1.20 (0.66, 2.19)
100–<160 μg/day	1.23 (0.79, 1.90)	1.25 (0.80, 1.99)	1.15 (0.67, 1.98)	1.17 (0.67, 2.05)
160–220 μg/day	Ref.	Ref.	Ref.	Ref.
>220–<400 μg/day	1.32 (0.83, 2.10)	1.31 (0.82, 2.10)	1.16 (0.66, 2.06)	1.12 (0.62, 2.01)
≥400 μg/day	1.53 (0.90, 2.60)	1.47 (0.86, 2.51)	1.21 (0.63, 2.30)	1.03 (0.53, 2.02)
Dietary and supplemental iodine intake				
<100 μg/day	1.72 (1.06, 2.79)	1.74 (1.07, 2.83)	1.35 (0.73 (2.49)	1.39 (0.74, 2.63)
100–<160 μg/day	1.23 (0.78, 1.94)	1.26 (0.80, 1.99)	1.38 (0.78, 2.45)	1.44 (0.80, 2.59)
160–220 μg/day	Ref.	Ref.	Ref.	Ref.
>220–<400 μg/day	0.94 (0.60, 1.48)	0.93 (0.59, 1.47)	1.35 (0.77, 2.39)	1.31 (0.73, 2.35)
≥400 μg/day	1.29 (0.78, 2.14)	1.22 (0.73, 2.04)	1.32 (0.70, 2.50)	1.12 (0.58, 2.17)

Models were adjusted for child sex, maternal age at birth, maternal race/ethnicity, education, pre-pregnancy depression, parity, and previous treatment for a thyroid disease. Anhedonia was based on items 1 and 2 of the 10-item EPDS (Edinburg depression scale), and those with a score of ≥1 were categorized with anhedonia symptoms and 0 with no anhedonia symptoms. Global depressive symptoms were based on a score ≥ 10 on the 10-item EPDS depression scale. Reference for iodine intake was based on the IOM, EAR (160 μg/day), and RDA (220 μg/day) for pregnant women in the US. Bold estimates indicate statistical significance at a Bonferroni corrected p-value < 0.025.

3.2.3. Iodine Intake and Anhedonia and Depressive Subscales Symptom Scores—Antepartum

Dietary iodine intake appears to be associated with greater odds of antepartum anhedonia for intake levels lower and greater than the recommended thresholds in unadjusted and adjusted models. When compared to the reference of 160–220 μg/day, those with intake of 100–<160 μg/day had higher adjusted odds of antepartum anhedonia symptoms, OR = 1.17 (95% CI: 0.72, 1.90). Likewise, those with the highest dietary intake levels ≥ 400 μg/day had higher adjusted odds of antepartum anhedonia of OR = 1.29 (95% CI: 0.72, 2.30). These estimates for low and high prenatal iodine intake levels are suggestive of associations in the detrimental direction to maternal mental health, although not statistically significant at the $p < 0.05$ threshold, likely due to the modest sample size. The estimates were similar for the combined dietary and supplemental iodine but with slightly attenuated estimates (Table 2). We found no meaningful associations between dietary and dietary/supplemental iodine intake with the 7-item depressive symptom subscale score during pregnancy (Supplementary Table S4).

3.2.4. Postpartum

Low and high dietary iodine intakes (relative to the reference of 160–220 μg/day) were associated with greater unadjusted and adjusted odds of 6-month postpartum anhedonia symptoms. Specifically, women with intake levels classified as <100 μg/day, 100–<160 μg/day, >220–<400 μg/day, and ≥400 μg/day had higher adjusted odds of 6-month postpartum anhedonia of 1.74 (95% CI: 1.08, 2.79), 1.25 (95% CI: 0.80, 1.99), 1.31 (95% CI: 0.82, 2.10), and 1.47 (95% CI: 0.86, 2.51), respectively, as compared to women in the reference intake level. We found similar trends for dietary and supplemental iodine but with slightly smaller magnitudes (Table 3). We found no meaningful associations between dietary and dietary/supplemental iodine intake with the 7-item depressive symptom subscale score 6 months postpartum (Supplementary Table S4).

Results of complete case analysis were similar in magnitude and direction for both the prenatal, n = 705 (Supplementary Table S1) and the postpartum period, n = 544 (Supplementary Table S2). Results of the global depressive symptom score with a cutoff score of ≥13 are presented in Supplementary Table S3.

4. Discussion

Our findings suggest an association (U-shaped) of dietary/supplemental iodine intake both below and above the IOM recommended intake thresholds for pregnant women with worse mental health outcomes in the postpartum period. For both the global depressive and anhedonia subscale symptoms, our findings were more compelling in the postpartum period than during pregnancy. Indeed, our findings suggest that a higher intake level might be needed during pregnancy to accommodate the needs of the mother and developing fetus while intake in the recommended IOM range, the EAR (160 μg/day) and RDA (220 μg/day) appear sufficient to mitigate poorer maternal health outcomes after birth, specifically depressive and anhedonia symptoms 6 months postpartum. Notably, our estimates of PPD (based on an EPDS ≥ 10) of 20% is similar to reports of 17–20% [1,38] previously reported among pregnant women.

Abnormalities in thyroid function are more prevalent after delivery, with up to 7% of all new mothers experiencing thyroid dysfunction postpartum, compared with a prevalence of 3–4% in the general population [39]. Mood disorders are common in individuals with thyroid conditions (hyper or hyperthyroidism) and autoimmune thyroiditis. Thyroid autoimmunity during pregnancy and in the weeks after childbirth is associated with an increased risk of developing PPD [13,14,40]. Iodine is important for thyroid hormone secretion and the proper functioning of the thyroid gland [41]. Although most patients with depression do not have overt thyroid disease, subclinical hypothyroidism is found in 15% to 20%, and it is the most common thyroid dysfunction in patients with mood disorders [41]. Thyroid dysfunction may thus be a mechanism by which this association occurs, and an explanation for the modest effect sizes may be an indication of iodine intake levels being a distal/upstream risk factor as opposed to more proximal thyroid dysfunction indicators such as high levels of hormones like TSH reported to be associated with worse maternal mental health in the postpartum period.

Studies have found that appropriate iodine supplementation during pregnancy can reduce thyroid volume, decrease serum thyroglobulin level, inhibit the increase in serum TSH level, and reduce the risk of low FT4 levels [20], precursors for poor maternal mental health outcomes. Unlike some prior studies, we found little discrepancy in maternal mental health outcomes for dietary iodine alone when compared to dietary and supplemental iodine at the recommended intake levels, albeit our findings were not always consistent between these two iodine intake pathways. The non-consistent results for iodine from food and iodine from food and supplements in our study may be explained by differences in the effect of long-term habitual iodine intake from food as compared to supplemental iodine. The impact of iodine from supplements depends on habitual iodine intake from food, timing of introduction, dose, frequency, and duration of use [42], which we were unable to consider fully in our data analysis. In mild-to-moderate iodine deficiency, the body adapts to low iodine intake, for example, by increasing the size of the thyroid gland. When iodine intake is increased by supplements or by salt iodization, it may take months to adapt to the new intake level, which can lead to a temporary inhibition of thyroid hormone production [43]. Duration of supplement use was not asked of PRISM cohort participants, but if supplements were used intermittently or for a short duration, it is possible that mothers may not have fully adapted to new intake levels. Another likely explanation for our findings is reverse causation, given that women with underlying psychopathology may be prone to using multivitamin supplements that can abruptly increase iodine levels and, as a side effect trigger, thyroid function imbalances known to affect mood [20]. Differences in the direction of effects for antepartum and postpartum mood states may also be due to physiological differences between pregnancy and the postpartum period.

The results herein point to the importance of considering depressive and anhedonia symptoms in pregnant women and women in the postpartum period, especially given supplement use drops sharply during the postpartum period. Indeed, our findings appear to be driven more by anhedonia. Given that anhedonia questions are a subset of the 10-item EPDS depression scale, the depressive symptom results may have also been driven by anhedonia. When we analyzed the data looking at depressive symptoms without considering the anhedonia questions, the associations were less compelling (Supplementary Table S4).

Strengths and Limitations

We acknowledge both the strengths and potential weaknesses of this study. These analyses are the first to examine these associations in a multi-ethnic, socioeconomically diverse U.S. sample, adding to the literature supporting an association between iodine intake in pregnancy and mood disorders in the antepartum and postpartum periods. We further add to the prior literature by considering both depressive and anhedonia symptoms assessed using the validated and widely used EPDS. Prenatal iodine intake was measured with a widely used and validated FFQ for assessing average habitual dietary intake in pregnant women, and we incorporated intake from both dietary sources and supplements. Nonetheless, the use of FFQs may result in underreporting of iodine intake. Future work should consider adding 24 h dietary recalls or food records as well as biomarkers of bioavailable iodine such as repeated urinary iodine concentrations [44,45] or cumulative prenatal iodine stores assessed with placenta [46] in relation to mood disorders in pregnancy and the postpartum period, particularly when evaluating intake above/below the suggested thresholds [47]. While we used a valid approach to characterizing anhedonia symptoms, scales developed specifically to assess anhedonia with an increased number of items (e.g., Specific Loss of Interest and Pleasure Scale (SLIPS) [48] and Temporal Experience of Pleasure Scale (TEPS) [49]) may provide greater precision in the assessment of this domain. However, it is not uncommon for symptoms of anhedonia to be assessed with a small number of items on a depression symptom scale. For instance, a single question on the 17-item Hamilton Depression Rating Scale, 4 items on the 21-item Beck Depression Inventory, and 4 items on the 30-item Inventory of Depressive Symptoms [50]. Higher scores on the EPDS scale provide an indication for the presence of depressive symptoms rather than the severity of depression or DSM-V depression diagnosis. Severity may be an important construct to study together with the anhedonia subtype, given evidence that the presence of anhedonia has been associated with increased depressive symptom severity and is a negative predictor of treatment response [2]. Recognized predisposing factors for depression include genetic susceptibility, previous psychiatric illnesses, adverse life events, marital disharmony, lack of a confiding relationship, housing problems, or other socioeconomic problems [51]. While we adjusted for many of these predisposing factors, others could not be considered as data were not available (e.g., genetics and other social conditions), thus leaving the possibility for residual confounding. These results warrant replication in other diverse populations with larger sample size cohorts to corroborate the growing evidence linking prenatal iodine intake and mood disorders in pregnancy and postpartum women, especially since iodine intake is modifiable and can be intervened upon. Larger sample size studies would also allow one to consider potential effect modifiers of these associations (e.g., race/ethnicity and socioeconomic status) and modification by multiple essential trace elements, notably, those that have been found to play pivotal roles in regulating neurodevelopment and mood depressive disorders, Se, Zn, Cu, and Mo (alongside iodine) [52].

5. Conclusions

Dietary/supplemental iodine intake lower and higher than the recommended threshold for pregnant women appears to adversely affect the mental health of women in this ethnically and socioeconomically diverse sample, particularly in the postpartum period, while intake levels higher than the recommended threshold appear beneficial to maternal mental health during pregnancy.

These results warrant future studies in other diverse populations with larger sample sizes to corroborate the growing evidence linking prenatal iodine intake and mood disorders in pregnant and postpartum women, especially since low iodine levels appear to be a risk factor amenable to behavioral, clinical, biomedical, and public health interventions.

Supplementary Materials: The following supporting information can be downloaded at: https://www.mdpi.com/article/10.3390/nu16111771/s1, Table S1: Prenatal Iodine intake and maternal pregnancy mental health symptoms scores; Table S2: Prenatal Iodine intake and maternal postpartum mental health symptoms scores; Table S3: Prenatal iodine intake and maternal pregnancy and 6-months postpartum global depression score; Table S4: Prenatal iodine intake and maternal pregnancy and 6-months postpartum depressive subscale scores; Table S5: Covariate balance between those participants included and excluded from current analyses.

Author Contributions: A.A.A. and R.J.W.: conceptualization, methodology, investigation, and writing—original draft. A.A.A.: statistical analysis. Y.-H.M.C., S.K., V.B. and R.J.W.: methodology and writing—review and editing. S.K.: exposure estimation. R.J.W.: supervision, project administration, and funding acquisition. All authors have read and agreed to the published version of the manuscript.

Funding: This work was supported by the National Institutes of Health (grant numbers R01 HL095606, R01 HL114396, and UG3 OD023337 supporting the cohort follow-up and data collection and statistical support through P30 ES023515 and UL1 TR004419). During the preparation of this manuscript, A.A.A. was supported by NIEHS, 5K12ES033594. None of the funding sources had any role in the study design, collection, analysis, or interpretation of the data, manuscript writing, or in the decision to submit the manuscript for publication.

Institutional Review Board Statement: This study was conducted according to the guidelines laid down in the Declaration of Helsinki, and all procedures involving research study participants were approved by the human studies committee at the Brigham and Women's Hospital and Icahn School of Medicine at Mount Sinai IRB# 12-00875, most recent approval 18 October 2023. All participants provided written consent in their primary language.

Informed Consent Statement: Informed consent was obtained from all participants involved in the study.

Data Availability Statement: The original contributions presented in the study are included in the article/Supplementary Material, further inquiries can be directed to the corresponding author.

Acknowledgments: The authors thank the participating families whose generous donation of time made this study possible.

Conflicts of Interest: The authors declare no conflicts of interest.

References

1. Shorey, S.; Chee, C.Y.I.; Ng, E.D.; Chan, Y.H.; Tam, W.W.S.; Chong, Y.S. Prevalence and incidence of postpartum depression among healthy mothers: A systematic review and meta-analysis. *J. Psychiatr. Res.* **2018**, *104*, 235–248. [CrossRef]
2. Gollan, J.K.; Yang, A.; Ciolino, J.D.; Sit, D.; Wisner, K.L. Postpartum anhedonia: Emergent patterns in bipolar and unipolar depression. *Psychiatry Res.* **2021**, *306*, 114274. [CrossRef]
3. Ma, Y.; Guo, C.; Luo, Y.; Gao, S.; Sun, J.; Chen, Q.; Lv, X.; Cao, J.; Lei, Z.; Fang, J. Altered neural activity in the reward-related circuit associated with anhedonia in mild to moderate Major Depressive Disorder. *J. Affect. Disord.* **2024**, *345*, 216–225. [CrossRef] [PubMed]
4. Mazza, M.; Marano, G. Is peripartum anhedonia a missing target? *Bipolar Disord.* **2024**, *26*, 289–290. [CrossRef] [PubMed]
5. Putnam, K.T.; Wilcox, M.; Robertson-Blackmore, E.; Sharkey, K.; Bergink, V.; Munk-Olsen, T.; Deligiannidis, K.M.; Payne, J.; Altemus, M.; Newport, J.; et al. Clinical phenotypes of perinatal depression and time of symptom onset: Analysis of data from an international consortium. *Lancet Psychiatry* **2017**, *4*, 477–485. [CrossRef]
6. Vliegen, N.; Casalin, S.; Luyten, P. The course of postpartum depression: A review of longitudinal studies. *Harv. Rev. Psychiatry* **2014**, *22*, 1–22. [CrossRef]
7. Mathers, C.D.; Loncar, D. Projections of global mortality and burden of disease from 2002 to 2030. *PLoS Med.* **2006**, *3*, e442. [CrossRef]
8. Eberhard-Gran, M.; Eskild, A.; Samuelsen, S.O.; Tambs, K. A short matrix-version of the Edinburgh Depression Scale. *Acta Psychiatr. Scand.* **2007**, *116*, 195–200. [CrossRef]
9. Conroy, S.; Pariante, C.M.; Marks, M.N.; Davies, H.A.; Farrelly, S.; Schacht, R.; Moran, P. Maternal psychopathology and infant development at 18 months: The impact of maternal personality disorder and depression. *J. Am. Acad. Child. Adolesc. Psychiatry* **2012**, *51*, 51–61. [CrossRef]
10. Leung, B.M.; Kaplan, B.J. Perinatal depression: Prevalence, risks, and the nutrition link—A review of the literature. *J. Am. Diet. Assoc.* **2009**, *109*, 1566–1575. [CrossRef]
11. Sun, Y.; Ferguson, M.; Reeves, M.M.; Kelly, J.T. Maternal Dietary Patterns and Risk of Postpartum Depression: A Systematic Review. *Matern. Child. Health J.* **2023**, *27*, 2077–2090. [CrossRef] [PubMed]
12. Bernal, J. Thyroid hormone receptors in brain development and function. *Nat. Clin. Pract. Endocrinol. Metab.* **2007**, *3*, 249–259. [CrossRef] [PubMed]
13. Dama, M.; Steiner, M.; Van Lieshout, R. Thyroid peroxidase autoantibodies and perinatal depression risk: A systematic review. *J. Affect. Disord.* **2016**, *198*, 108–121. [CrossRef] [PubMed]
14. Minaldi, E.; D'andrea, S.; Castellini, C.; Martorella, A.; Francavilla, F.; Francavilla, S.; Barbonetti, A. Thyroid autoimmunity and risk of post-partum depression: A systematic review and meta-analysis of longitudinal studies. *J. Endocrinol. Investig.* **2020**, *43*, 271–277. [CrossRef] [PubMed]
15. Sylvén, S.M.; Elenis, E.; Michelakos, T.; Larsson, A.; Olovsson, M.; Poromaa, I.S.; Skalkidou, A. Thyroid function tests at delivery and risk for postpartum depressive symptoms. *Psychoneuroendocrinology* **2013**, *38*, 1007–1013. [CrossRef]
16. Zimmermann, M.B. The Importance of Adequate Iodine during Pregnancy and Infancy. *World Rev. Nutr. Diet.* **2016**, *115*, 118–124. [PubMed]
17. Pearce, E.N.; Lazarus, J.H.; Moreno-Reyes, R.; Zimmermann, M.B. Consequences of iodine deficiency and excess in pregnant women: An overview of current knowns and unknowns. *Am. J. Clin. Nutr.* **2016**, *104* (Suppl. S3), 918s–923s. [CrossRef] [PubMed]
18. Institute of Medicine (US) Panel on Micronutrients. *Dietary Reference Intakes for Vitamin A, Vitamin K, Arsenic, Boron, Chromium, Copper, Iodine, Iron, Manganese, Molybdenum, Nickel, Silicon, Vanadium, and Zinc*; National Academies Press (US): Washington, DC, USA, 2001.
19. Brantsæter, A.L.; Garthus-Niegel, S.; Brandlistuen, R.E.; Caspersen, I.H.; Meltzer, H.M.; Abel, M.H. Mild-to-moderate iodine deficiency and symptoms of emotional distress and depression in pregnancy and six months postpartum—Results from a large pregnancy cohort. *J. Affect. Disord.* **2022**, *318*, 347–356. [CrossRef] [PubMed]
20. Moleti, M.; Di Bella, B.; Giorgianni, G.; Mancuso, A.; De Vivo, A.; Alibrandi, A.; Trimarchi, F.; Vermiglio, F. Maternal thyroid function in different conditions of iodine nutrition in pregnant women exposed to mild-moderate iodine deficiency: An observational study. *Clin. Endocrinol.* **2011**, *74*, 762–768. [CrossRef] [PubMed]
21. Wang, Z.; Li, C.; Teng, Y.; Guan, Y.; Zhang, L.; Jia, X.; Cui, D.; Li, J.; Guan, H. The Effect of Iodine-Containing Vitamin Supplementation during Pregnancy on Thyroid Function in Late Pregnancy and Postpartum Depression in an Iodine-Sufficient Area. *Biol. Trace Elem. Res.* **2020**, *198*, 1–7. [CrossRef]
22. Block, G.; Hartman, A.M.; Dresser, C.M.; Carroll, M.D.; Gannon, J.; Gardner, L. A data-based approach to diet questionnaire design and testing. *Am. J. Epidemiol.* **1986**, *124*, 453–469. [CrossRef]
23. Parrott, M.S.; Bodnar, L.M.; Simhan, H.N.; Harger, G.; Markovic, N.; Roberts, J.M. Maternal cereal consumption and adequacy of micronutrient intake in the periconceptional period. *Public Health Nutr.* **2009**, *12*, 1276–1283. [CrossRef]
24. Boucher, B.; Cotterchio, M.; Kreiger, N.; Nadalin, V.; Block, T.; Block, G. Validity and reliability of the Block98 food-frequency questionnaire in a sample of Canadian women. *Public Health Nutr.* **2006**, *9*, 84–93. [CrossRef] [PubMed]
25. Wirfält, A.K.; Jeffery, R.W.; Elmer, P.J. Comparison of food frequency questionnaires: The reduced Block and Willett questionnaires differ in ranking on nutrient intakes. *Am. J. Epidemiol.* **1998**, *148*, 1148–1156. [CrossRef]

26. Völgyi, E.; Carroll, K.N.; Hare, M.E.; Ringwald-Smith, K.; Piyathilake, C.; Yoo, W.; Tylavsky, F.A. Dietary patterns in pregnancy and effects on nutrient intake in the Mid-South: The Conditions Affecting Neurocognitive Development and Learning in Early Childhood (CANDLE) study. *Nutrients* **2013**, *5*, 1511–1530. [CrossRef] [PubMed]
27. Roseland, J.M.; Spungen, J.H.; Patterson, K.Y.; Ershow, A.G.; Gahche, J.J.; Pehrsson, P. USDA, FDA, and ODS-NIH Database for the Iodine Content of Common Foods. In *Release*; U.S. Department of Agriculture Agricultural Research Service: West Beltsville, MD, USA, 2022.
28. Ershow, A.G.; Haggans, C.J.; Roseland, J.M.; Patterson, K.Y.; Spungen, J.H.; Gahche, J.J.; Merkel, J.M.; Pehrsson, P.R. Databases of Iodine Content of Foods and Dietary Supplements-Availability of New and Updated Resources. *J. Acad. Nutr. Diet.* **2022**, *122*, 1229–1231. [CrossRef]
29. Pehrsson, P.R.; Roseland, J.M.; Patterson, K.Y.; Phillips, K.M.; Spungen, J.H.; Andrews, K.W.; Gusev, P.A.; Gahche, J.J.; Haggans, C.J.; Merkel, J.M.; et al. Iodine in Foods and Dietary Supplements: A Collaborative Database Developed by NIH, FDA and USDA. *J. Food Compost. Anal.* **2022**, *109*, 104369. [CrossRef]
30. Abt, E.; Kumar, S.; Weyant, R.J. Periodontal disease and medical maladies: What do we really know? *J. Am. Dent. Assoc.* **2022**, *153*, 9–13. [CrossRef]
31. Ershow, A.G.; Skeaff, S.A.; Merkel, J.M.; Pehrsson, P.R. Development of Databases on Iodine in Foods and Dietary Supplements. *Nutrients* **2018**, *10*, 100. [CrossRef]
32. Milagres, R.; Souza, E.C.G.; Peluzio, M.; Franceschini, S.; Duarte, M.S.L. Food Iodine Content Table compiled from international databases. *Rev. Nutr.* **2020**, *33*, e190222. [CrossRef]
33. Lautarescu, A.; Victor, S.; Lau-Zhu, A.; Counsell, S.J.; Edwards, A.D.; Craig, M.C. The factor structure of the Edinburgh Postnatal Depression Scale among perinatal high-risk and community samples in London. *Arch. Womens Ment. Health* **2022**, *25*, 157–169. [CrossRef] [PubMed]
34. Flom, J.D.; Chiu, Y.-H.M.; Tamayo-Ortiz, M.; Schnaas, L.; Curtin, P.C.; Wright, R.J.; O Wright, R.; Téllez-Rojo, M.M.; Rosa, M.J. Subconstructs of the Edinburgh Postpartum Depression Scale in a postpartum sample in Mexico City. *J. Affect. Disord.* **2018**, *238*, 142–146. [CrossRef] [PubMed]
35. Chiu, Y.-H.M.; Sheffield, P.E.; Hsu, H.-H.L.; Goldstein, J.; Curtin, P.C.; Wright, R.J. Subconstructs of the Edinburgh Postnatal Depression Scale in a multi-ethnic inner-city population in the U.S. *Arch. Womens Ment. Health* **2017**, *20*, 803–810. [CrossRef] [PubMed]
36. Levis, B.; Negeri, Z.; Sun, Y.; Benedetti, A.; Thombs, B.D. Accuracy of the Edinburgh Postnatal Depression Scale (EPDS) for screening to detect major depression among pregnant and postpartum women: Systematic review and meta-analysis of individual participant data. *BMJ (Clin. Res. Ed.)* **2020**, *371*, m4022. [CrossRef] [PubMed]
37. White, I.R.; Royston, P.; Wood, A.M. Multiple imputation using chained equations: Issues and guidance for practice. *Stat. Med.* **2011**, *30*, 377–399. [CrossRef] [PubMed]
38. Yonkers, K.A.; Vigod, S.; Ross, L.E. Diagnosis, pathophysiology, and management of mood disorders in pregnant and postpartum women. *Obstet. Gynecol.* **2011**, *117*, 961–977. [CrossRef]
39. Basraon, S.; Costantine, M.M. Mood disorders in pregnant women with thyroid dysfunction. *Clin. Obstet. Gynecol.* **2011**, *54*, 506–514. [CrossRef] [PubMed]
40. Siegmann, E.M.; Müller, H.H.O.; Luecke, C.; Philipsen, A.; Kornhuber, J.; Grömer, T.W. Association of Depression and Anxiety Disorders with Autoimmune Thyroiditis: A Systematic Review and Meta-analysis. *JAMA Psychiatry* **2018**, *75*, 577–584. [CrossRef] [PubMed]
41. Hendrick, V.; Altshuler, L.; Whybrow, P. Psychoneuroendocrinology of mood disorders. The hypothalamic-pituitary-thyroid axis. *Psychiatr. Clin. N. Am.* **1998**, *21*, 277–292. [CrossRef]
42. Bath, S.C. The effect of iodine deficiency during pregnancy on child development. *Proc. Nutr. Soc.* **2019**, *78*, 150–160. [CrossRef]
43. Abel, M.H.; Korevaar, T.I.M.; Erlund, I.; Villanger, G.D.; Caspersen, I.H.; Arohonka, P.; Alexander, J.; Meltzer, H.M.; Brantsaeter, A.L. Iodine Intake is Associated with Thyroid Function in Mild to Moderately Iodine Deficient Pregnant Women. *Thyroid* **2018**, *28*, 1359–1371. [CrossRef]
44. Rasmussen, L.B.; Ovesen, L.; Bülow, I.; Jørgensen, T.; Knudsen, N.; Laurberg, P.; Perrild, H. Dietary iodine intake and urinary iodine excretion in a Danish population: Effect of geography, supplements and food choice. *Br. J. Nutr.* **2002**, *87*, 61–69. [CrossRef]
45. Andersen, S.; Karmisholt, J.; Pedersen, K.M.; Laurberg, P. Reliability of studies of iodine intake and recommendations for number of samples in groups and in individuals. *Br. J. Nutr.* **2008**, *99*, 813–818. [CrossRef] [PubMed]
46. Burns, R.; Azizi, F.; Hedayati, M.; Mirmiran, P.; O'Herlihy, C.; Smyth, P.P. Is placental iodine content related to dietary iodine intake? *Clin. Endocrinol.* **2011**, *75*, 261–264. [CrossRef]
47. Murphy, S.P.; Guenther, P.M.; Kretsch, M.J. Using the dietary reference intakes to assess intakes of groups: Pitfalls to avoid. *J. Am. Diet. Assoc.* **2006**, *106*, 1550–1553. [CrossRef] [PubMed]
48. Winer, E.S.; Veilleux, J.C.; Ginger, E.J. Development and validation of the Specific Loss of Interest and Pleasure Scale (SLIPS). *J. Affect. Disord.* **2014**, *152–154*, 193–201. [CrossRef] [PubMed]
49. Gard, D.E.; Gard, M.G.; Kring, A.M.; John, O.P. Anticipatory and consummatory components of the experience of pleasure: A scale development study. *J. Res. Personal.* **2006**, *40*, 1086–1102. [CrossRef]
50. Treadway, M.T.; Zald, D.H. Reconsidering anhedonia in depression: Lessons from translational neuroscience. *Neurosci. Biobehav. Rev.* **2011**, *35*, 537–555. [CrossRef] [PubMed]

51. Guintivano, J.; Manuck, T.; Meltzer-Brody, S. Predictors of Postpartum Depression: A Comprehensive Review of the Last Decade of Evidence. *Clin. Obstet. Gynecol.* **2018**, *61*, 591–603. [CrossRef] [PubMed]
52. Fu, J.; Wang, Q.; Wang, N.; Li, S.; Zhang, H.; Zhu, Y.; Guo, H.; Wang, F.; He, L.; Xia, S.; et al. Serum and urinary essential trace elements in association with major depressive disorders: A case-control study. *Front. Psychiatry* **2023**, *14*, 1297411. [CrossRef]

nutrients

MDPI

Article

A Study of Fluid Intake, Hydration Status, and Body Composition of Pregnant Women in Their Third Trimester, and Relationships with Their Infant's Birth Weight in China: A Prospective Cohort Study

Yongye Song [1,2], Fan Zhang [3], Xing Wang [1,2], Guotian Lin [4], Limin He [3], Zhixiong Lin [5], Na Zhang [1,2,*] and Guansheng Ma [1,2]

[1] Department of Nutrition and Food Hygiene, School of Public Health, Peking University, 38 Xue Yuan Road, Haidian District, Beijing 100191, China; songyongye@bjmu.edu.cn (Y.S.); wangxing_98@126.com (X.W.); mags@bjmu.edu.cn (G.M.)

[2] Laboratory of Toxicological Research and Risk Assessment for Food Safety, Peking University, 38 Xue Yuan Road, Haidian District, Beijing 100191, China

[3] International School of Public Health and One Health, Hainan Medical University, 3 Xue Yuan Road, Longhua District, Haikou 571199, China; zhangfan@hainmc.edu.cn (F.Z.); banxia75@163.com (L.H.)

[4] School of Health Medicine, University of Sanya, 191 Xue Yuan Road, Jiyang District, Sanya 572022, China; linguotian123@163.com

[5] Haikou Hospital of the Maternal and Child Health, 6 Wen Tan Road, Guo Xing Avenue, Qiongshan District, Haikou 570203, China; zgyglzx@163.com

* Correspondence: zhangna@bjmu.edu.cn; Tel./Fax: +86-10-8280-5266

Abstract: Background: Water intake and hydration status may potentially influence maternal and child health. However, there is little research regarding this topic. Objectives: This study aimed to investigate pregnant women's total fluid intake (TFI) levels, hydration status, and body composition and further explore their relationship with infant birth weight. Methods: A 7-day, 24 h fluid intake recorded was applied to determine participants' TFI levels. Morning urine samples were collected and tested to evaluate their hydration status. Maternal body compositions in their third trimester and infant birth weights were measured. Results: A total of 380 participants completed the study. The TFI was insufficient for pregnant women during their third trimester (median = 1574 mL), with only 12.1% of participants meeting the recommended adequate fluid intake level for pregnant women living in China (1.7 L per day). With the increasing TFI values, the urine osmolality decreased, which showed statistical significance among the four groups ($\chi^2 = 22.637$, $p < 0.05$). The participants displayed a poor hydration status. Meanwhile, the percentage of participants who were in dehydrated status decreased ($\chi^2 = 67.618$, $p < 0.05$), while body water content and basal metabolic rate increased with the increase in TFI levels ($\chi^2 = 20.784$, $p < 0.05$; $\chi^2 = 14.026$, $p < 0.05$). There were positive linear relationships between plain water intake, the basal metabolic rate of pregnant women and their infant birth weight (SE = 0.153, $p < 0.05$; SE = 0.076, $p < 0.05$). Conclusions: Water intake was insufficient, and poor hydration status was common among pregnant women in China. There may be potential relationships between plain water intake, basal metabolic rate, and infant birth weight.

Keywords: fluid intake; hydration status; body composition; pregnant women; birth weight

1. Introduction

Water accounts for approximately 60~70% of a healthy adult's body weight [1]. It exerts an enormous function in maintaining electrolyte homeostasis, retaining stable body temperature, and lubricating organs, joints, muscles, and tissues [2,3]. There exist three pathways for water input: water intake from beverages, water intake from food, and endogenous water. The four ways of water elimination from the body refer to water excreted through the kidneys in the form of urine, water excreted through skin evaporation in the form of sweat, water excreted through pulmonary respiration, and water excreted through the intestine in the form of feces [4,5]. As a result, the daily intake and discharge of water are maintained at around 2500 mL. Hydration status is linked to the balance of water input and water elimination in the human body [4]. Pregnancy is a special and complex period during which women are subjected to anatomical and physiological changes. It is of great importance to meet the increased maternal metabolic demands. Apart from that, it is essential for meeting the requirements of fetal development [6]. Growing evidence has demonstrated that maternal nutrition has a direct effect on body composition and weight at birth. In addition, it has a long-lasting influence on health status and metabolic responses in adulthood [7,8].

During pregnancy, blood volume significantly increases [9]. In addition, oxygen consumption increases by 30%, metabolic rate by 15%, and tidal volume by 30~50% [10,11]. Additionally, an increase occurs in the glomerular filtration rate (GFR) and effective renal plasma flow (RPF) [12]. As a result, total body water content roughly increases by 6.5~8 L [6,13]. Body water distribution during pregnancy affects the hydration status, as a study showed that, except for pregnancy elements (placenta, infant, and uterus), the added hydration is mainly extracellular [14]. Additionally, human chorionic gonadotropin (HCG) levels increase during pregnancy, leading to changes in water homeostasis and osmolality [15]. They may also be related to regulatory system changes and hormone-level fluctuations [16]. Plasma osmolality decreases during pregnancy, and changes also occur in the osmolality threshold for vasopressin release [17]. This leads to increased activity in sympathetic and renin–angiotensin–aldosterone pathways, which is critical for water homeostasis [18]. A significant increase in the plasma vasopressin enzyme may explain the changes in water homeostasis in the third trimester of pregnancy [16]. In addition, body water distribution will be affected, as the extracellular and plasma volume of pregnant women increased by 50~70%, accompanied by significant accumulation of sodium retention shared by the mother and fetus. During pregnancy, a water imbalance can even predict gestational hypertension [19], pre-eclampsia [20], low birth weight, and poor pregnancy outcomes [21,22].

Total water intake consists of two parts, namely, the fluid intake from water and beverages (accounting for approximately 50%) and the water intake from food (accounting for approximately 40%) [1]. Daily TFI is defined as the amount of water and beverages consumed, with water from food being excluded. The recommended adequate fluid intake level for pregnant women in China is 1.7 L per day (excluding water intake from food) [23]. However, previous studies have found that women during pregnancy generally suffer from insufficient fluid intake. A water intake investigation was conducted on 300 pregnant Indonesian women using the 7-day, 24 h fluid intake record. The results showed that approximately 42% of participants were under Indonesia's recommended adequate fluid intake level (2048 mL/d) [24]. A previous study found that the median TFI level among Chinese pregnant women in the second trimester was 1485 mL [25]. Thus, the fluid intake of women needs to be improved during their pregnancy.

A low birth weight refers to a newborn weighing less than 2500 g [26]. A large prospective cohort study in China showed that the low-birth-weight incidence rate was 14.5% [27]. Low birth weight is a key determinant of the health status and development of newborns, which can increase the morbidity and mortality of newborns. It is also closely related to the risk of chronic diseases, including hypertension, diabetes, obesity, and cardiovascular and cerebrovascular diseases in adulthood [28,29]. A study was carried out in Canada among 196 pairs of mothers and live singleton newborns whose gestational ages were 37 weeks or more. The body composition of 196 women between 4 and 12 h postpartum was measured. In this study, compared with the mother's gestational weight gain, total body water content was a major determinant of birth weight variability [22]. A prospective study conducted in America followed 105 healthy women who delivered of-term infants [30]. Body composition was evaluated eight times during their pregnancy. The result showed that body water content was considered an independent predictor of infant birth weight. A case-control study performed in America indicated that fluid intake was associated with low birth weight. Women with lower fluid intake levels during pregnancy developed lower birth weights of their infants [31]. Twenty-nine pregnant women and their full-term infants were followed in a longitudinal study in Poland. However, the result showed no significant correlation between maternal water intake and infant birth weight [18]. The nutrition required during different trimesters of pregnancy is not invariable, but it is a dynamic process. Conclusions regarding body composition, particularly total body water, are still inconsistent in the literature [19,20,32]. Nevertheless, abnormal fluid might be the cause of maternal and fetal pathologies, including intrauterine growth restriction or hypertensive complications during pregnancy [33,34].

Therefore, the aims of this study were the following: (1) to determine and assess the TFI levels and body compositions of women in their third trimester of pregnancy; (2) to assess the urine biomarkers and evaluate the hydration status; and (3) to explore the relationships between maternal fluid intake, body composition, and infant birth weight. The results can provide accurate and meaningful references for promoting the fluid intake level for pregnant Chinese women in their third trimester. Moreover, these can provide possible ways to improve infants' birth weights.

2. Materials and Methods

2.1. Study Design

A convenience sampling method was adopted in this study. Recruitment was performed according to the inclusion and exclusion criteria. Pregnant women who attended outpatient clinics at the Haikou Maternal and Child Health Hospital from August 2020 to March 2021 were enrolled.

2.2. Sample-Size Calculation

The variable used for the sample-size calculation was the incidence of low birth weight. The relevant study in China reported that the incidence of low birth weight was 14.5% [27]. The sample size was determined on the basis of the following formula: $n = {Z_{1-\alpha/2}}^2 p (1-p)/e^2$. In the formula, we set $\alpha = 0.05$ and $Z_{1-\alpha/2} = 1.96$. Moreover, "e" was the error bound and was set as 4%. The required sample size was 298. Considering a dropout rate of 20%, 372 participants need to be recruited.

2.3. Participants

The criteria for inclusion in the study were as follows: first, maternity screening conducted before 28 weeks gestation; being aged between 21 and 35 years old; a singleton pregnancy; being in a good health condition before enrollment; routine prenatal examinations at the hospital where the study was conducted (Haikou Hospital of The Maternal and Child Health); and having the ability to complete questionnaires independently. The following exclusion criteria were applied: smoker; habitual alcohol consumer (>20 g/day) [35]; any fluid intake intervention; engagement in rigorous physical activity; or the presence of endocrine diseases, urinary system diseases, digestive system diseases, cardiovascular diseases, or cognitive disorders; diabetes mellitus; or any other pre-existing diseases before pregnancy.

2.4. Ethics

The study protocol underwent a thorough review and get approval by the Ethical Review Committee of the Hainan Medical University (with an identification code of 2018-4). The study protocol has been registered on the Chinese Clinical Trial Registry website under the trial registration number Chi CTR 800019284. The study adhered to the principles of the Declaration of Helsinki. Participants were informed of the background, purpose, duration, steps, and potential issues at the beginning of the study.

2.5. Study Procedure

This prospective cohort study was carried out from August 2020 to March 2021. Maternal socio-economics, socio-demographics, and other basic information, including the participants' pregnancy, childbearing, disease, and drug-usage histories, was collected after recruitment. Meanwhile, participants' heights, weights, and body compositions were measured in the third trimester of pregnancy. The 7-day, 24 h fluid intake record was used to observe the fluid intake patterns of these participants in their third trimester. Their first morning urine samples were collected by themselves. The samples were tested within 2 h by professional laboratory technicians on day 4 during the 7 consecutive days. Infant birth weight was measured within 1 h after delivery. The temperature and humidity data for this period were acquired from the China Meteorological Administration statement. The timeline for study duration, data collection, and collected indicators is presented (Table 1).

Table 1. Indicators and different time points for collection in this study.

	The Third Trimester of Pregnancy							Delivery
	Day 1	Day 2	Day 3	Day 4	Day 5	Day 6	Day 7	
Individual information	√ *							
Physical measurements	√							
Body-composition measurements	√							
7-day 24 h fluid intake record	√	√	√	√	√	√	√	
Fasting blood samples				√				
Morning urine samples and relevant biomarkers				√				
Temperature and humidity	√	√	√	√	√	√	√	
Infant birth weight								√

Note: *, means the data was collected on that day.

2.6. Physical Measurements

For height and weight, investigators were uniformly trained prior to the study. Participants were measured using uniform instruments (DHM-300; Huaju, Yiwu, Zhejiang, China). The values were measured twice according to the standardized method. Height values were accurate to 0.1 cm and weight values were accurate to 0.1 kg, respectively (BMI is calculated as weight (kg)/height squared (m^2)). The average values were calculated and reported.

2.7. Tests of Blood Pressure and Blood Glucose

For blood pressure measurements, an electronic upper-arm sphygmomanometer (U10L; Omron, Dalian, China) was used by trained investigators to measure the participants' blood pressure. The standard process was used for measurement in this study [36]. Participants were asked not to perform intense exercise for 1 h before the measurement and to stay calm for 5 min. Eating or drinking beverages containing caffeine was also not allowed. They were asked to remove heavy clothing and sit in an upright and relaxing position. For blood pressure measurement, a cuff was wrapped around the participant's left arm 1 to 2 cm above the medial joint of the elbow. The readings of blood pressure were accurate to 2 mmHg. Two consecutive measurements were taken, and the average values of both the systolic and diastolic blood pressure measurements were recorded.

For blood glucose, the participants' blood glucose was determined with elbow venous blood using an automatic biochemical analyzer (AU5800, Beckman, Brea, CA, USA) by laboratory physicians. Blood glucose levels during the fasting state of the participants were measured in the study.

2.8. Body-Composition Measurements

Participants' body compositions were measured by uniformly trained investigators using a human-fat-measuring instrument (BC-601; TANITA; Tokyo, Japan). Bioelectrical impedance analysis (BIA) was the instrument's method. Impedances at different segments were measured, including the right arm, left arm, right leg, left leg, and trunk for all frequencies. Due to the different electrical characteristics of body tissues, the volume of conductive tissues was determined according to the electrical resistances of various tissue parts of the human body. Thus, the body composition was estimated. Participants were required to discharge their night soil and urine before measurements and wear lightweight clothing, with their socks, shoes, and any metal jewelry removed.

In the meantime, it is necessary for them to be prepared with clean soles. Information was imported into the instrument by investigators, such as the participants' ages, genders, and heights. When the value on the screen was reset to zero, participants were instructed to stand on the instrument. Their palms and soles contacted the electrode surface. Their torsos and upper limbs were maintained at an angle of approximately 30°. Participants were required to remain quiet and not move during the measurement process. The results were displayed on the screen automatically when the measurements were finished. The results included data on body water content, bone mineral content, percent of body fat, skeletal muscles, and basal metabolic rate.

2.9. Assessment of Daily Total Fluid Intake (TFI)

Daily total water intake levels refer to the sum of daily total fluid intake (TFI) and daily water intake from food. TFI refers to the fluid intake level from water and beverages, with water from food excluded. The amount of water intake from food was not assessed in the present study.

A "7-day 24-h fluid intake record" was applied to observe the fluid intake level [37–40]. This record has been validated and employed in many studies, which are authoritatively and widely applied to record fluid intake in various countries [41–43]. Expert consensus has been reached, as the record has been subjected to expert consultation and repeated argumentation [40,44]. Fluid intake types were classified according to the classification criteria [45]. The included types were plain water, dairy products, and sugar-sweetened beverages. Plain water refers to tap, packaged, mineral, and purified water. Dairy products included pure milk, yogurt, and other dairy products with no sugar added during the production. Sugar-sweetened beverages (SSBs) refer to beverages with the addition of sugar during production, including carbonated, fruit and vegetable juice, protein, sugary coffee, plant-based, flavored, and special-purpose beverages. Each participant was provided with a uniformly customized cup. A cup with a scale was used to estimate the amount of fluid intake each time. Fluid intake levels and types for 7 consecutive days were recorded in detail. The capacity of the cup was 400 mL, with the cup scale accurate to 10 mL.

2.10. Tests Conducted for Urine Biomarkers

For urine osmolality, values were achieved from participants' first morning urine. The samples were collected in this study to test urine biomarkers. Sterile disposable urine-sample cups were used for urine collection. Urine osmolality was measured by an osmotic pressure molar concentration meter (SMC 30C; Tianhe, Tianjin, China) with the freezing-point method. The process of the test was in accordance with the Standard Operating Procedure. Urine osmolality values were then applied to evaluate the hydration status of the participants.

For urine specific gravity (USG), it was tested with an automatic urinary sediment analyzer (FUS-200; Dirui; Changchun, China). The uric dry-chemistry method was applied to urine testing, and color development was achieved by replacing hydrogen ions with cations. The urine samples were delivered to the laboratory and tested within 2 h of collection.

2.11. Evaluation and Definition of Hydration Status

With reference to current studies [38,46], urine osmolality was used for the assessment and classification of participants' hydration status. Based on urine osmolality values, participants were categorized into three groups in terms of their hydration status: groups with a dehydrated status, normal hydrated status, and optimal hydrated status. The classification of hydration status determination using urine osmolality is presented below (Table 2).

Table 2. Thresholds for determining hydration status based on urine osmolality.

Definition of Hydration Status	Urine Osmolality Values (mOsm/kg)
Dehydrated status	urine osmolality > 800 [47,48]
Normal hydrated status	500 < urine osmolality ≤ 800 [4]
Optimal hydrated status	urine osmolality ≤ 500 [49]

2.12. Measurement of Infant Birth Weight

Infant birth weight was measured within 1 h after delivery. The measurement was taken using a weight-measuring device (HLZ-20; Hualizheng, Tianjin, China) by professional obstetricians while the infant wore light clothing. The measurement value was accurate to within 0.1 g.

2.13. Temperature and Humidity

The present study was implemented in Haikou city. Daily minimum and maximum temperatures were recorded during the 7 consecutive days. The data were provided by the Meteorological Administration of China. The median temperature was considered as the day's temperature, and the average temperature over the seven days was calculated. What is more, humidity was recorded during the study period.

2.14. Quality Control

A unified procedure was developed, and all the investigators were uniformly trained before the study. A research guide was designed, including the research protocol, questionnaire, methodology, and timeline, and sample and indicators to be collected. The reasons for and the time for dropping out were also collected in a comprehensive way. During the entire research process, all procedures were subjected to strict supervision by quality control staff. Trained investigators guided participants to complete the questionnaire. Double checks were performed on the completeness and logicality of the questionnaires. If any errors were found, the participants were contacted to correct the records until they met the requirements. Prior to data entry, each item in the questionnaire or record was verified, and the incorrect records were deleted.

2.15. Statistical Methods

Data entry was completed using the EpiData 3.1 software. This process was performed using the double-entry method and the database was created. The SPSS Statistics 26.0 (IBM Crop., Armok, NC, USA) was applied for statistical analysis. The continuous variables were subjected to normality tests. The medians (M) were used to report and analyze abnormal distribution data. The interquartile ranges of the interval limited by the 25th and 75th percentiles (Q_1~Q_3) were also shown. A one-way ANOVA was used to compare differences in the normally distributed data among the four groups. The Kruskal–Wallis H test was applied for comparison of differences in the abnormal distribution data. The proportions of participants meeting the adequate fluid intake (AI) level in China, fluid intake amount and percent, and hydration status among the four groups were compared by chi-square test. Multiple comparisons were performed using the Student–Newman–Keuls (SNK) method ($p < 0.05$). The Spearman correlation was used to test the correlations between total drinking and plain water intake. Adjusted analyses were carried out using multivariable linear regression models to analyze the linear relationships between different types of fluid intake and infant birth weight. All tests were two-sided, and $p < 0.05$ was considered statistically significant.

3. Results

3.1. Participants' Characteristics and the Environment

In total, 380 pregnant women who were in compliance with the inclusion criteria were recruited for our study. Finally, 380 participants completed the study, resulting in a completion rate of 100%. More detailed characteristics of the 380 participants are summarized in Table 3.

Table 3. Characteristics of participants.

	LFI_1 (n = 95)	LFI_2 (n = 95)	HFI_1 (n = 95)	HFI_2 (n = 95)	Total (n = 380)	*p*
Age (year) [a]	30.0 (26.0~32.0)	29.0 (26.5~31.0)	28.0 (26.0~31.0)	28.0 (26.0~31.5)	29.0 (26.0~32.0)	0.791
Height (cm) [a]	156.5 (154.3~160.0)	156.0 (153.0~159.0)	157. (153.0~161.0)	158.0 (154.8~161.0)	156.5 (153.5~160.0)	0.101
Weight (kg) [a]	60.5 (54.2~65.8)	60.7 (54.2~67.8)	58.5 (54.1~63.2)	58.4 (55.1~62.6)	59.3 (54.2~65.0)	0.187
BMI (kg/m^2) [a]	24.4 (22.9~26.9) [b]	24.6 (22.6~26.9) [c]	23.8 (22.4~26.4) [b]	23.2 (22.1~25.1) [d]	24.1 (22.4~26.3)	0.023 *
Blood pressure [a]						
Systolic (mmHg) [a]	117 (107~123)	115 (108~122)	117 (110~123)	115 (105~120)	115 (108~122)	0.308
Diastolic (mmHg) [a]	74 (67~79)	75 (68~80)	74 (69~77)	71 (66~77)	74 (68~78)	0.174
Blood glucose (mmol/L) [a]	3.7 (3.4~4.3)	3.7 (3.4~4.2)	3.5 (3.3~4.2)	3.7 (3.3~4.7)	3.7 (3.3~4.4)	0.166

Note: [a] Values were shown as median (Q_1~Q_3) and compared using the Kruskal–Wallis test, whose degrees of freedom (df) were 3. *, means the *p*-value was less than 0.05, indicating that there was a significant difference. [(b–d)]: The same letter indicates no statistically significant differences between the two groups; different letters indicate significant differences for $p < 0.05$. BMI: body mass index. LFI_1: low fluid intake 1; LFI_2: low fluid intake 2; HFI_1: high fluid intake 1; HFI_2: high fluid intake 2.

According to the quartiles of participants' TFI levels, they were categorized into four groups, namely, the LFI_1 (low fluid intake 1), LFI_2 (low fluid intake 2), HFI_1 (high fluid intake 1), and HFI_2 (high fluid intake 2), (Q_1: 1200~1487 mL, Q_2: 1488~11573 mL, Q_3: 1574~1641 mL, and Q_4: 1642~1950 mL). Among the factors investigated, no significant differences in the factors of age, height, weight, and blood pressure were observed between the four groups (all $p > 0.05$). However, significant differences were observed between the BMIs among the four groups ($F = 9.500$, $p < 0.05$).

The average value of temperature was 27.6 ± 3.3 °C, with an average humidity of 78.3 ± 7.9% RH in Hainan during the study period.

3.2. Measurement of TFI of Participants with Different TFI Levels

Among the 380 participants, the median value of TFI was 1574 mL. Approximately 85.2% of the participants were below China's recommendation for an adequate fluid intake level (1.7 L per day for pregnant women). The most common source for participants' fluid intake was plain water, as it represented 94.3% of daily TFI. Dairy products were the second largest contributor to TFI, accounting for 4.1%. The median dairy product intake level was 59 mL. SSBs (sugar-sweetened beverages) accounted for a small proportion of TFI (Table 4).

Table 4. Composition of fluid intake of participants with different TFI levels.

	LFI_1 (n = 95)	LFI_2 (n = 95)	HFI_1 (n = 95)	HFI_2 (n = 95)	Total (n = 380)	*p*
Daily TFI (mL) [a]	1421 (1374~1456) [c]	1534 (1511~1557) [d]	1607 (1590~1623) [e]	1697 (1600~1747) [f]	1574 (1488~1641)	<0.001 *
Percentage meeting Chinese fluid AI level (%) [b]	0 (0.0) [c]	0 (0.0) [c]	0 (0.0) [c]	46 (48.4) [d]	46 (12.1)	<0.001 *
TFI sources						
Plain water						
Amount (mL) [a]	1349 (1304~1391) [c]	1447 (1412~1478) [d]	1506 (1455~1551) [e]	1579 (1544~1631) [f]	1467 (1397~1549)	<0.001 *
Percent (%) [a]	95.3 (93.1~96.9) [c]	94.4 (92.1~96.2) [d]	93.5 (91.4~96.2) [e]	93.6 (90.5~95.4) [e]	94.3 (91.6~96.2)	0.002 *
Dairy products						
Amount (mL) [a]	47 (27~79) [c]	57 (34~86) [d]	63 (36~88) [d]	70 (43~94) [e]	59 (33~89)	0.044 *
Percent (%) [a]	4.0 (2.0~5.8)	3.9 (2.3~6.2)	4.2 (2.3~6.9)	4.6 (2.6~6.0)	4.1 (2.3~6.0)	0.783
SSBs						
Amount (mL) [a]	0 (0~31) [c]	21 (0~61) [d]	27 (0~69) [d]	43 (0~83) [e]	24 (0~64)	<0.001 *
Percent (%) [a]	0.0 (0.0~2.3) [c]	1.4 (0.0~3.9) [d]	1.7 (0.0~4.3) [e]	2.5 (0.0~4.7) [f]	1.5 (0.0~3.9)	0.001 *

Note: [a] Values presented as median (Q_1~Q_3) and compared using the Kruskal–Wallis test, whose degrees of freedom (df) were 3; [b] values represent n (percentage) which were compared using the chi-squared test. * values mean significant differences existed as the *p*-value was less than 0.05. [(c–f)]: The same letter indicates no statistically significant differences between the two groups; different letters indicate significant differences for $p < 0.05$. AI represents recommendations for adequate intake levels. The AI recommendation for TFI levels for pregnant women set by the Chinese Nutrition Society is 1.7 L per day. LFI_1: low fluid intake 1; LFI_2: low fluid intake 2; HFI_1: high fluid intake 1; and HFI_2: high fluid intake 2. TFI: total fluid intake; SSBs: sugar-sweetened beverages.

3.3. Measurement of Urine Biomarkers of Participants with Different TFI Levels

The data indicated that the increase in TFIs decreased urine osmolality from the LFI_1 to HFI_2 groups and significantly differed between the four groups ($\chi^2 = 22.637$, $p < 0.05$). There were 15.0% of participants who were in an optimal hydration status in the third trimester when assessed by urine osmolality. The median USG value of the participants was 1.015.

Hydration status improved with the increase of TFI and differed significantly between the four groups ($\chi^2 = 67.618$, $p < 0.05$). USG, urine pH, urine creatinine, and uric acid values differed significantly between the four groups ($\chi^2 = 19.092$, $p < 0.05$; $\chi^2 = 9.791$, $p < 0.05$; $\chi^2 = 5.939$, $p < 0.05$; $\chi^2 = 10.680$, $p < 0.05$; and $\chi^2 = 14.030$, $p < 0.05$). No significant differences in urea values were observed between the four groups ($p > 0.05$) (Table 5).

Table 5. Urine indexes for participants with different TFI levels.

	LFI_1 (n = 95)	LFI_2 (n = 95)	HFI_1 (n = 95)	HFI_2 (n = 95)	Total (n = 380)	p
Urine osmolality (mOsm/kg) [a]	689 (597~767) [c]	672 (569~753) [c]	664 (560~763) [c]	562 (356~733) [d]	666 (554~763)	<0.001 *
Hydration status						
Optimal hydrated status (n,%) [b]	6 (6.3%)	4 (4.2%)	4 (4.2%)	15 (15.8%)	29 (7.6%)	
Normal hydrated status (n,%) [b]	53 (55.8%)	79 (83.2%)	88 (92.6%)	74 (77.9%)	294 (77.4%)	<0.001 *
Dehydrated status (n,%) [b]	36 (37.9%)	12 (12.6%)	3 (3.2%)	6 (6.3%)	57 (15.0%)	
Urine specific gravity (USG) [a]	1.020 (1.015~1.026) [c]	1.020 (1.015~1.023) [c]	1.018 (1.010~1.021) [c]	1.010 (1.010~1.020) [d]	1.015 (1.010~1.023)	<0.001 *
Urine pH [a]	6.0 (5.0~6.5) [c]	6.0 (5.0~6.5) [d]	6.0 (5.0~6.5) [c]	6.0 (5.9~7.0) [e]	6.0 (5.5~6.5)	0.020 *
Urea (mmol/L) [a]	4.2 (3.5~5.0)	3.9 (3.4~4.6)	4.0 (3.3~4.7)	3.9 (3.3~4.4)	4.0 (3.3~4.7)	0.115
Urine creatinine (mmol/L) [a]	59.2 (52.3~66.3) [c]	58.5 (51.8~63.7) [d]	56.6 (52.3~63.7) [d]	54.6 (52.6~58.0) [e]	56.6 (52.2~56.3)	0.014 *
Uric acid (mmol/L) [a]	277 (229~321) [c]	276 (231~305) [c]	267 (221~3.7) [c]	237 (209~281) [d]	265 (223~307)	0.003 *

Note: [a] Values presented as median (Q_1~Q_3) and compared using the Kruskal–Wallis test, whose degrees of freedom (df) were 3; [b] Values presented as n (percentage) and compared using the chi-square test. * Values mean significant differences existed, as a p-value of less than 0.05 was considered significant. [(c–e)]: The same letter indicates no statistically significant differences between the two groups; different letters indicate significant differences for $p < 0.05$. LFI_1: low fluid intake 1; LFI_2: low fluid intake 2; HFI_1: high fluid intake 1; and HFI_2: high fluid intake 2.

3.4. Measurement of Body Compositions of Participants with Different TFI Levels

The basal metabolic rate and body water content differed significantly among the four groups ($\chi^2 = 20.784$, $p < 0.05$; $\chi^2 = 14.026$, $p < 0.05$). Participants with higher TFI levels had higher values of basal metabolic rate and body water content. No statistically significant differences were identified in the skeletal muscle, bone mineral content, or percent body fat (all $p > 0.05$) (Table 6).

Table 6. Body compositions of participants with different TFI levels.

	LFI_1 (n = 95)	LFI_2 (n = 95)	HFI_1 (n = 95)	HFI_2 (n = 95)	Total (n = 380)	p
Skeletal muscle (kg) [a]	43.0 (39.4~44.9)	50.4 (39.8~45.0)	49.2 (40.3~45.0)	50.8 (41.0~45.1)	49.4 (40.1~45.0)	0.262
Bone mineral content (kg) [a]	2.1 (2.0~2.2)	2.1 (2.0~2.3)	2.1 (2.0~2.2)	2.1 (2.0~2.3)	2.1 (2.0~2.3)	0.572
Basal metabolic rate (kcal) [a]	2173 (1972~2302) [b]	2202 (2108~2357) [c]	2253 (2086~2395) [d]	2314 (2153~2515) [e]	2241 (2086~2394)	<0.001 *
Percent body fat (%) [a]	27.4 (25.5~29.2)	28.3 (26.7~29.9)	28.0 (24.9~29.9)	28.6 (26.5~30.1)	28.1 (25.8~29.9)	0.262
Body water content (%) [a]	48.6 (46.4~52.0) [b]	50.4 (46.8~53.5) [c]	49.2 (46.9~53.2) [b]	50.8 (48.0~54.2) [d]	49.4 (46.9~53.2)	0.003 *

Note: [a] Values presented as median (Q_1~Q_3) and compared using the Kruskal–Wallis test, whose degrees of freedom (df) were 3. * values mean significant differences existed, as a p-value of less than 0.05 was considered significant. [(b–e)]: The same letter indicates no statistically significant differences between the two groups; different letters indicate significant differences for $p < 0.05$. LFI_1: low fluid intake 1; LFI_2: low fluid intake 2; HFI_1: high fluid intake 1; and HFI_2: high fluid intake 2.

3.5. Relationships between Fluid Intake Types, Maternal Body Composition, and Infant Birth Weight

The sample consisted of 380 singleton births in this study, with a mean birth weight of 3206 ± 342 g. The mean values of infant birth weight in the four groups from LFI_1 to HFI_2 were 3231 ± 332, 3183 ± 365, 3285 ± 347, and 3125 ± 306 g, respectively. The four groups varied significantly in infant birth weight ($\chi^2 = 3.885$, $p < 0.05$).

Linear regression models were applied to explore linear relationships between different fluid intake types, participants' body compositions, and their infants' birth weights. To begin with, fluid intake and body-composition variables were input into a linear regression model (Model 1). The method of backward elimination was used in the model fitting. A collinearity diagnosis and variable adjustment were applied to improve the goodness of fit and stability of the model. As a result, two models were fitted to the data: Model 1 presented a linear regression analysis in which fluid intake and body-composition variables were entered, and Model 2 was the model after adjustment. Due to the correlation between TFI and plain water intake (conducted using the Spearman test, r = 0.866, $p < 0.001$), the variable of TFI was not included in Model 1. Potential confounding factors were selected and included in the two regression models based on previous analyses, including maternal weight and BMI.

The analysis showed linear relationships between plain water intake, basal metabolic rate, and infant birth weight (SE = 0.153, $p < 0.05$; SE = 0.076, $p < 0.05$). There were no linear relationships between dairy product intake, SSB intake, skeletal muscle, body water content, percent of body fat, or infant birth weight (all $p > 0.05$) (Table 7).

Table 7. Associations between fluid intake levels and body composition with infant birth weight among participants.

Variables	Dependent Variable	Unstandardized Coefficient		Standardized Coefficient	*p*	VIF
		B	SE	*β*		
Model 1						
Plain water (mL)	Infant birth weight	0.384	0.160	0.129	0.017 *	1.113
Dairy products (mL)		0.400	0.469	0.045	0.395	1.056
SSBs (mL)		0.007	0.394	0.001	0.985	1.037
Skeletal muscle (kg)		0.693	1.705	0.006	0.913	1.026
Bone mineral content (kg)		94.089	81.539	0.063	0.249	1.118
Body water content (%)		2.999	3.250	0.049	0.357	1.427
Percent body fat (%)		0.078	1.705	0002	0.964	1.022
Basal metabolic rate (kcal)		0.194	0.090	0.131	0.032 *	1.085
Model 2						
Plain water (mL)	Infant birth weight	0.395	0.153	0.133	0.011 *	1.038
Basal metabolic rate (kcal)		0.208	0.076	0.140	0.007 *	1.038

Note: Linear regression models were applied to explore the linear relationship between different types of maternal fluid intake and infant birth weight. *, A *p*-value of less than 0.05 was considered significant. Infant birth weight was the dependent variable in the two models. B: unstandardized coefficients; SE: standard error of the coefficients; β: standardized coefficients; VIF: variance inflation factors; and SSBs: sugar-sweetened beverages.

4. Discussion

Our present study investigated TFI levels and types of pregnant women during their third trimester. Maternal body compositions were also measured. Related urine indicators were collected and assessed to evaluate their hydration status. Furthermore, the relationships between different types of fluid intake, maternal body compositions, and infant birth weights were analyzed. The results indicated that most pregnant women in their third trimester had insufficient TFI, with only 12.1% of participants meeting the Chinese water AI level (1.7 L/day for pregnant women). A study performed on 583 Chinese pregnant women revealed that TFI levels in the third trimester were 1446 mL, lower than the results obtained from our study (1574 mL) [50]. Notably, the retrospective questionnaire was used in the previous one, while a more accurate 7-day, 24 h real-time fluid intake record was used in our study. Previous studies revealed that the different methods can result in a deviation of up to 500 mL per day [51,52]. Compared with studies conducted in other countries, TFI levels among Chinese women were lower than those gained in a study among 132 French pregnant women in their third trimester (1937 mL/d) in 2014 [53].

Plain water was the primary type, with the highest intake level in this study accounting for 94.3% of TFI. This was similar to the findings from other studies [25,54].

Urine osmolality is the most accurate indicator to reflect kidney function of concentration and dilution, and it is also the most widely used to evaluate hydration status [55,56]. In this study, the proportion of the participants with a dehydration status was 15.0%, evaluated with urine osmolality. A previous study among pregnant women revealed that over 50% of overweight and obese women in America experienced dehydration status during pregnancy [57]. A study examined 38 pregnant women in West Jakarta during their second trimester; surprisingly, 20 participants had a dehydrated status, resulting in a dehydration rate of 52.6% [58]. It is clear that the hydration status of the participants in our present study is better than that of pregnant women from other countries. Correlation analysis revealed that negative correlations existed between urine osmolality, USG, urine pH, urine acid, and TFIs. There was a positive correlation between TFI, plain water, dairy products, SSBs, and hydration status. This suggests the possibility of urine biomarkers as indicators to reveal fluid intake and hydration status. Urine, an important pathway for water excretion, is crucial in maintaining hydration status. A total of 573 volunteers in Spain, Germany, and Greece participated in an eight-day study, which showed that TFI was negatively associated with urine specific gravity and color [59]. These basic findings were consistent with research showing that biomarkers in morning urine distinguished between high-level and low-level daily water intakes [60].

In our present study, participants with higher TFI levels had higher basal metabolic rates and body water content ($\chi^2 = 20.784$, $p < 0.05$; $\chi^2 = 14.026$, $p < 0.05$). This was in line with the result showing that water intake increases fat oxidation. This was under the condition when blood carbohydrate and insulin concentrations were kept stable, and when the fluid type was not caloric beverages, and the hydration status was not altered. Water intake is associated with increased energy consumption in the short term [61]. Another study reported that 500 mL of plain water intake resulted in higher energy consumption than the same volume (500 mL) of saline [62]. The result was also in line with the previous study, which noted the relationship between water intake behaviors and body water content. A study performed on 358 young Spanish women revealed that TFI was positively correlated with body water content ($r = 0.196$, $p = 0.002$; $r = 0.180$, $p = 0.006$). It also suggested that higher TFI was related to lower weight, body fat mass, and waist circumference [63]. Moreover, another study revealed a positive correlation between TFI normalized via body weight and body water content, while there was the inverse with BMI and fat body mass [64]. In a study conducted in America, researchers assessed the body compositions of 440 pregnant women and found that total body water content could be a powerful predictor of deterioration of pre-eclampsia [20]. Thus, adequate fluid intake is required during pregnancy to promote a better body water condition and ensure maternal and fetal health. A linear relationship was found between plain water intake and infant birth weight ($t = 2.074$; $p < 0.05$). This is consistent with a study that found that a low level of fluid intake during pregnancy was a risk factor for low birth weight [31]. A prospective cohort study on 2039 pregnant women in America showed that, after confounding adjustment, infant birth weight increased with the increase in the maternal TFI level during pregnancy [65]. Infant birth weight correlated with body adipose tissue increases in early pregnancy [18]. Fat-free mass and total body water content have been shown to be associated with birth weight, and total body water gain was positively linked to birth weight from studies conducted in different countries [13,66–68]. In our study, no linear relationship existed between body water content and infant birth weight ($p > 0.05$). It is worth noting that maternal dietary and nutritional statuses have an essential effect on the programming of the body [69]. Maternal and infant health may be influenced by these confounding factors in this study, and the association and mechanism are still unclear. Meanwhile, no linear relationship existed between the percent of body fat and infant birth weight ($p > 0.05$). This was similar to a previous study indicating that infant birth weight was positively correlated with maternal fat-free mass [70]. These findings suggest that increasing body fat mass during pregnancy may not protect infants from low birth weight to a certain extent. The results showed that participants with higher basal metabolic rates were associated with higher infant birth weight. A previous study showed that extra energy is in demand during pregnancy for supporting fetal development, maternal tissue increase, and maternal energy-metabolism change [71].

Our study has some strengths and limitations. Regarding the strengths, this is the first Chinese study to explore TFI, maternal body compositions in the third trimester during pregnancy, and their relationships with infant birth weight in China. Additionally, detailed data on fluid intake types were collected in this study. Thus, this led to further analysis of the correlations between different types of fluid and infant birth weight. What is more, a 7-day, 24 h fluid intake record in real-time was performed, which significantly reduced the inaccuracy associated with retrospective recording. In addition, multiple body composition indicators during pregnancy were detected, and their relationships with infant birth weight were analyzed. Last but not least, potential confounders have been part of our models, such as BMI and weight. The robustness of our results was enhanced by this comprehensive analysis. However, there are also notable limitations. First, only morning urine osmolality was obtained, lacking the 24 h urine osmolality. As circadian fluctuations influence urine biomarkers, this may result in some bias in evaluating hydration status throughout the day [72]. Secondly, only the TFI levels of participants were explored in our present study because of the unavailability of data on water intake levels from food. The result cannot be applied comprehensively to reflect pregnant women's total water intake level. Additionally, only infant birth weight was measured, while height, head circumference, and hip circumference were not. This leads to a lack of comprehensive assessment of infant growth status. Therefore, studies attempting to explore the long-term effects of TFI and hydration status during pregnancy and lactation on maternal and child health are needed in the future.

5. Conclusions

Water intake was insufficient among pregnant women during the third trimester, with only 12.1% of participants meeting the recommended adequate fluid intake for pregnant women living in China (1.7 L). The participants displayed a poor hydration status. There may be potential relationships between plain water intake, basal metabolic rate, and infant birth weight. Further studies should focus on the long-term dynamic monitoring of fluid intake during pregnancy and postnatal to effectively analyze the influence on maternal and child health.

Author Contributions: Y.S. was involved in the original drafting and revising of the manuscript, as well as contributing to the data analysis. G.M. and N.Z. supervised the implementation of the study and were responsible for finalizing the manuscript. N.Z. and F.Z. designed the study and were responsible for project administration, quality management, control of the study implementation, and data collection. X.W. was responsible for testing study samples and formal analysis. L.H., Z.L. and G.L. were the main coordinators and implementers of the project and were responsible for recruitment, fieldwork, data collection, and testing of study samples. Y.S., N.Z. and X.W. were responsible for report writing. All authors have read and agreed to the published version of the manuscript.

Funding: This work received support from Danone Institute China (No. DIC2018-11 and No. DIC2019-06), an independent non-profit organization (Danone.institute@danone-institute.org.cn). Neither funder played any role in study design, study implementation, data analysis, decision to publish, or manuscript preparation.

Institutional Review Board Statement: The study adhered to the guidelines of the Declaration of Helsinki. It was approved by the Ethical Review Committee of the Hainan Medical University on 9 November 2018. The ethical approval project identification code is 2018-4. The study protocol has been registered on the Chinese Clinical Trial Registry website with trial registration number Chi CTR800019284.

Informed Consent Statement: Before the beginning of the study, participants read and voluntarily signed the informed consent forms. The written consent was obtained from all the participants.

Data Availability Statement: The data can be obtained from the corresponding authors on reasonable request. As the data was currently explored and further analyzed, it will not be disclosed publicly at this stage.

Acknowledgments: The authors would like to thank all the participants and co-investigators who contributed to this research. In addition, Yongye Song wants to thank Guansheng Ma and Na Zhang for their patience, care, and support.

Conflicts of Interest: The authors have no competing interests to declare.

Abbreviations

AI	Adequate intake
BMI	Body mass index
SSB	Sugar-sweetened beverage
TFI	Total fluid intake
USG	Urine specific gravity

References

1. Chinese Nutrition Society. *Chinese Dietary Reference Intakes 2023*; Science Press: Beijing, China, 2023.
2. Jéquier, E.; Constant, F. Water as an essential nutrient: The physiological basis of hydration. *Eur. J. Clin. Nutr.* **2010**, *64*, 115–123. [CrossRef]
3. Häussinger, D. The role of cellular hydration in the regulation of cell function. *Biochem. J.* **1996**, *313 Pt 3*, 697–710. [CrossRef]
4. Ma, G. Hydration status and health. *Chin. J. Prev. Med.* **2019**, *53*, 337–341.
5. Baron, S.; Courbebaisse, M.; Lepicard, E.M.; Friedlander, G. Assessment of hydration status in a large population. *Br. J. Nutr.* **2015**, *113*, 147–158. [CrossRef] [PubMed]
6. Tan, E.K.; Tan, E.L. Alterations in physiology and anatomy during pregnancy. *Best Pract. Res. Clin. Obstet. Gynaecol.* **2013**, *27*, 791–802. [CrossRef] [PubMed]
7. Fall, C.H.D. Evidence for the intra-uterine programming of adiposity in later life. *Ann. Hum. Biol.* **2011**, *38*, 410–428. [CrossRef] [PubMed]
8. Aoyama, T.; Li, D.; Bay, J.L. Weight gain and nutrition during pregnancy: An analysis of clinical practice guidelines in the Asia-Pacific region. *Nutrients* **2022**, *14*, 1288. [CrossRef]
9. Bernstein, I.M.; Ziegler, W.; Badger, G.J. Plasma volume expansion in early pregnancy. *Obstet. Gynecol.* **2001**, *97*, 669–672. [PubMed]
10. Rees, G.B.; Pipkin, F.B.; Symonds, E.M.; Patrick, J.M. A longitudinal study of respiratory changes in normal human pregnancy with cross-sectional data on subjects with pregnancy-induced hypertension. *Am. J. Obstet. Gynecol.* **1990**, *162*, 826–830. [CrossRef] [PubMed]
11. Crapo, R.O. Normal cardiopulmonary physiology during pregnancy. *Clin. Obstet. Gynecol.* **1996**, *39*, 3–16. [CrossRef] [PubMed]
12. Lindheimer, M.D.; Davison, J.M.; Katz, A.I. The kidney and hypertension in pregnancy: Twenty exciting years. *Semin. Nephrol.* **2001**, *21*, 173–189. [CrossRef] [PubMed]
13. Larciprete, G.; Valensise, H.; Vasapollo, B.; Altomare, F.; Sorge, R.; Casalino, B.; De Lorenzo, A.; Arduini, D. Body composition during normal pregnancy: Reference ranges. *Acta Diabetol.* **2003**, *40* (Suppl. S1), S225–S232. [CrossRef] [PubMed]
14. Cheek, D.B.; Petrucco, O.M.; Gillespie, A.; Ness, D.; Green, R.C. Muscle cell growth and the distribution of water and electrolyte in human pregnancy. *Early Hum. Dev.* **1985**, *11*, 293–305. [CrossRef] [PubMed]
15. Davison, J.M.; Lindheimer, M.D. Volume homeostasis and osmoregulation in human pregnancy. *Baillieres Clin. Endocrinol. Metab.* **1989**, *3*, 451–472. [CrossRef] [PubMed]
16. Cheung, K.L.; Lafayette, R.A. Renal physiology of pregnancy. *Adv. Chronic Kidney Dis.* **2013**, *20*, 209–214. [CrossRef] [PubMed]
17. Davison, J.M.; Gilmore, E.A.; Dürr, J.; Robertson, G.L.; Lindheimer, M.D. Altered osmotic thresholds for vasopressin secretion and thirst in human pregnancy. *Am. J. Physiol.* **1984**, *246*, F105–F109. [CrossRef] [PubMed]
18. Kozłowska, A.; Jagielska, A.M.; Okręglicka, K.M.; Oczkowski, M.; Przekop, D.; Szostak-Węgierek, D.; Nitsch-Osuch, A.; Wielgoś, M.; Bomba-Opoń, D. *Maternal Nutritional and Water Homeostasis as a Presage of Fetal Birth Weight*; Pokorski, M., Ed.; Advances in Biomedicine; Springer International Publishing: Cham, Switzerland, 2019; pp. 89–99.
19. Valensise, H.; Andreoli, A.; Lello, S.; Magnani, F.; Romanini, C.; De Lorenzo, A. Multifrequency bioelectrical impedance analysis in women with a normal and hypertensive pregnancy. *Am. J. Clin. Nutr.* **2000**, *72*, 780–783. [CrossRef] [PubMed]
20. Yasuda, R.; Takeuchi, K.; Funakoshi, T.; Maruo, T. Bioelectrical impedance analysis in the clinical management of preeclamptic women with edema. *J. Perinat. Med.* **2003**, *31*, 275–280. [CrossRef]

21. Ghezzi, F.; Franchi, M.; Balestreri, D.; Lischetti, B.; Mele, M.C.; Alberico, S.; Bolis, P. Bioelectrical impedance analysis during pregnancy and neonatal birth weight. *Eur. J. Obstet. Gynecol. Reprod. Biol.* **2001**, *98*, 171–176. [CrossRef] [PubMed]
22. Sanin, A.L.; Reza-López, S.; Levario-Carrillo, M. Relation between maternal body composition and birth weight. *Biol. Neonatol.* **2004**, *86*, 55–62. [CrossRef]
23. Chinese Nutrition Society. *Dietary Guidelines for Chinese Residents: 2022*; People's Medical Publishing House: Beijing, China, 2022.
24. Bardosono, S.; Prasmusinto, D.; Hadiati, D.R.; Purwaka, B.T.; Morin, C.; Pohan, R.; Sunardi, D.; Chandra, D.N.; Guelinckx, I. Fluid intake of pregnant and breastfeeding women in Indonesia: A cross-sectional survey with a seven-day fluid specific record. *Nutrients* **2016**, *8*, 651. [CrossRef] [PubMed]
25. Song, Y.; Zhang, F.; Lin, G.; Wang, X.; He, L.; Li, Y.; Zhai, Y.; Zhang, N.; Ma, G. A study of the intake, hydration status, and health effects among pregnant women in their second trimester in China: A cross-sectional study. *Nutrients* **2023**, *15*, 1739. [CrossRef] [PubMed]
26. World Health Organization. *International Statistical Classification of Diseases and Related Health Problems*; World Health Organization: Geneva, Switzerland, 2015.
27. Liu, X.; An, H.; Li, N.; Li, Z.; Zhang, Y.; Le, Z.; Li, H.; Liu, J.; Ye, R. Preconception Hemoglobin Concentration and Risk of Low Birth Weight and Small-for-Gestational-Age: A Large Prospective Cohort Study in China. *Nutrients* **2022**, *14*, 271. [CrossRef] [PubMed]
28. Blencowe, H.; Krasevec, J.; de Onis, M.; Black, R.E.; An, X.; Stevens, G.A.; Borghi, E.; Hayashi, C.; Estevez, D.; Cegolon, L.; et al. National, regional, and worldwide estimates of low birthweight in 2015, with trends from 2000: A systematic analysis. *Lancet Glob. Health* **2019**, *7*, e849–e860. [CrossRef] [PubMed]
29. Fall, C.H.D. Fetal malnutrition and long-term outcomes. *Nestle Nutr. Inst. Workshop Ser.* **2013**, *74*, 11–25. [PubMed]
30. Villar, J.; Cogswell, M.; Kestler, E.; Castillo, P.; Menendez, R.; Repke, J.T. Effect of fat and fat-free mass deposition during pregnancy on birth weight. *Am. J. Obstet. Gynecol.* **1992**, *167*, 1344–1352. [CrossRef] [PubMed]
31. Savitz, D.A.; Andrews, K.W.; Pastore, L.M. Drinking water and pregnancy outcome in central North Carolina: Source, amount, and trihalomethane levels. *Environ. Health Perspect.* **1995**, *103*, 592–596. [CrossRef] [PubMed]
32. Martin, A.; O'Sullivan, A.J.; Brown, M.A. Body composition and energy metabolism in normotensive and hypertensive pregnancy. *Br. J. Obstet. Gynaecol.* **2001**, *108*, 1263–1271.
33. Levario-Carrillo, M.; Rodríguez, N.; Tufiño-Olivares, E.; Jiménez, M.D.R.; Delgado-Monge, M.C.; Reza-López, S. Body composition of women with newborns who are small for gestational age. *Neonatology* **2009**, *95*, 15–22. [CrossRef] [PubMed]
34. Levario-Carrillo, M.; Avitia, M.; Tufiño-Olivares, E.; Trevizo, E.; Corral-Terrazas, M.; Reza-López, S. Body composition of patients with hypertensive complications during pregnancy. *Hypertens. Pregnancy* **2006**, *25*, 259–269. [CrossRef] [PubMed]
35. Pross, N.; Demazières, A.; Girard, N.; Barnouin, R.; Metzger, D.; Klein, A.; Perrier, E.; Guelinckx, I. Effects of changes in water intake on mood of high and low drinkers. *PLoS ONE* **2014**, *9*, e94754. [CrossRef]
36. Ministry of Health of the PRC. *Anthropometric Measurements Method in Health Surveillance*; Standards Press of China: Beijing, China, 2013.
37. Zhang, J.; Zhang, N.; Liu, S.; Du, S.; Ma, G. Young adults with higher salt intake have Inferior hydration status: A cross-sectional study. *Nutrients* **2022**, *14*, 287. [CrossRef] [PubMed]
38. Zhang, J.; Zhang, N.; Liu, S.; Du, S.; He, H.; Ma, G. The comparison of water intake patterns and hydration biomarkers among young adults with different hydration statuses in Hebei, China. *Nutr. Metab.* **2021**, *18*, 2. [CrossRef] [PubMed]
39. Zhang, N.; Zhang, J.; Wang, X.; Li, Y.; Yan, Y.; Ma, G. Behaviors of Water Intake, Hydration Status, and Related Hydration Biomarkers among Physically Active Male Young Adults in Beijing, China: A Cross-Sectional Study. *Int. J. Clin. Pract.* **2022**, *2022*, 9436186. [CrossRef]
40. Zhang, J.; Zhang, N.; Liang, S.; Wang, Y.; Liu, S.; Liu, S.; Du, S.; He, H.; Xu, Y.; Cai, H.; et al. The amounts and contributions of total drinking fluids and water from food to total water intake of young adults in Baoding, China. *Eur. J. Nutr.* **2019**, *58*, 2669–2677. [CrossRef] [PubMed]
41. Ma, G.; Zhang, Q.; Liu, A.; Zuo, J.; Zhang, W.; Zou, S.; Li, X.; Lu, L.; Pan, H.; Hu, X. Fluid intake of adults in four Chinese cities. *Nutr. Rev.* **2012**, *70* (Suppl. S2), 105–110. [CrossRef] [PubMed]
42. Zhang, N.; Morin, C.; Guelinckx, I.; Moreno, L.A.; Kavouras, S.A.; Gandy, J.; Martinez, H.; Salas-Salvadó, J.; Ma, G. Fluid intake in urban China: Results of the 2016 *Liq.In*[7] national cross-sectional surveys. *Eur. J. Nutr.* 2018; 57, 77–88.
43. Zhang, N.; He, H.; Li, Y.; Yan, Y.; Zhang, J.; Ma, G. Analysis of the amount and types of fluid intake among male college students in spring. *Chin. J. Sch. Health* **2020**, *41*, 329–332.
44. Shahnazi, M.; Tagavi, S.; Hajizadeh, K.; Khalili, A.F. The effects of intravenous hydration on amniotic fluid index in pregnant women with preterm premature rupture of membranes: A randomized clinical trial. *J. Caring Sci.* **2013**, *2*, 47–52. [PubMed]
45. Technical Working Committee of China Beverage Industry Association. General Standard for Beverage. In *General Administration of Quality Supervision, Inspection and Quarantine of the People's Republic of China*; China National Standardization Administration: Beijing, China, 2015.
46. Perrier, E.T.; Buendia-Jimenez, I.; Vecchio, M.; Armstrong, L.E.; Tack, I.; Klein, A. Twenty-four-hour urine osmolality as a physiological index of adequate water intake. *Dis. Markers* **2015**, *2015*, 231063. [CrossRef] [PubMed]
47. Suh, H.; Summers, L.G.; Seal, A.D.; Colburn, A.T.; Mauromoustakos, A.; Perrier, E.T.; Bottin, J.H.; Kavouras, S.A. Afternoon urine osmolality is equivalent to 24 h for hydration assessment in healthy children. *Eur. J. Clin. Nutr.* **2020**, *74*, 884–890. [CrossRef] [PubMed]

48. Bar-David, Y.; Urkin, J.; Landau, D.; Bar-David, Z.; Pilpel, D. Voluntary dehydration among elementary school children residing in a hot arid environment. *J. Hum. Nutr. Diet. Off. J. Br. Diet. Assoc.* **2009**, *22*, 455–460. [CrossRef] [PubMed]
49. Kavouras, S.A. Hydration, dehydration, underhydration, optimal hydration: Are we barking up the wrong tree? *Eur. J. Nutr.* **2019**, *58*, 471–473. [CrossRef]
50. Zhencheng, X.; Lin, X.; Lu, X.; Teng, Y.; Dai, N.; Fuling, W.; Guo, J.; Ding, Y.; Wu, J.; Wang, Z. Water intake and its influence factors among pregnant and lactating women in some areas of China in 2020. *J. Hyg. Res.* **2022**, *51*, 367–373.
51. Bardosono, S.; Monrozier, R.; Permadhi, I.; Manikam, N.R.M.; Pohan, R.; Guelinckx, I. Total fluid intake assessed with a 7-day fluid record versus a 24-h dietary recall: A crossover study in Indonesian adolescents and adults. *Eur. J. Nutr.* **2015**, *54* (Suppl. S2), 17–25. [CrossRef] [PubMed]
52. Martinez, H. Fluid consumption by Mexican women during pregnancy and first semester of lactation. *BioMed Res. Int.* **2014**, *2014*, 603282. [CrossRef] [PubMed]
53. Albouy-Llaty, M.; Dupuis, A.; Grignon, C.; Strezlec, S.; Pierre, F.; Rabouan, S.; Migeot, V. Estimating drinking-water ingestion and dermal contact with water in a French population of pregnant women: The EDDS cohort study. *J. Expo. Sci. Environ. Epidemiol.* **2015**, *25*, 308–316. [CrossRef] [PubMed]
54. Ding, Y.; Xie, Z.; Lu, X.; Luo, H.; Pan, H.; Lin, X.; Wu, J.; Wang, Z. Water intake in pregnant women in China, 2018: The report of a survey. *Nutrients* **2021**, *13*, 2219. [CrossRef] [PubMed]
55. MacPherson, S.; Arbuckle, T.E.; Fisher, M. Adjusting urinary chemical biomarkers for hydration status during pregnancy. *J. Expo. Sci. Environ. Epidemiol.* **2018**, *28*, 481–493. [CrossRef] [PubMed]
56. Li, H.; Liang, H.; Zhou, Y. Osmole of blood and urinary-the most well index for condensing and diluting function of kidney. *J. Pract. Med. Technol.* **2003**, *15*, 20–21.
57. Rosinger, A.Y.; Bethancourt, H.J.; Pauley, A.M.; Latona, C.; John, J.; Kelyman, A.; Leonard, K.S.; Hohman, E.E.; McNitt, K.; Gernand, A.D.; et al. Variation in urine osmolality throughout pregnancy: A longitudinal, randomized-control trial among women with overweight and obesity. *Eur. J. Nutr.* **2022**, *61*, 127–140. [CrossRef] [PubMed]
58. Mulyani, E.Y.; Hardinsyah; Briawan, D.; Santoso, B.I.; Jus'At, I. Effect of dehydration during pregnancy on birth weight and length in West Jakarta. *J. Nutr. Sci.* **2021**, *10*, e70.
59. Malisova, O.; Athanasatou, A.; Pepa, A.; Husemann, M.; Domnik, K.; Braun, H.; Mora-Rodriguez, R.; Ortega, J.F.; Fernandez-Elias, V.E.; Kapsokefalou, M. Water Intake and Hydration Indices in Healthy European Adults: The European Hydration Research Study (EHRS). *Nutrients* **2016**, *8*, 204. [CrossRef] [PubMed]
60. Hahn, R.G. Quantifying the daily intake of water from morning and spot urine samples; retrospective analysis of a clinical trial in volunteers. *BMC Nutr.* **2023**, *9*, 3. [CrossRef] [PubMed]
61. Stookey, J.J.D. Negative, Null and Beneficial Effects of Drinking Water on Energy Intake, Energy Expenditure, Fat Oxidation and Weight Change in Randomized Trials: A Qualitative Review. *Nutrients* **2016**, *8*, 19. [CrossRef]
62. Boschmann, M.; Steiniger, J.; Franke, G.; Birkenfeld, A.L.; Luft, F.C.; Jordan, J. Water drinking induces thermogenesis through osmosensitive mechanisms. *J. Clin. Endocrinol. Metab.* **2007**, *92*, 3334–3337. [CrossRef] [PubMed]
63. García, A.I.L.; Moráis-Moreno, C.; de Lourdes Samaniego-Vaesken, M.; Puga, A.M.; Partearroyo, T.; Varela-Moreiras, G. Influence of Water Intake and Balance on Body Composition in Healthy Young Adults from Spain. *Nutrients* **2019**, *11*, 1923. [CrossRef] [PubMed]
64. García, A.I.L.; Moráis-Moreno, C.; de Lourdes Samaniego-Vaesken, M.; Puga, A.M.; Varela-Moreiras, G.; Partearroyo, T. Association between Hydration Status and Body Composition in Healthy Adolescents from Spain. *Nutrients* **2019**, *11*, 2692. [CrossRef] [PubMed]
65. Wright, J.M.; Hoffman, C.S.; Savitz, D.A. The relationship between water intake and foetal growth and preterm delivery in a prospective cohort study. *BMC Pregnancy Childbirth* **2010**, *10*, 48. [CrossRef] [PubMed]
66. Kramer, M.S. Determinants of low birth weight: Methodological assessment and meta-analysis. *Bull. World Health Organ.* **1987**, *65*, 663–737. [PubMed]
67. Lederman, S.A.; Paxton, A.; Heymsfield, S.B.; Wang, J.; Thornton, J.; Pierson, R.N., Jr. Maternal body fat and water during pregnancy: Do they raise infant birth weight? *Am. J. Obstet. Gynecol.* **1999**, *180*, 235–240. [CrossRef] [PubMed]
68. Butte, N.F.; Ellis, K.J.; Wong, W.W.; Hopkinson, J.M.; Smith, E.O. Composition of gestational weight gain impacts maternal fat retention and infant birth weight. *Am. J. Obstet. Gynecol.* **2003**, *189*, 1423–1432. [CrossRef] [PubMed]
69. Kwon, E.J.; Kim, Y.J. What is fetal programming?: A lifetime health is under the control of in utero health. *Obstet. Gynecol. Sci.* **2017**, *60*, 506–519. [CrossRef] [PubMed]
70. Kent, E.; O'Dwyer, V.; Fattah, C.; Farah, N.; O'Connor, C.; Turner, M.J. Correlation between birth weight and maternal body composition. *Obstet. Gynecol.* **2013**, *121*, 46–50. [CrossRef] [PubMed]
71. Minami, M.; Naw Awn, J.P.; Noguchi, S.; Eitoku, M.; Muchanga, S.M.J.; Mitsuda, N.; Komori, K.; Yasumitsu-Lovell, K.; Maeda, N.; Fujieda, M.; et al. Gestational weight gain mediates the effects of energy intake on birth weight among singleton pregnancies in the Japan Environment and Children's Study. *BMC Pregnancy Childbirth* **2022**, *22*, 568. [CrossRef] [PubMed]
72. Perrier, E.; Demazières, A.; Girard, N.; Pross, N.; Osbild, D.; Metzger, D.; Guelinckx, I.; Klein, A. Circadian variation and responsiveness of hydration biomarkers to changes in daily water intake. *Eur. J. Appl. Physiol.* **2013**, *113*, 2143–2151. [CrossRef] [PubMed]

nutrients

MDPI

Article

Prediction of Gestational Diabetes Mellitus in the First Trimester of Pregnancy Based on Maternal Variables and Pregnancy Biomarkers

Antigoni Tranidou [1], Ioannis Tsakiridis [1], Aikaterini Apostolopoulou [2], Theodoros Xenidis [1], Nikolaos Pazaras [2], Apostolos Mamopoulos [1], Apostolos Athanasiadis [1], Michail Chourdakis [2] and Themistoklis Dagklis [1,*]

[1] 3rd Department of Obstetrics and Gynecology, School of Medicine, Faculty of Health Sciences, Aristotle University of Thessaloniki, 54642 Thessaloniki, Greece; antigoni.tranidou@gmail.com (A.T.); iotsakir@gmail.com (I.T.); xenidistheodoros@yahoo.com (T.X.); amamop@auth.gr (A.M.); apostolos3435@gmail.com (A.A.)

[2] Laboratory of Hygiene, Social & Preventive Medicine and Medical Statistics, School of Medicine, Faculty of Health Sciences, Aristotle University of Thessaloniki, 54124 Thessaloniki, Greece; katapost@yahoo.gr (A.A.); nikpazaras@hotmail.com (N.P.); mhourd@gapps.auth.gr (M.C.)

* Correspondence: dagklis@auth.gr

Abstract: Gestational diabetes mellitus (GDM) is a significant health concern with adverse outcomes for both pregnant women and their offspring. Recognizing the need for early intervention, this study aimed to develop an early prediction model for GDM risk assessment during the first trimester. Utilizing a prospective cohort of 4917 pregnant women from the Third Department of Obstetrics and Gynecology, Aristotle University of Thessaloniki, Greece, the study sought to combine maternal characteristics, obstetric and medical history, and early pregnancy-specific biomarker concentrations into a predictive tool. The primary objective was to create a series of predictive models that could accurately identify women at high risk for developing GDM, thereby facilitating early and targeted interventions. To this end, maternal age, body mass index (BMI), obstetric and medical history, and biomarker concentrations were analyzed and incorporated into five distinct prediction models. The study's findings revealed that the models varied in effectiveness, with the most comprehensive model combining maternal characteristics, obstetric and medical history, and biomarkers showing the highest potential for early GDM prediction. The current research provides a foundation for future studies to refine and expand upon the predictive models, aiming for even earlier and more accurate detection methods.

Keywords: gestational diabetes mellitus; GDM; early screening; prediction; first trimester; pregnancy

1. Introduction

The number of pregnancies diagnosed with gestational diabetes mellitus (GDM) shows a steadily rising trend worldwide, parallel to the increasing maternal age (MA) and prevalence of obesity [1,2]. In addition to the synergistic effect of hormonal changes that occur during pregnancy, risk factors for GDM include higher parity and personal history of previous GDM [3,4]. Results from a meta-analysis report that GDM risk may be decreased by avoiding significant weight gain during pregnancy [5]. In addition, in a recent network meta-analysis, Wu et al. studied overweight and obese individuals. Their findings revealed two effective strategies for limiting gestational weight gain; physical activity alone and physical activity combined with a proper diet. These approaches were especially beneficial for reducing the risk of GDM in the study participants [6]. Moreover, current evidence shows that excessive gestational weight gain among individuals with pre-pregnancy obesity category 2 during the first half of pregnancy is associated with higher odds for GDM occurrence, while, in the normal weight pre-pregnancy individuals, a weight gain beyond 8 kg, in the first trimester of gestation, is associated with higher incidence of GDM [7].

This metabolic dysregulation has been gaining increasing focus as GDM is associated with a higher risk of adverse perinatal outcomes, including preeclampsia, macrosomia, shoulder dystocia, preterm delivery, cesarean delivery and neonatal hyperinsulinemia [8,9]. Furthermore, the risk of future metabolic disorders for both the mother and the infant are increased; they include maternal higher risk for cardiovascular disease, metabolic syndrome, type 2 diabetes mellitus (T2DM), as well as ophthalmic, psychiatric or renal disease. In children, there is increased risk for T2DM, excess adiposity, impaired neurodevelopment, neuropsychiatric, and ophthalmic disease [10–12].

The state of the art in GDM prediction has evolved significantly over recent years. Advanced statistical and machine learning models have been increasingly applied to improve the accuracy and timeliness of GDM prediction [13]. Despite these advancements, the heterogeneity in populations studied, differences in diagnostic criteria, and variability in predictor variables used across studies pose challenges in standardizing and adopting these models universally [14]. Concurrently, systematic reviews focusing on routine screening methods have highlighted the importance of traditional risk factors and clinical markers in predicting GDM. These studies underscore the effectiveness of integrating clinical data from routine antenatal care with prediction models to enhance early detection and management of GDM [15].

Notably, screening for GDM differs across national and international guidelines and depends on preexisting risk factors [16]. It is not uncommon that metabolic dysregulation may be present prior to conception; the underlying insulin resistance increases the odds for developing GDM in these women [17]. Accordingly, some women may experience GDM earlier in the course of their pregnancy, especially in the presence of aggravating factors such as excess adipose tissue [18]. Hence, regardless of the onset of metabolic alterations, it is critical for pregnant women to undergo prenatal care that allows timely identification of GDM. Towards this end, a number of studies have implemented early prediction models based on various biometric indicators like adiponectin/leptin ratio [19], inflammation markers like C-reactive protein (CRP) [20], as well as anthropometric parameters, e.g., age, weight, obstetric history [21], with each of the models achieving variable degrees of predictability, probably attributable to the different ethnic groups, the data available for each study group, the diversity of adjusted factors and various diagnostic standards.

The significance of computing the risk associated with GDM at early stages of pregnancy is highlighted, as timely intervention may be crucial for the prevention of adverse pregnancy outcomes. Thus, the aim of this study was to assess the risk factors and create a prediction model for GDM in the first trimester of pregnancy.

2. Materials and Methods

The data used in this study are prospectively (August 2020–December 2022) collected as part of an ongoing cohort study on diabetes in pregnancy, named "BORN2020". All attendees were recruited at the Third Department of Obstetrics and Gynecology, School of Medicine, Faculty of Health Sciences, Aristotle University of Thessaloniki, Greece. Women were recruited at their first trimester antenatal visit at 11^{+0}–13^{+6} weeks of gestation. Eligibility criteria were the following: (i) age > 18 years old, (ii) absence of preexisting diabetes (type 1 or 2), (iii) pregnancies that did not end as miscarriage or termination before 28 weeks of gestation; this criterion was applied to ensure inclusion of only those pregnancies where GDM screening was viable and relevant, and (iv) pregnancies continuing beyond 28 weeks of gestation, to ensure that GDM screening was performed. A total of 4532 women were initially recruited. Of these, 335 women were subsequently excluded due to miscarriage or termination before 28 weeks of gestation. This exclusion was necessary to focus our analysis on viable pregnancies where GDM screening is typically performed. Therefore, the final cohort for the study comprised 4917 women.

Participants' data included the following information: maternal age (MA), body mass index (BMI) before pregnancy, smoking status, method of conception, obstetric history and history of thyroid disease or chronic hypertension. Chronic hypertension was identified based on participants' self-reported medical history, validated by medical records, and defined as blood pressure $\geq$ 140/90 before the 20th week of pregnancy. Furthermore, serum PAPP-A and free β-hCG were assessed as part of routine screening for Down's syndrome. Mean uterine artery pulsatility index (UtA-PI) was measured by transabdominal pulsed wave Doppler ultrasonography, as part of routine screening for preeclampsia.

With regards to GDM screening, the Hellenic Society of Obstetricians and Gynecologists recommends universal screening at 24–28 weeks of gestation, using GDM diagnostic criteria that are based on the results of the "Hyperglycemia and Adverse Pregnancy Outcome" (HAPO) study [22]. Specifically, after fasting for at least 8 h, women are tested for glucose levels and then they are given 75 g of oral glucose and tested again at one and two hours. GDM is diagnosed when at least one of the following cutoffs is met: fasting blood glucose $\geq$ 92 mg/dL, blood glucose concentration 1 h after OGTT $\geq$ 180 mg/dL and/or blood glucose concentration 2 h post OGTT $\geq$ 153 mg/dL.

The study received approval by the Bioethics Committee of Aristotle University of Thessaloniki, Greece (6.231/29 July 2020). Written consent was obtained from all participants.

Statistical Analysis

Regarding univariate feature analyses of maternal characteristics, medical and obstetric history and measured variables, the following methods were applied: in case of continuous variables, the Shapiro–Wilk test was used to determine normality, the F-test was used to determine variance equality, and the t-test, Wilcoxon test, or Mann–Whitney test was used to test the validity of the hypothesis. For binary variables the Fisher's exact test was applied.

Values of fβ-hCG and PAPP-A were converted into multiples of the median (MoM). The UtA-PI was expressed as a z-score. The correlation between maternal characteristics, obstetric history, pregnancy biomarkers and the probability of subsequently developing GDM was examined using multivariate logistic regression analysis. Five models were tested to detect GDM early. The models were created based on data readily available in routine care practice. The features of each model were selected based on clinical characteristics proposed in previous studies [21,23,24], and thus, different categories were formed by the available data (maternal characteristics, obstetric history, biomarkers and measured variables) with regards to known risk factors for GDM development. An addition to our models, not extensively reported in the previous literature, was the computation of fβ-hCG. The detection rates at fixed false-positive rates (FPR) of 5%, 10%, 15%, and 20% were provided, as well as the area under the ROC curve (AUROC). Bootstrapping was used to compute confidence intervals for the detection rate of each model, given the specific fixed false positive rate. The differences in AUROC across the five prediction models were evaluated. The R programming language was used for all statistical implementations (v4.2.1).

3. Results

Overall, 4917 women were eligible based on the study selection criteria. Of these, 474 (9.64%) developed GDM and 4443 women (90.4%) did not. The median MA of the GDM population was higher in the GDM group compared to the non-GDM group ($p < 0.0001$), while 39% (n = 183) of women with GDM and 26% (n = 1138) of women without GDM were >35 years old ($p < 0.0001$). Pre-pregnancy BMI was higher in the GDM group vs. the non-GDM group ($p < 0.0001$). Moreover, conception via ART was higher in the GDM group ($p < 0.0001$), and smoking during pregnancy was also higher in the GDM group ($p = 0.03$). In addition, chronic hypertension ($p = 0.02$), thyroid disease ($p = 0.01$), history of preeclampsia ($p = 0.003$) and history of previous cesarean section ($p = 0.001$) were higher in the GDM women compared to the non-GDM individuals. Finally,

PAPP-A levels ($p = 0.04$) and also the UtA-PI z-score ($p = 0.03$) were lower in the GDM individuals. Maternal characteristics and available biomarkers are presented in Table 1.

Table 1. Maternal characteristics of women with and without gestational diabetes.

Maternal Characteristics	GDM (N = 474)	Non-GDM (N = 4443)	*p* Value
MA (years) 25%, 50%, 75%	33.5 30, 33.5, 36.9	31.8 28.4, 31.8, 35	<0.0001
MA > 35 (n%)	183 (38.6)	1138 (25.6)	<0.0001
BMI pre (kg/m^2)	25 22.2, 25, 30.5	22.7 20.7, 22.7, 25.7	<0.0001
Conception via ART (n%)	44 (9.3)	209 (4.7)	<0.0001
Smoking during pregnancy (n%)	67 (14.1)	481 (10.8)	0.03
Chronic Hypertension (n%)	5 (1.05)	12 (0.27)	0.02
Thyroid disease (n%)	55 (11.6)	356 (8.01)	0.01
SLE/APS (n%)	3 (0.63)	23 (0.51)	0.73
Obstetric history			
Preeclampsia (n%)	28 (5.9)	136 (3.06)	0.003
SGA (n%)	2 (0.42)	34 (0.76)	0.57
PCS (n%)	105 (22.2)	719 (16.2)	0.001
Parity (n%)	202 (42.6)	1807 (40.7)	0.43
Measured variables			
fβ-hCG MoM	0.46, 0.9, 1.27	0.65, 0.97, 1.47	0.11
PAPP-A MoM	0.9, 1.07, 1.26	0.94, 1.09, 1.26	0.04
UtA-PI z-score	−0.50, 0.20, 0.88	−0.24, 0.28, 0.88	0.03

BMI pre: Body Mass Index before pregnancy; Conception ART: conception with assisted reproductive technologies; fβ-hCG: free-beta subunit human chorionic gonadotropin; GDM: gestational diabetes mellitus; PAPP-A: plasma protein-A; PCS: previous caesarian section; Thyroid disease: Hypothyroidism, Hyperthyroidism, Hashimoto's disease; SLE/APS: Systemic lupus erythematosus/Antiphospholipid syndrome; SGA: small for gestational age; UtA-PI: uterine artery pulsatility index.

In the multivariate analysis, as shown in Table 2, several models were evaluated for their ability to predict GDM:

Model 1: MA and pre-pregnancy BMI were independent contributors for GDM (aOR: 1.08; 95% CI: 1.05–1.09; $p < 0.0001$ and aOR: 1.10; 95% CI: 1.08–1.12; $p < 0.0001$, respectively).

Model 2: Similar to Model 1, MA and pre-pregnancy BMI were associated with higher incidence of GDM (aOR: 1.07; 95% CI: 1.04–1.09; $p < 0.0001$ and aOR: 1.10; 95% CI: 1.08–1.12; $p < 0.0001$, respectively).

Model 3: Added history of preeclampsia to the factors in Model 2, identifying it as an independent contributing factor for GDM (aOR: 1.80; 95% CI: 1.12–2.81; $p = 0.01$), while higher parity was associated with reduced incidence of GDM (aOR: 0.72: 95% CI: 0.56–0.92; $p = 0.009$).

Model 4: Included MA (aOR: 1.08; 95% CI: 1.06–1.10; $p < 0.0001$), levels of PAPP-A (aOR: 0.83; 95% CI: 0.70–0.98; $p = 0.03$) and UtA-PI (aOR: 0.89; 95% CI: 0.80–0.98; $p = 0.02$) were independent contributors for GDM.

Model 5: the combination of all the available data showed that MA, pre-pregnancy BMI and history of preeclampsia were strongly correlated with increased risk GDM (aOR: 1.07; 95% CI: 1.05–1.09; $p < 0.0001$, aOR: 1.10; 95% CI: 1.08–1.12; $p < 0.0001$ and aOR: 1.78; 95% CI: 1.11–2.80; $p = 0.01$, respectively), while higher parity was found to be associated with reduced rates of GDM (aOR: 0.73; 95% CI: 0.57–0.85; $p = 0.01$).

Table 2. Maternal characteristics, maternal medical and obstetric history and measured variables of present pregnancy associated with gestational diabetes.

	Multivariate Regression Analysis, aOR, 95% CI									
	Model 1	***p* Value**	**Model 2**	***p* Value**	**Model 3**	***p* Value**	**Model 4**	***p* Value**	**Model 5**	***p* Value**
MA (years)	1.08 (1.05, 1.09)	<0.0001	1.07 (1.04, 1.09)	<0.0001	1.07 (1.05, 1.10)	<0.0001	1.08 (1.06, 1.10)	<0.0001	1.07 (1.05, 1.09)	<0.0001
BMI pre	1.10 (1.08, 1.12)	<0.001	1.10 (1.08, 1.12)	<0.0001	1.10 (1.08, 1.12)	<0.0001			1.10 (1.08, 1.12)	<0.0001
Conception ART			1.44 (0.98, 2.07)	0.052					1.36 (0.91, 1.10)	0.11
Smoking during pregnancy	1.23 (0.92, 1.63)	0.15							1.27 (0.94, 1.70)	0.10
Thyroid disease			1.25 (0.90, 1.69)	0.16					1.25 (0.90, 1.70)	0.15
Chronic hypertension			1.64 (0.49, 4.75)	0.38					1.32 (0.40, 3.91)	0.62
SLE/APS			1.20 (0.28, 3.54)	0.76					1.14 (0.27, 3.40)	0.83
Preeclampsia History					1.80 (1.12, 2.81)	0.01			1.78 (1.11, 2.80)	0.01
SGA History					0.49 (0.08, 1.68)	0.33			0.51 (0.08, 1.78)	0.37
PCS History					1.24 (0.91, 1.67)	0.16			1.21 (0.89, 1.64)	0.21
Parity					0.72 (0.56, 0.92)	0.009			0.73 (0.57, 0.85)	0.01
fβ-hCG MoM							0.95 (0.83, 1.07)	0.41	0.97 (0.86, 1.09)	0.63
PAPP-A MoM							0.83 (0.70, 0.98)	0.03	0.86 (0.72, 1.01)	0.07
UtA-PI z-score							0.89 (0.80, 0.98)	0.02	0.94 (0.85, 1.04)	0.22

aOR: adjusted odds ratio; CI: confidence interval; MA: maternal age; BMI pre: Body Mass Index before conception; Conception ART: conception with assisted reproductive technologies; Thyroid disease: Hypothyroidism, Hyperthyroidism, Hashimoto's disease; SLE/APS: Systemic lupus erythematosus/Antiphospholipid syndrome; SGA: small for gestational age; PCS: previous caesarian section; MoM: multiples of the median; fβ-hCG: free-beta subunit human chorionic gonadotropin; PAPP-A: plasma protein-A; UtA-PI: uterine artery pulsatility index.

Model Performance and Comparison

As shown in Table 3, the AUROCs of each model was used to assess performance:

Model 1: AUROC of 0.672, using maternal characteristics and smoking.

Model 2: Similar to AUROC of Model 2 that used maternal characteristics and maternal medical history (0.672).

Model 3: Slight improvement of the AUROC (0.675) with the use of obstetric history.

Model 4: Lower predictability when pregnancy biomarkers were employed (AUROC of 0.606).

Model 5: Slightly higher AUROC (0.678) compared to other models.

Models 1, 2, 3, and 5 have similar performance and the difference of their AUROCs is not statistically significant. Model 4 is the only model that is statistically different from Models 1, 2, 3, and 5. In Table 4, the detection rates for all models at 5%, 10%, 15% and 20% fixed FPR are presented, while Figure 1 presents the ROC curves of the five models that were employed.

Table 3. Comparison of prediction models for gestational diabetes. Each cell in the Model Comparison section presents the difference of AUROCs between the model in the row and the model in the column, along with the 95% CI for this difference.

			Model Comparison—Difference of AUROCs (95% CI for the Difference)				
Screening Model for GDM	AUROC (95% CI)	SE	Model 1	Model 2	Model 3	Model 4	Model 5
Model 1	0.672 (0.65–0.70)	0.0141	-	−0.0005 (−0.006, 0.004)	−0.003 (−0.01, 0.006)	0.07 (0.04, 0.09) *	−0.006 (−0.02, 0.004)
Model 2	0.672 (0.65–0.70)	0.0141	-	-	−0.003 (−0.01, 0.007)	0.07 (0.04, 0.09) *	−0.006 (−0.02, 0.004)
Model 3	0.675 (0.65–0.70)	0.0141	-	-	-	0.07 (0.04, 0.09) *	−0.003 (−0.01, 0.004)
Model 4	0.606 (0.58–0.63)	0.0143	-	-	-	-	−0.07 (−0.10, −0.05) *
Model 5	0.678 (0.65–0.70)	0.0140	-	-	-	-	-

AUROC: area under the curve; SE: standard errors; Model 1: maternal characteristics (maternal age, BMI before pregnancy), smoking during pregnancy; Model 2: maternal characteristics, maternal medical history (thyroid disease, chronic hypertension conception via assisted reproductive technology); Model 3: maternal characteristics, obstetric history (history of preeclampsia, small for gestational age neonate, previous cesarean delivery, parity); Model 4: maternal characteristics, pregnancy biomarkers (free-beta subunit human chorionic gonadotropin, plasma protein-A) and measured variables (uterine artery pulsatility index); Model 5 is a comprehensive model combining all elements of the previous models, including maternal characteristics, smoking during pregnancy, maternal medical history, conception with assisted reproductive technologies, obstetric history, and pregnancy biomarkers. * $p < 0.05$ for the difference in AUROC comparison between the models.

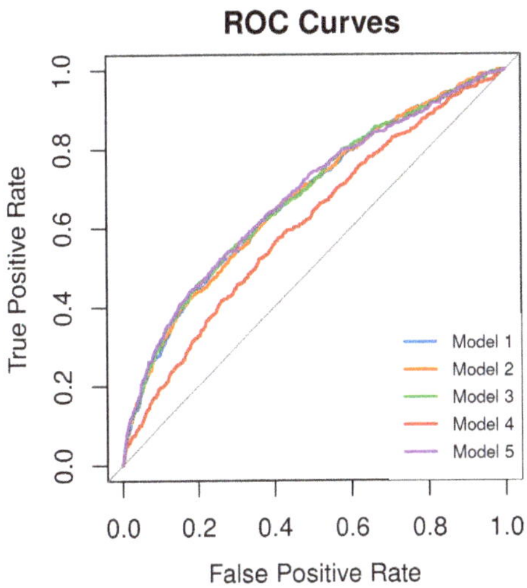

Figure 1. ROC curves of the 5 models for early screening of GDM. Model 1: maternal characteristics (maternal age, BMI before pregnancy), smoking during pregnancy; Model 2: maternal characteristics, maternal medical history (thyroid disease, chronic hypertension conception via assisted reproductive technology; Model 3: maternal characteristics, obstetric history (history of preeclampsia, small for gestational age neonate, previous cesarean delivery, parity); Model 4: maternal characteristics, pregnancy biomarkers (free-beta subunit human chorionic gonadotropin, plasma protein-A) and measured variables (uterine artery pulsatility index); Model 5 is a comprehensive model combining all elements of the previous models, including maternal characteristics, smoking during pregnancy, maternal medical history, conception with assisted reproductive technologies, obstetric history, and pregnancy biomarkers.

Table 4. Detection and fixed false positive rates for the predictive models for gestational diabetes.

Detection Rate	Fixed False Positive Rate			
	5%	10%	15%	20%
Model 1	12.26 (5.45, 21.18)	23.79 (14.98, 34.35)	33.04 (24.55, 43.69)	39.1 (29.57, 48.70)
Model 2	11.45 (5.38, 22.01)	24.38 (15.39, 34.5)	32.97 (23.61, 44.5)	39.5 (29.91, 49.81)
Model 3	11.32 (6.03, 20.84)	22.01 (12.64, 32.07)	33.83 (24.53, 43.69)	41.82 (32.72, 51.21)
Model 4	10.65 (4.09, 21.36)	17.58 (9.84, 27.5)	23.54 (14.13, 35.11)	31.71 (20.77, 42.77)
Model 5	12.24 (7.04, 23.46)	20.19 (11.1, 31.51)	30.68 (21.99,41.67)	41.12 (33.24, 50.8)

Model 1: maternal characteristics, smoking during pregnancy; Model 2: maternal characteristics, maternal medical history, conception with assisted reproductive technologies; Model 3: maternal characteristics, obstetric history; Model 4: maternal characteristics, pregnancy biomarkers; Model 5 is a comprehensive model combining all elements of the previous models, including maternal characteristics, smoking during pregnancy, maternal medical history, conception with assisted reproductive technologies, obstetric history, and pregnancy biomarkers.

4. Discussion

Results from this study showed the following: (i) The incidence of GDM in our population was 9.6%; (ii) In the first trimester of pregnancy, for the models combining maternal characteristics with obstetric history (i.e., Models 3 and 5), the following variables were independent risk factors for GDM: maternal age, pre-pregnancy BMI and history of preeclampsia. This underscores the importance of these factors in early intervention strategies. Mirabelli et al. further emphasize the significant impact of maternal preconception BMI over age as a risk factor for GDM, suggesting that interventions targeting preconception weight management might be particularly effective in areas with high GDM prevalence [25]; (iii) the predictive model combining maternal characteristics (MA, pre-pregnancy BMI), maternal medical and obstetric history, as well as pregnancy biomarkers, for early GDM screening (Model 5) had the highest predictive value. This finding highlights the potential of integrated models in improving early detection and management of GDM, which is crucial for reducing associated risks; Lastly, (iv) the inclusion of fβ-hCG in the multivariate model for GDM prediction (Model 4) had the lowest performance compared to the other models. This result indicates that not all biomarkers are equally predictive for GDM, emphasizing the need for critical selection and combination of variables in model development.

The variations between the national and international recommendations on screening for GDM were recently reviewed in a comparative analysis by Tsakiridis et al. [16]. In particular, the American College of Obstetricians and Gynecologists (ACOG), as well as the Australasian Diabetes in Pregnancy Society (ADIPS), the Society of Obstetricians and Gynecologists of Canada (SOGC), and the International Federation of Gynecology and Obstetrics (FIGO) suggest screening at 24–28 weeks of gestation for all pregnant women that have no other risk factors, while in contrast, the National Institute for Health and Care Excellence (NICE) recommends screening at 24–28 weeks only for those who have risk factors. The Endocrine Society (ES) recommends universal screening at the beginning of the first trimester for all pregnant women and if negative, repeat testing at 24–28 weeks of gestation. The FIGO guideline recommends this latter approach of screening only in nations with a higher risk of developing GDM.

In a systematic review, the authors identified the constraints of the available performance models implemented for the prediction of GDM [26]. The biomarkers addressed for the prediction of GDM demonstrate that their predictive ability is constrained, and conflicting results have been reported. Moreover, studies on the added value of readily available biomarkers to noninvasive models are rare. Another meta-analysis highlighted the need for implementing more sophisticated risk prediction algorithms and more research on precise (bio)markers [15]. Our study aimed to identify possible markers for early GDM prediction, with the use of different combinations of the available biomarkers and non-invasive measures as compared to those referred in literature. Data were collected during routine care screening, while the population included participants with and without known risk factors for GDM.

The incidence of GDM in our population is consistent with previous European studies [27,28]. In addition, a recent meta-analysis indicated that the overall weighted prevalence of GDM in a total of 24 European countries was 10.9% [29]. The highest prevalence of GDM was observed in Eastern Europe (31.5%), while the lowest was recorded in Northern Europe with 8.9%. The corresponding values for Western and Southern Europe were 10.7% and 12.3%, respectively.

Several risk factors have been identified for the development of GDM. In our study, GDM was associated with higher MA and increased pre-pregnancy BMI, as has been described in previous studies [30,31]. Yong et al. reported that in women of older age that started their pregnancy while being overweight or obese, the risk for GDM increased by 2.5 times, while gaining excess weight during pregnancy aggravated these odds [31]. Moreover, in a study conducted by Buerger et al., the authors evaluated the risk for GDM in singleton and twin pregnancies [32]. The odds were higher with advancing MA, increased weight and birthweight z-score from previous pregnancy, in both cases. The risk remained higher in cases where there was personal history of GDM or for individuals with a first- or second-degree family history of diabetes and for women that conceived with the use of medications for ovulation induction. The authors applied this information in the development of a screening model for GDM; therefore, setting the FPR at 10% and 20% for singleton pregnancies, the detection rates were 42.8% and 58%, respectively. The screening accuracy of the model by Buerger et al. may be overestimated as the authors declare that their large sized control group may have included women with undiagnosed GDM, as OGTT was not applied in all pregnancies [32]. Likewise, in a predictive model used by Shen at al., which computed the maternal characteristics and obstetric history of pregnant women in screening for GDM, at FPR of 10% and 20%, the detection rates were 35.6% and 53%, respectively [21]. Moreover, when the authors compared maternal characteristics, obstetric history and preeclampsia biomarkers, the AUROC of the model yielded more accuracy (0.738). But as mentioned by the authors, the results may be biased towards underestimating the risk for GDM because the OGTT screening was based on a targeted screening strategy. The FPR at 10% and 20% in this case yielded detection rates at 36.7% and 51.5%, respectively.

Furthermore, the use of UtA-PI has been previously studied. More specifically, Chatzakis et al. investigated the phenotype subgroups of GDM in relation to preeclampsia and UtA-PI percentiles and reported significant differences among the three distinguished phenotypes [33]. The first phenotype included individuals with abnormal fasting blood glucose levels, the second included women with abnormal blood glucose levels after one or two hours following the OGGT, while the third phenotype included a combination of the other two phenotypes. The third phenotype was associated with a higher uterine artery resistance and higher incidence of preeclampsia. The correlation between GDM and preeclampsia is well established in the literature [34]. In our study, the UtA-PI was associated with increased risk for GDM. However, the model that used this index achieved the lowest predictability. Furthermore, in a meta-analysis by Talasaz et al., the prognostic value of plasma protein-A (PAPP-A) was found of low predictive value when used alone. However, if used collectively with other tests, it may have a better prognostic result [35]. In the current study, lower levels of PAPP-A were detected in the GDM population in comparison to the non-GDM individuals. The incorporation of PAPP-A in Model 4, which combined maternal characteristics and measured variables showed that low levels of PAPP-A were associated with 17% lower chance for GDM incidence (aOR: 0.83, 95% CI [0.70, 0.98], $p = 0.03$). As per our study findings, the incidence of previous cesarean delivery was associated with GDM. This finding is in accordance with previous studies [36]. Particularly, according to Xiong et al., among other risk factors for GDM, prior cesarean section increased the risk for GDM by 18% [37].

The strengths of this study include the representative sample size, the prospective systematic method to collect obstetric and medical history, the implementation of universal GDM screening with the same diagnostic criteria and the implementation of biomarkers (fβ-hCG, PAPP-a and UtA-PI) in the model to assess its use for the early diagnosis of those at risk for developing GDM. One of the limitations of our study is that we did not have consistent information on family history of GDM or GDM occurrence in previous pregnancy which are important predictors for GDM and this may have underestimated the accuracy of our prediction models. Moreover, all data were collected from a single center and thus, the prediction models lack external verification. As a future work we plan to gather data in collaboration with other settings, to confirm the accuracy of the prediction models implemented in this study.

5. Conclusions

In conclusion, our study has demonstrated the utility of comprehensive models in early GDM screening, with Model 5 showing the highest predictability. These findings are significant for clinical practice, offering a potential pathway for early intervention and improved outcomes. However, the study also highlights the complexity of the early prediction of GDM and the need for ongoing research. Future research should focus on validating these models in diverse populations and settings to enhance their generalizability and clinical utility. Additionally, the exploration of new biomarkers and risk factors, as well as the application of advanced statistical and machine learning techniques, could further refine GDM prediction models. The main goal is to develop a universally applicable, non-invasive, and accurate prediction model that can be readily implemented in the early course of pregnancy.

By critically reflecting on the study's findings and outlining a clear path for future research, this study contributes to the evolving landscape of GDM prediction and underscores the importance of continued innovation and critical evaluation in this field.

Author Contributions: T.D., I.T., A.A. (Aikaterini Apostolopoulou) and A.T. recruited the population of the study. T.D., I.T., A.M., T.X. and A.A. (Apostolos Athanasiadis) performed all clinical evaluations of the study population. A.T. performed the statistical analysis in R language. N.P., T.D., I.T. and M.C. reviewed the statistical analysis. T.D., I.T. and M.C. critically reviewed the whole text and statistical analysis. All authors have read and agreed to the published version of the manuscript.

Funding: This research received no external funding.

Institutional Review Board Statement: The study was conducted in accordance with the Declaration of Helsinki and was approved by the Bioethics Committee of the Aristotle University of Thessaloniki was obtained (6.231/29 July 2020).

Informed Consent Statement: Informed consent was obtained from all subjects involved in the study.

Data Availability Statement: The data presented in this study are not publicly available due to privacy restrictions.

Acknowledgments: We would like to express our gratitude to Evangelia Varagka, Aikaterini Pelagou, and Sofia Daliani for their help in organizing and collecting the data of the population under investigation.

Conflicts of Interest: The authors declare no conflicts of interest.

References

1. Wang, M.C.; Shah, N.S.; Petito, L.C.; Gunderson, E.P.; Grobman, W.A.; Matthew, J.O.; Khan, S.S. Gestational diabetes and overweight/obesity: Analysis of nulliparous women in the US, 2011–2019. *Am. J. Prev. Med.* **2021**, *61*, 863–871. [CrossRef] [PubMed]
2. Agha, M.; Agha, R. The rising prevalence of obesity: Part A: Impact on public health. *Int. J. Surg. Oncol.* **2017**, *2*, e17. [CrossRef] [PubMed]
3. Li, Y.; Ren, X.; He, L.; Li, J.; Zhang, S.; Chen, W. Maternal age and the risk of gestational diabetes mellitus: A systematic review and meta-analysis of over 120 million participants. *Diabetes Res. Clin. Pract.* **2020**, *162*, 108044. [CrossRef] [PubMed]

4. Abu-Heija, A.T.; Al-Bash, M.R.; Al-Kalbani, M.A. Effects of maternal age, parity and pre-pregnancy body mass index on the glucose challenge test and gestational diabetes mellitus. *J. Taibah Univ. Med. Sci.* **2017**, *12*, 338–342. [CrossRef] [PubMed]
5. Brunner, S.; Stecher, L.; Ziebarth, S.; Nehring, I.; Rifas-Shiman, S.L.; Sommer, C.; von Kries, R. Excessive gestational weight gain prior to glucose screening and the risk of gestational diabetes: A meta-analysis. *Diabetologia* **2015**, *58*, 2229–2237. [CrossRef] [PubMed]
6. Wu, S.; Jin, J.; Hu, K.-L.; Wu, Y.; Zhang, D. Prevention of gestational diabetes mellitus and gestational weight gain restriction in overweight/obese pregnant women: A systematic review and network Meta-analysis. *Nutrients* **2022**, *14*, 2383. [CrossRef] [PubMed]
7. Tranidou, A.; Magriplis, E.; Tsakiridis, I.; Pazaras, N.; Apostolopoulou, A.; Chourdakis, M.; Dagklis, T. Effect of Gestational Weight Gain during the First Half of Pregnancy on the Incidence of GDM, Results from a Pregnant Cohort in Northern Greece. *Nutrients* **2023**, *15*, 893. [CrossRef]
8. Billionnet, C.; Mitanchez, D.; Weill, A.; Nizard, J.; Alla, F.; Hartemann, A. Gestational diabetes and adverse perinatal outcomes from 716,152 births in France in 2012. *Diabetologia* **2017**, *60*, 636–644. [CrossRef]
9. Baskind, M.; DiMeglio, L.A.; Cabana, M.D. Diabetes in Pregnancy. In *Orthopaedics for the Newborn and Young Child: A Practical Clinical Guide*; Springer International Publishing: Cham, Switzerland, 2023; pp. 405–413.
10. Farahvar, S.; Walfisch, A.; Sheiner, E. Gestational diabetes risk factors and long-term consequences for both mother and offspring: A literature review. *Expert Rev. Endocrinol. Metab.* **2019**, *14*, 63–74. [CrossRef]
11. Tranidou, A.; Dagklis, T.; Tsakiridis, I.; Siargkas, A.; Apostolopoulou, A.; Mamopoulos, A.; Goulis, D.G. Risk of developing metabolic syndrome after gestational diabetes mellitus-a systematic review and meta-analysis. *J. Endocrinol. Investig.* **2021**, *44*, 1139–1149. [CrossRef]
12. Wicklow, B.; Retnakaran, R. Gestational Diabetes Mellitus and Its Implications across the Life Span. *Korean Diabetes J.* **2023**, *47*, 1516082861. [CrossRef] [PubMed]
13. Mennickent, D.; Rodríguez, A.; Farías-Jofré, M.; Araya, J.; Guzmán-Gutiérrez, E. Machine learning-based models for gestational diabetes mellitus prediction before 24–28 weeks of pregnancy: A review. *Artif. Intell. Med.* **2022**, *132*, 102378. [CrossRef] [PubMed]
14. Meertens, L.J.E.; Scheepers, H.C.J.; van Kuijk, S.M.J.; Roeleveld, N.; Aardenburg, R.; van Dooren, I.M.A.; Langenveld, J.; Zwaan, I.M.; Spaanderman, M.E.A.; van Gelder, M.M.H.J.; et al. External validation and clinical utility of prognostic prediction models for gestational diabetes mellitus: A prospective cohort study. *Acta Obstet. Gynecol. Scand.* **2020**, *99*, 891–900. [CrossRef] [PubMed]
15. Farrar, D.; Simmonds, M.; Bryant, M.; Lawlor, D.A.; Dunne, F.; Tuffnell, D.; Sheldon, T.A. Risk factor screening to identify women requiring oral glucose tolerance testing to diagnose gestational diabetes: A systematic review and meta-analysis and analysis of two pregnancy cohorts. *PLoS ONE* **2017**, *12*, e0175288. [CrossRef] [PubMed]
16. Ioannis, T.; Sonia, G.; Apostolos, M.; Anargyros, K.; Apostolos, A.; Dionysia, F.; Themistoklis, D. Diagnosis and management of gestational diabetes mellitus: An overview of national and international guidelines. *Obstet. Gynecol. Surv.* **2021**, *76*, 367–381.
17. Catalano, P. Trying to understand gestational diabetes. *Diabet. Med.* **2014**, *31*, 273–281. [CrossRef]
18. Bozkurt, L.; Göbl, C.S.; Pfligl, L.; Leitner, K.; Bancher-Todesca, D.; Luger, A.; Baumgartner-Parzer, S.; Pacini, G.; Kautzky-Willer, A. Pathophysiological characteristics and effects of obesity in women with early and late manifestation of gestational diabetes diagnosed by the International Association of Diabetes and Pregnancy Study Groups criteria. *J. Clin. Endocrinol. Metab.* **2015**, *100*, 1113–1120. [CrossRef]
19. Thagaard, I.N.; Krebs, L.; Holm, J.-C.; Lange, T.; Larsen, T.; Christiansen, M. Adiponectin and leptin as first trimester markers for gestational diabetes mellitus: A cohort study. *Clin. Chem. Lab. Med. (CCLM)* **2017**, *55*, 1805–1812. [CrossRef]
20. Kononova, O.; Pristrom, A.; Vasilkova, V.; Mokhort, T. C-reactive protein and gestational diabetes mellitus. *Endocr. Abstr. Biosci.* **2013**, *32*, 604. [CrossRef]
21. Shen, L.; Sahota, D.S.; Chaemsaithong, P.; Tse, W.T.; Chung, M.Y.; Ip, J.K.H.; Leung, T.Y.; Poon, L.C.Y. First trimester screening for gestational diabetes mellitus with maternal factors and biomarkers. *Fetal Diagn. Ther.* **2022**, *49*, 256–264. [CrossRef]
22. Coustan, D.R.; Lowe, L.P.; Metzger, B.E.; Dyer, A.R. The Hyperglycemia and Adverse Pregnancy Outcome (HAPO) study: Paving the way for new diagnostic criteria for gestational diabetes mellitus. *Am. J. Obstet. Gynecol.* **2010**, *202*, 654.e1–654.e6. [CrossRef] [PubMed]
23. Sweeting, A.N.; Wong, J.; Appelblom, H.; Ross, G.P.; Kouru, H.; Williams, P.F.; Sairanen, M. A first trimester prediction model for gestational diabetes utilizing aneuploidy and pre-eclampsia screening markers. *J. Matern. Fetal Neonatal Med.* **2018**, *31*, 2122–2130. [CrossRef] [PubMed]
24. Tenenbaum-Gavish, K.; Sharabi-Nov, A.; Binyamin, D.; Møller, H.J.; Danon, D.; Rothman, L.; Hadar, E.; Idelson, A.; Vogel, I.; Koren, O.; et al. First trimester biomarkers for prediction of gestational diabetes mellitus. *Placenta* **2020**, *101*, 80–89. [CrossRef] [PubMed]
25. Mirabelli, M.; Tocci, V.; Donnici, A.; Giuliano, S.; Sarnelli, P.; Salatino, A.; Greco, M.; Puccio, L.; Chiefari, E.; Foti, D.P.; et al. Maternal Preconception Body Mass Index Overtakes Age as a Risk Factor for Gestational Diabetes Mellitus. *J. Clin. Med.* **2023**, *12*, 2830. [CrossRef]
26. Lamain-de Ruiter, M.; Kwee, A.; Naaktgeboren, C.A.; Franx, A.; Moons, K.G.; Koster, M.P. Prediction models for the risk of gestational diabetes: A systematic review. *Diagn. Progn. Res.* **2017**, *1*, 3. [CrossRef] [PubMed]
27. Dłuski, D.F.; Ruszała, M.; Rudziński, G.; Pożarowska, K.; Brzuszkiewicz, K.; Leszczyńska-Gorzelak, B. Evolution of Gestational Diabetes Mellitus across Continents in 21st Century. *Int. J. Environ. Res. Public Health* **2022**, *19*, 15804. [CrossRef]

28. Wang, H.; Li, N.; Chivese, T.; Werfalli, M.; Sun, H.; Yuen, L.; Hoegfeldt, C.A.; Powe, C.E.; Immanuel, J.; Karuranga, S.; et al. IDF diabetes atlas: Estimation of global and regional gestational diabetes mellitus prevalence for 2021 by International Association of Diabetes in Pregnancy Study Group's Criteria. *Diabetes Res. Clin. Pract.* **2022**, *183*, 109050. [CrossRef]
29. Paulo, M.S.; Abdo, N.M.; Bettencourt-Silva, R.; Al-Rifai, R.H. Gestational diabetes mellitus in Europe: A systematic review and meta-analysis of prevalence studies. *Front. Endocrinol.* **2021**, *12*, 691033. [CrossRef]
30. Dong, B.; Yu, H.; Wei, Q.; Zhi, M.; Wu, C.; Zhu, X.; Li, L. The effect of pre-pregnancy body mass index and excessive gestational weight gain on the risk of gestational diabetes in advanced maternal age. *Oncotarget* **2017**, *8*, 58364. [CrossRef]
31. Yong, H.Y.; Shariff, Z.M.; Yusof, B.N.M.; Rejali, Z.; Tee, Y.Y.S.; van der Beek, E.M. Independent and combined effects of age, body mass index and gestational weight gain on the risk of gestational diabetes mellitus. *Sci. Rep.* **2020**, *10*, 8486. [CrossRef]
32. Buerger, O.; Elger, T.; Varthaliti, A.; Syngelaki, A.; Wright, A.; Nicolaides, K.H. First-trimester screening for gestational diabetes mellitus in twin pregnancies. *J. Clin. Med.* **2021**, *10*, 3814. [CrossRef] [PubMed]
33. Chatzakis, C.; Sotiriadis, A.; Demertzidou, E.; Eleftheriades, A.; Dinas, K.; Vlahos, N.; Eleftheriades, M. Prevalence of preeclampsia and uterine arteries resistance in the different phenotypes of gestational diabetes mellitus. *Diabetes Res. Clin. Pract.* **2023**, *195*, 110222. [CrossRef] [PubMed]
34. Östlund, I.; Haglund, B.; Hanson, U. Gestational diabetes and preeclampsia. *Eur. J. Obstet. Gynecol. Reprod. Biol.* **2004**, *113*, 12–16. [CrossRef] [PubMed]
35. Talasaz, Z.H.; Sadeghi, R.; Askari, F.; Dadgar, S.; Vatanchi, A. First trimesters Pregnancy-Associated Plasma Protein-A levels value to Predict Gestational diabetes Mellitus: A systematic review and meta-analysis of the literature. *Taiwan. J. Obstet. Gynecol.* **2018**, *57*, 181–189. [CrossRef]
36. Ben-Haroush, A.; Yogev, Y.; Hod, M. Epidemiology of gestational diabetes mellitus and its association with Type 2 diabetes. *Diabet. Med.* **2004**, *21*, 103–113. [CrossRef]
37. Xiong, X.; Saunders, L.D.; Wang, F.L.; Demianczuk, N.N. Gestational diabetes mellitus: Prevalence, risk factors, maternal and infant outcomes. *Int. J. Gynecol. Obstet.* **2001**, *75*, 221–228. [CrossRef]

nutrients

MDPI

Article

Can Pre-Pregnancy Body Mass Index and Maternal Exercise Affect Birth and Neonatal Outcomes—A Cross Sectional Study

Anna Weronika Szablewska [1,*], Jolanta Wierzba [2], Rita Santos-Rocha [3,4] and Anna Szumilewicz [5]

1 Department of Obstetric and Gynaecological Nursing, Institute of Nursing and Midwifery, Medical University of Gdansk, Debinki 7, 80-211 Gdansk, Poland
2 Department of Pediatric and Internal Medicine Nursing, Institute of Nursing and Midwifery, Medical University of Gdansk, Debinki 7, 80-211 Gdansk, Poland; kwierz@gumed.edu.pl
3 ESDRM Department of Physical Activity and Health, Sport Sciences School of Rio Maior, Polytechnic Institute of Santarém, 2040-413 Rio Maior, Portugal; ritasantosrocha@esdrm.ipsantarem.pt
4 CIPER Interdisciplinary Centre for the Study of Human Performance, Faculty of Human Kinetics (FMH), University of Lisbon, 1495-751 Lisbon, Portugal
5 Department of Physical Culture, Gdansk University of Physical Education and Sport, 80-336 Gdansk, Poland; anna.szumilewicz@awf.gda.pl
* Correspondence: anna.szablewska@gumed.edu.pl; Tel.: +48-509-586-094

Abstract: There has been a dramatic worldwide increase in the prevalence of obesity or overweight and physical inactivity in women of reproductive age. Growing evidence suggests that pre-pregnancy maternal abnormal body mass index (BMI) and lower physical activity level are associated with poor maternal health and perinatal outcomes. The aim of this study was to assess how self-perceived exercise and pre-pregnancy BMI are associated with preterm birth, low birth weight, and type of birth. We conducted a retrospective cross-sectional study of 394 Polish women in the postpartum period. We used a questionnaire with the structure of the medical interview. To analyze factors related to birth outcomes, we used the Pearson's Chi-squared test of independence and odds ratio (OR), with a corresponding 95% confidence interval (CI), followed by a multiple logistic regression. Women who reported being physically active before pregnancy ($p = 0.00$) and during pregnancy ($p = 0.03$) were more likely to give birth on time and had a lower incidence of very-premature and extremely premature births compared to inactive women. Importantly, they were more likely to have vaginal birth ($p = 0.03$). Pre-pregnancy BMI influenced the week of delivery, i.e., inadequate, too-high BMI contributed to an increase in the percentage of premature births [OR (95% CI) = 1.19 (1.06; 1.34)]. The findings indicate that promoting physical activity and weight management remains a priority in public health policy, and women of childbearing age should be encouraged to adopt or maintain an active and healthy lifestyle during pregnancy in order to avoid sedentary- and obesity-associated risks affecting birth and newborns' health.

Keywords: preterm birth; pre-pregnancy BMI; exercise; birth outcomes

1. Introduction

The recent data have shown that regular physical activity during pregnancy and before pregnancy has a positive effect on the physical and psychological condition of the future mother, fetal development, parturition, and functioning during the postpartum period [1–6]. What is more, physical activity started in pregnancy may have impact on a lifelong change to a health-promoting lifestyle. Research has also proved that the prenatal physical activity of mothers has a long-term effect on the health of the children, including a reduction in the risk of obesity in later life [7,8].

The presence of abnormal body weight before pregnancy and in the first trimester of pregnancy is a crucial risk factor of preterm birth (PTB) and low birth weight (LBW) [9,10]. The global preterm birth rate has remained constant for over 20 years, amounting to

9.6–11% [11–13]. On the other hand, data from the World Health Organization (WHO) show that in recent years an increase in the number of premature births has been observed in many countries (mainly in industrialized countries). Prematurity and low birth weight are one of the most important and still valid challenges of modern medicine, and are also a socio-economic problem. It is important to emphasize that the incidence of preterm birth is a multi-faceted and multifactorial aspect. Its occurrence is influenced by maternal, fetal, genetic, infectious, and environmental factors. In many cases, the cause of preterm birth remains unknown, making it an unresolved and still current problem in perinatology [14]. It is also important to note that the factors determining the incidence of preterm births change over the years and vary according to geographical location [15]. Preterm babies require interdisciplinary, specialist treatment, diagnostics, and rehabilitation, sometimes lasting their entire life. The literature data show that approximately 15 million premature babies are born in the world each year [11,16,17].

In many studies, researchers have mentioned that abnormal pre-pregnancy BMI is a very important independent risk factor of PTB. This value also determines the recommended maternity weight gain during pregnancy. The data obtained in this way are considered the most important indicators of the nutritional status of a pregnant woman [18]. Abnormal BMI is also associated with an increased risk of gestational diabetes, pre-eclampsia and eclampsia, pregnancy-induced hypertension (PIH), and other perinatal abnormalities [19–21]. The consequences of the increase in the frequency of premature childbirths and low birth weight have led to a critical analysis of the factors that may affect their occurrence and effects (social, medical, psychological, and economic). Focusing on a specific population of Polish women adds a unique dimension to this field. By delving into a distinct demographic, our research contributes to a better understanding of the relationship between physical activity, BMI, and birth outcomes within the context of the Polish population. Additional exploration of how pre-pregnancy BMI influences the week of pregnancy completion (using categories), particularly the association with an increased percentage of premature births (which is still an unsolved problem), provides valuable insights.

Aim

The aim of this study was to assess how pre-pregnancy BMI and self -perceived maternal exercise are associated with preterm birth, low birth weight, and other newborn and birth outcomes.

2. Materials and Methods

2.1. Study Design

The present study was a multi-center, retrospective, cross-sectional study among a group of 394 Polish women (in the Polish population, ethnic minorities represent a relatively small percentage of the total population, so we did not distinguish ethnic groups) in the postpartum period and after singleton pregnancy; of which, 153 women delivered preterm (22–37 weeks) (38.8%) and 241 had a full-term birth (38–42 weeks) (61.2%). We used a questionnaire with the structure of the medical interview. Also, medical history, especially maternal and neonatal outcomes, were analyzed (see the Supplementary Materials). We followed the STROBE guidelines for cross-sectional studies [22]. All procedures were performed in accordance with the principles outlined in the Declaration of Helsinki of the World Medical Association (WMA) and approved by the Bioethics Commission of the Gdansk Medical University, no. NKBB/393/2015 for studies involving humans.

2.2. Setting

The study was conducted in 2 hospitals of tertiary referral centers (the Poland classification system establishes levels of maternal care that pertain to level I of perinatal care: the care of a physiologically progressing pregnancy, labor and the puerperium, and a healthy newborn (possibly short-term pregnancy pathology); level II of perinatal care: the care of intermediate-level pathological pregnancies; and level III of perinatal care: the care of the most severe pregnancy pathology) in the northern region of Poland. The period of data collection and patient eligibility was from 1 January 2016 to 1 January 2018.

2.3. Participants

All participants were informed of the study objectives and provided their voluntary consent to participate, by marking consent to participate in the survey in the questionnaire and consent for access to medical records (it was one of the inclusion criteria). The parents were informed that taking part in the research would not affect their child's diagnostic and therapeutic process and that the child would not be exposed to additional procedures. The children's mothers, as their legal carers, also consented to access to the documentation concerning the newborn child.

The principal investigator had a personal conversation with each mother of the children, explaining all concerns about the conduct of the study and the recruitment process. Mothers were invited to the study during their stay in the maternity ward after delivery or during a visit to the newborn in the neonatal intensive care unit (if the baby's mother was not invited to participate after delivery and the baby's condition required prolonged hospitalization). The children's parents had the right to ask questions. Each child and mother included in the study were given an identification number, based on data from the medical records (such as mode of pregnancy completion, duration of pregnancy, maternal weight gain during pregnancy, the newborn's birth weight and Apgar score, anthropometric data of the mother before pregnancy) that were completed, to minimize information bias.

The study included 394 mothers aged 19 to 44 years (hospitalized in the maternity wards of hospitals) and their children born, alive, between 22 and 42 weeks' gestation, who met the inclusion criteria (hospitalized in the neonatology and neonatal intensive care unit of the associated units or in their mothers room in the system).

Approximately 5000 mothers received an invitation to take part in the study. Only 10% responded, and 136 participants were subsequently excluded from the study due to not meeting the eligibility criteria (as a result the rate of preterm birth was 38.8%). We conducted the study at the level III reference medical centers, where the rate of premature births was assumed to be higher than in other hospitals, due to the access to specialized equipment. Nevertheless, for our study, this increased rate of preterm birth compared to the general population appeared to be beneficial, providing access to a larger group of newborns born prematurely. This allowed for more accurate statistical analysis and more accurate inferences. The participants' flow through the study is presented in Figure 1.

2.4. Inclusion and Exclusion Criteria

The inclusion criteria were mothers having a single, alive birth after 22 weeks of pregnancy, those that gave birth at the public hospitals, and those understanding the Polish language.

We excluded multiple gestations (assuming that it could be a potential reason for preterm birth and low birth weight), lack of consent to access medical records, obtaining an incomplete interview questionnaire, death of a newborn in the perinatal period, stillbirth, and gestational age of the newborn below 22 weeks (in the case of alive births).

2.5. Variables and Data Sources

2.5.1. Maternal Variables

Understanding the importance of pre-pregnancy exercise on the pregnancy and newborn outcomes, we included two subcategories of the study women in terms of their exercise habits:

Self-perceived exercise before pregnancy—exercise performed by the mother 6 months before becoming pregnant, excluding normal home- and work-related activity, but including active transportation, and autonomous and supervised physical exercise. As "exercise" we considered all forms of physical activity that were planned, structured, repetitive, and performed with the goal of improving health or fitness [23]. We noted these data from the survey addressed to mothers. This variable was categorized as YES or NO.

Self-perceived exercise during pregnancy (new exercise, started after becoming pregnant)—exercise started after becoming pregnant and performed by the mother during pregnancy, excluding normal home and work-related activity, but including active transportation, and autonomous and supervised physical exercise. We noted these data from survey addressed to mothers. This variable was categorized as YES or NO.

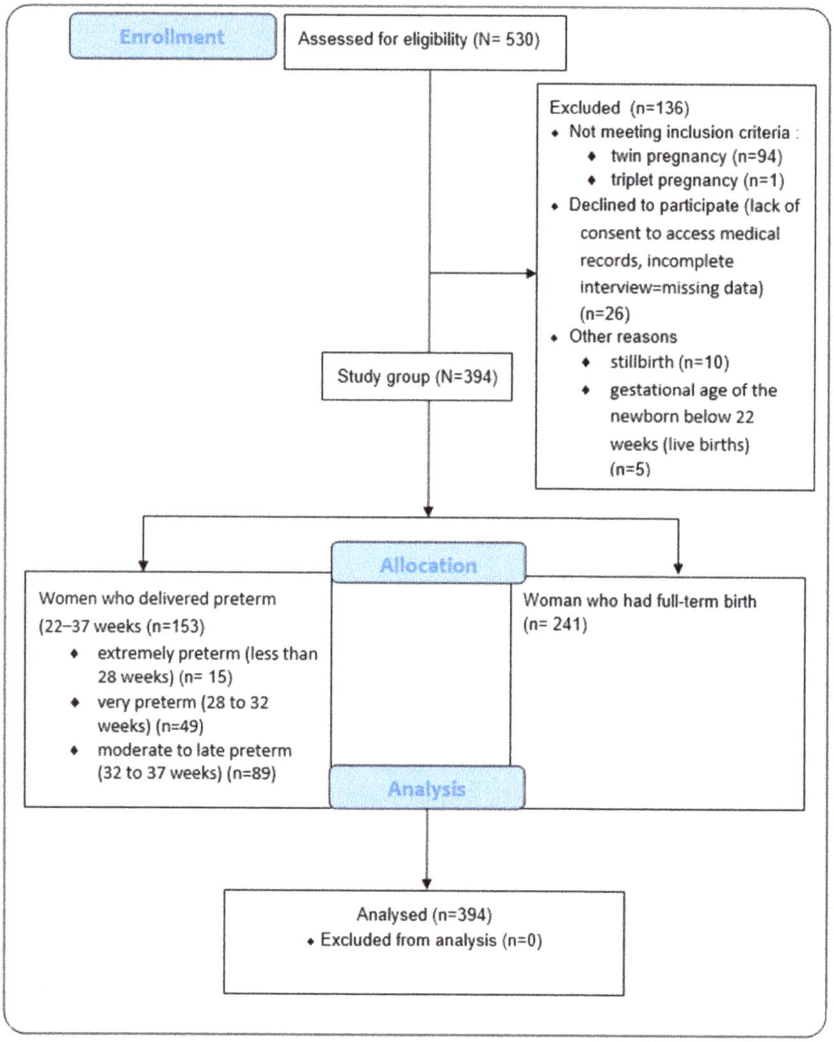

Figure 1. The flow of participants through the study.

Pre-pregnancy BMI category—this value was calculated by taking a mother's weight (before becoming pregnant or in the first weeks of pregnancy-data obtained from pregnancy chart), in kilograms, divided by their height, in meters squared, or BMI = weight (in kg)/height^2 (in m^2). The number generated from this equation was marked as the individual's pp-BMI number. These classifications for BMI are in use by the National

Institute of Health (NIH) and the World Health Organization (WHO) for White, Hispanic, and Black individuals [24]. The BMI number and classifications are listed below:

- Overweight and obesity—BMI greater than or equal to 25.0 and greater than 30 kg/m^2;
- Normal weight—BMI greater than or equal to 18.5 to 24.9 kg/m^2;
- Underweight—BMI under >18.5 kg/m^2;

We connected these two categories (overweight and obesity) because of the small group of obese mothers.

Maternal weight gain (WG) (kg)—this was calculated by recommendations for total and rate of Weight Gain During Pregnancy, by Pre-pregnancy Body Mass Index (pp-BMI), data from the Institute of Medicine/National Research Council [25]:

- Overweight and obesity (25.0–29.9 and 30.0 or higher)—7.0–11.5 and 5.0–9.0 kg
- Normal weight (18.5–24.9)—11.5–16.0 kg
- Underweight (less than 18.5)—12.5–18.0 kg

Methods of labor—the method of pregnancy completion was recorded from the participants' medical records. Vaginal delivery, caesarean section, or operative delivery (vacuum, forceps delivery) were considered. Perineal episiotomy and degrees of perineal tears were not analyzed in cases of vaginal delivery.

2.5.2. Newborn Variables

Gestational age at delivery (number of weeks category)—the newborn's age at birth, determined by the week of gestation according to Neagele's rule or, if there was a discrepancy between the gestation date and the first-trimester ultrasound, according to the first-trimester ultrasound. The information on the week of pregnancy completion was recorded from the medical records and verified by the medical staff.

Particular consideration was given to completion of the pregnancy prematurely (PTB, preterm birth), i.e., between 22 and 27 weeks' gestation. The subcategories of preterm births, according to the WHO, by gestational age were used [26,27]:

a. Extremely preterm birth (less than 28 weeks);
b. Very preterm birth (between 28 and 32 weeks);
c. Moderate and late preterm birth (32 to 37 weeks).

The proposed subdivision was taken into account due to the different proportion of preterm births in each category, with the largest group being late preterm births, which also has an impact on the prognosis and further development of the newborn. It is also important to underline here that the gestational age at delivery categories were related to the referral of the patient to the appropriate reference center (hospital reference levels), which is crucial issue in planning the care of pregnant women.

Newborn's birth weight (in grams)—the birth weight of the neonate is an important clinical criterion. Many times, the birth weight of a neonate born prematurely corresponds to that of a full-term neonate, i.e., between 2500 g and 4000 g. It also happens that a neonate born on time is born with a low birth weight, which can be indicative of hypotrophy. We noted these data from medical records, and qualified newborns for subcategories of newborn weight [28].

Division of neonates by birth weight:

a. Hypertrophic neonate, too large for gestational age (LGA, large for gestational age), defined as macrosomia-neonatal weight above 4000 g;
b. Eutrophic neonate, weight appropriate for gestational age (AGA, appropriate for gestational age)—body weight between 2500 g and 4000 g;
c. Hypotrophic neonate, too small for gestational age (SGA)—body weight below the 10th centile for gestational age or less than 2500 g;
d. Low birth weight (LBW) neonate—weight between 2500 g and 1500 g;
e. Very-low birth weight newborn (VLBW)—weight between 1499 g and 1000 g;
f. Extremely low birth weight (ELBW)—weight between 1000 g and 750 g;

g. Incredibly low birth weight newborn (ILBW, or incredibly low birth weight)—weight less than 749 g.

Preterm birth is the leading cause of low birth weight in both developing and highly developed countries. These pathologies (LBW and PTL) most often occur together. In our work we described normal weight and compared the results with LGA, LBW, VLBW, ELBW, and ILBW because of the potential negative influence of this factor on the babies; according to previous studies, they were more likely to die during their first month of life and those who survived face lifelong consequences, including a higher risk of stunted growth, lower IQ, and adult-onset chronic conditions such as obesity, diabetes, and cardiovascular disease (CVD) [28].

Apgar score in 1st minute (0–10 points)—As an indicator of the general condition immediately after birth, the Apgar scale was chosen as a universal and easily obtainable parameter [29] from the records (given that the clinical material and the analysis of the records concerned different institutions, and the analysis was intended to compare neonates born full-term and prematurely). We noted these data from newborn medical records.

2.6. Statistical Analysis

The data were analyzed using statistical software: the Statistica 12.0 version (advanced package) and PQStat v 1.8.0.476. Pearson's Chi-squared test of independence was used to present the differences in the rates of full term vs. preterm deliveries and the differences in the birth weight categories in subgroups of active and inactive women. With the same test, we analyzed the rates of various modes of delivery in subgroups of women with the different pre-pregnancy BMI. Logistic regression analysis was performed (analyzed variables: group; mother's weight at pregnancy; mother's pp-BMI; weight gain in pregnancy). Multiple regression analysis was performed in order to analyze the strength of the relationship between maternal BMI and newborn variables (newborn' birth weight, Apgar score). The level of significance adopted was 0.05. Sample size was computed using G-power 3.1. (correlations: two independent Pearson, effect size q = 0.5; α error of probability $p = 0.05$; power = 0.95; allocation ratio N2/N1 = 2; result: sample size group 1 = 68; sample size group 2 = 135; total sample size = 203, using variable: maternal exercise before pregnancy). The calculated sample size was smaller than our final study group; however, due to access to more women after childbirth, we decided to analyze larger data, which in turn allowed for subgroup analysis.

3. Results

A total of 394 women participated in the study: 153 women who delivered preterm (22–37 weeks-study group) and 241 who had a full-term birth (38–42 weeks-control group). Demographic characteristics, maternal data, and pregnancy outcomes are shown in Tables 1 and 2.

Table 1. Demographic characteristics of study participants ($n = 394$).

Characteristics	N	%
Maternal age (years)		
<24	37	9.4%
25–29	118	30.0%
30–34	153	38.8%
>35	86	21.8%
Place of residence		
rural	79	20.1%
City below 20,000 residents	12	3.0%
City 20–100,000 residents	47	11.9%
City 100–200,000 residents	31	7.9%
City with over 200,000 residents	225	57.1%

Table 1. *Cont.*

Characteristics	*N*	%
Education		
Primary school	36	9.1%
High school	89	22.6%
University degree	269	68.3%
Marital status		
Single	52	13.2%
Married	289	73.4%
Cohabiting	53	13.4%

Table 2. Maternal data and birth outcomes.

Gestational Age at Delivery (Weeks)		
Extremely preterm (less than 28 weeks)	15	3.8%
Very preterm (28 to 32 weeks)	49	12.4%
Moderate to late preterm (32 to 37 weeks)	89	22.6%
Full-term pregnancy	241	61.2%
Mode of childbirth		
Vaginal birth, VB	207	52.5%
Caesarean section, CS	182	46.2%
Vacuum/forceps delivery	5	1.3%
Maternal exercise before pregnancy		
Yes	133	33.8%
No	261	66.2%
Maternal exercise during pregnancy		
Yes	59	15.0%
No	335	85.0%
Pre-pregnancy BMI category		
Overweight and obesity (25.0 to <30)	121	30.7%
Normal weight (18.5 to 24.9)	255	64.7%
Underweight (<18.5)	18	4.6%
Maternal weight gain [kg]		
<−5; 0)	5	1.3%
<0>	3	0.7%
(0; 7>	48	12.2%
(8; 14>	191	48.5%
(15; 21>	117	29.7%
(22; 32>	30	7.6%
Newborn's birth weight		
Incredibly low birth weight, ILBW	5	1.3%
Extremely low birth weight, ELBW	15	3.8%
Very-low birth weight, VLBW	28	7.1%
Low birth weight, LBW	55	14.0%
Normal weight, AGA	253	64.2%
Large for gestational age, LGA	38	9.6%
Apgar score in 1st minute		
0–3 points	11	2.8%
4–7 points	47	11.9%
8–10 points	336	85.3%

We found that 25.1% women with normal weight (BMI 18.5 to 24.9) had EWG, excessive gestational weight gain; 40.0% had AWG, appropriate weight gain; and 34.9% LWG, too little weight gain (recommended WG 11.5–16.0 kg). Women who were overweight and obesity (BMI 25.0 to <30) had EWG in 62.0%, AWG in 20.6%, and LWG in 17.4% (recommended WG 7.0–11.5 kg). Women who were underweight (>18.5) had EWG in 5.5%, AWG in 66.7%, and LWG in 27.8% (recommended WG 12.5–18.0 kg).

In our research, we assessed self-perceived exercise before pregnancy and we compared the results with the week of pregnancy category. Chi-squared Pearson's test showed statistically significant differences between the groups ($p = 0.05$). In the group of women who were active, 69.9% ($n = 93$) delivered full term, 19.5% ($n = 26$) had moderate to late preterm birth, 9.0% ($n = 12$) had very preterm birth, and 1.4% ($n = 1$) had extremely preterm birth. In the group of women who were not active, 56.7% ($n = 148$) delivered full term, 24.1% ($n = 63$) had moderate to late preterm birth, 14.2% ($n = 37$) had very preterm birth, and 5.0% ($n = 13$) had extremely preterm birth. The results are shown in Figure 2 and Supplementary Table S7.

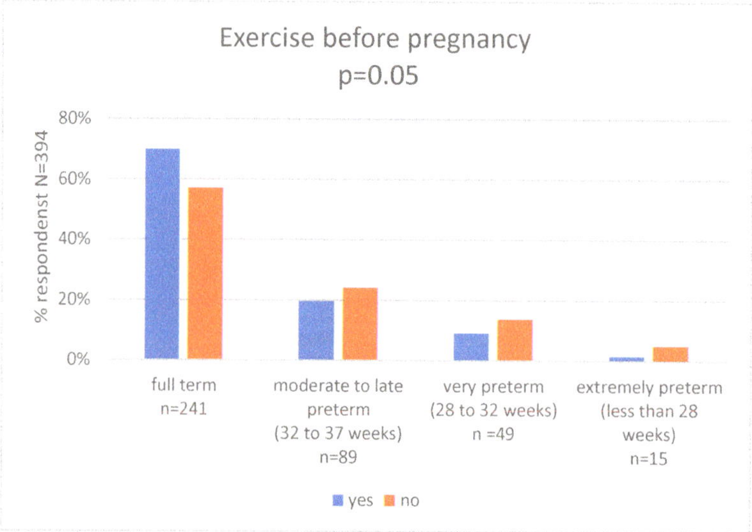

Figure 2. Exercise before pregnancy and gestational age at delivery (weeks).

We also asked women about self-perceived maternal exercise during pregnancy (new exercise, started after becoming pregnant) and we compared the results with that of the gestational age at delivery (weeks) category. Pearson's chi-squared test showed statistically significant differences between the groups ($p < 0.001$). In the group of women who started to be active during pregnancy, 83.0% ($n = 50$) delivered full term, 11.9% ($n = 7$) had moderate to late preterm birth, 5.1% ($n = 3$) had very preterm birth, and 0.0% ($n = 0$) had extremely preterm birth. In the group of women who were not active, 57.6% ($n = 192$) delivered full term, 24.5% ($n = 82$) had moderate to late preterm birth, 13.4% ($n = 46$) had very preterm birth, and 4.5% ($n = 15$) had extremely preterm birth. The results are shown in Figure 3 and Supplementary Table S8.

In the next step, we assessed self-perceived maternal exercise during pregnancy and we compared results with the newborn birth weight category. Pearson's chi-squared test showed statistically significant differences between the groups ($p = 0.03$). In the group of women who were active, 10.2% ($n = 6$) newborns had LGA, 79.6% ($n = 47$) newborns had a normal birth weight, 5.1% ($n = 3$) had low birth weight (LBW), 5.1% ($n = 3$) had very-low birth weight (VLBW), 0.0% ($n = 0$) had extremely (ELBW), and 0.0% ($n = 0$) had incredible low birth weight (ILBW). In the group of women who were not active, 9.2% ($n = 31$) newborns had LGA, 61.8% ($n = 207$) newborns had a normal birth weight, 15.5% ($n = 52$) had low birth weight (LBW), 7.5% ($n = 25$) had very-low birth weight (VLBW), 4.5% ($n = 15$) had extremely (ELBW), and 1.5% ($n = 5$) had incredible low birth weight (ILBW). The results are shown in Figure 4 and Supplementary Table S9.

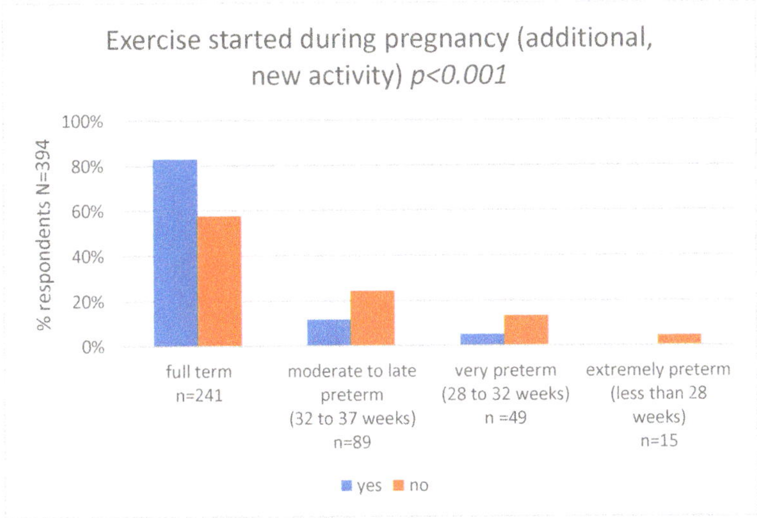

Figure 3. Exercise started during pregnancy and gestational age at delivery (weeks).

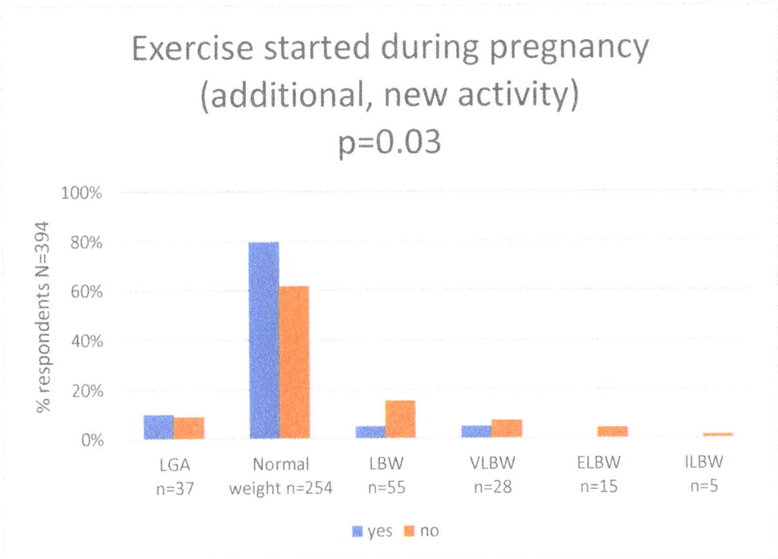

Figure 4. Exercise started during pregnancy and newborn birth weight (g). (LGA—large for gestational age (more than 4000 g), LBW—low birth weight (less than 2500 g), VLBW—very-low birth weight (less than 1500 g), ILBW—incredibly low birth weight (less than 750 g)).

We also wanted to know how pre-pregnancy BMI affected the mode of birth. Pearson's chi-squared test showed statistically significant differences between the groups ($p = 0.03$). Of the women who had normal weight before pregnancy, 56.5% ($n = 144$) had a VB, 42.3% ($n = 108$) had a CS, and 1.2% ($n = 3$) had forceps or vacuum delivery. Of the women who were obese or overweight, 41.3% ($n = 50$) had VB, 57.0% ($n = 69$) had CS. and 1.7% ($n = 2$) had an assisted vaginal birth. Of the mothers who were underweight, 72.2% ($n = 13$) had

VB and 27.8% ($n = 5$) had a CS or had an instrumental delivery. The data are shown in Figure 5 and Supplementary Table S10.

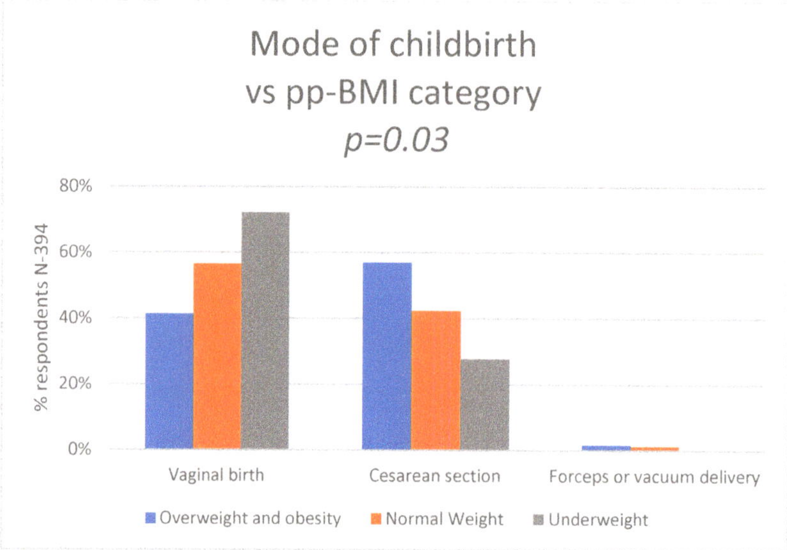

Figure 5. Mode of the childbirth vs. pre-pregnancy BMI category.

The variables were collected on an interval scale. On the basis of the knowledge gained after running a multivariate regression model simulation of the various selected variables, we planned to predict how the duration of pregnancy is related singly (week of delivery) with the specified variables during this simulation. Based on the interpretation of the obtained results, we can assume that some of the variables do not have a significant impact on the gain and may be redundant.

We built a multiple linear regression model by selecting the following variables: pp-BMI (pp-BMI), newborn's birth weight (NBW), and APGAR (1st minute). As a result, the coefficients of the regression equation and measures were calculated to assess the quality of the model. Based on the estimated value of the b-factor, the relationship between week of pregnancy completion (WPC) and all the independent variables can be described with the equation:

$$WPC = 26.366 - 0.062.56\ (\text{pp-BMI}) + 0.003\ (NBW) + 0.531\ (APGAR) + [1.962]$$

The model fits well, as evidenced by a small standard error estimate SE = 1.96; high value of the coefficient multiple determination $R^2 = 0.780825$; corrected coefficient multiple determination $R^2adj = 0.78$; and the result of the F test of the analysis of variance: $p < 0.000$.

Interpretation of the model: if the mother's pp-BMI increases by 10 kg/m^2, the time to complete pregnancy will be shortened by an average of 4 days, assuming ceteris paribus. If the pregnancy is lengthened by 3.5 days, the Apgar index increases by 1 point, assuming ceteris paribus. If the time to complete the pregnancy increases by 3 weeks, the weight of the child at birth increases by 1000 g, assuming ceteris paribus. Additionally, 78.08% of the total variability in the time of completion of pregnancy was explained by the model (interpretation for the R^2 index value). Note that the multivariate regression equation only applies to the study population under unchanged conditions (ceteris paribus).

The fit quality of the model was not high (R^2Pseudo = 0.03, R^2Nagelkerke = 0.05, and R^2Coxa − Snella = 0.04). At the same time, the model was statistically significant ($p = 0.001$ of the likelihood-ratio test) and, therefore, the independent variables in the model were statistically significant. The Hosmer–Lemeshow test result indicates no statistical significance ($p = 0.09$). However, in the case of the Hosmer–Lemeshow test, the lack of significance is desirable because it indicates the similarity of the size of the observed groups and the predicted probability.

The risk of premature delivery depends on the above-mentioned variables as described by the OR: variable maternal BMI before pregnancy OR [95% CI] = 1.19 [1.06; 1.34]. The risk of preterm labor increases with increasing maternal BMI before pregnancy.

In the Supplementary Materials (Supplementary Tables S2–S6 and S11) we present a logistic regression model (analyzed variables: group; mother's weight at pregnancy; mother's pp-BMI; weight gain in pregnancy). In the Figure 6 we presented categories of gestational age at delivery vs maternal pp-BMI.

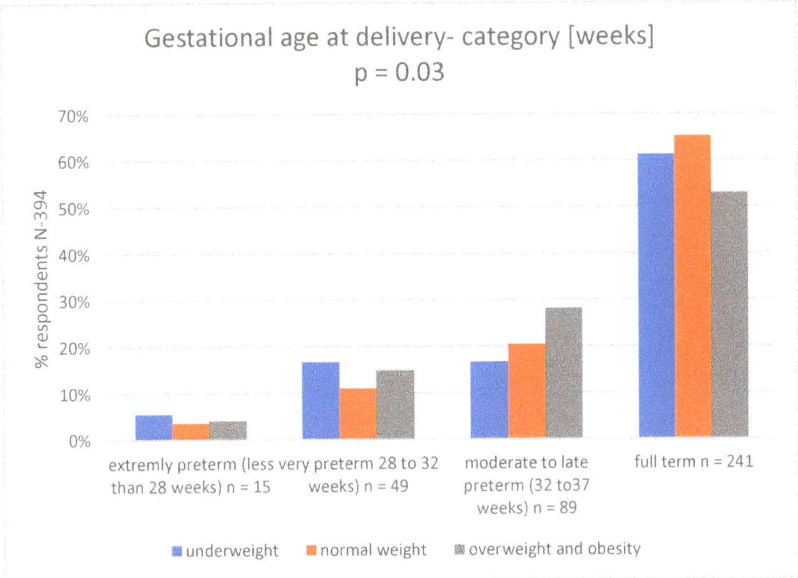

Figure 6. Gestational age at delivery category (weeks) vs. maternal pp-BMI4.

4. Discussion

The principal objective of this study was to identify the associations of self-perceived maternal exercise undertaken before and during pregnancy, pp-BMI, and selected birth and newborn's outcomes.

The most important findings of this work are that maternal exercise before and during pregnancy and normal maternal pp-BMI can positively affect birth outcomes, leading to a reduced risk of PTB and births of children with low birth weight.

Worldwide, there has been a dramatic increase in the prevalence of obesity and overweight in women of reproductive age. Growing evidence suggests that abnormal pre-pregnancy body mass index (pp-BMI) is associated with poor maternal and perinatal outcomes [19,30]. Proper diet and physical activity have the potential to reduce weight gain and alter pregnancy outcomes [31]. The effect of these interventions across pregnant women and woman of reproductive age may have implications for clinical management and the provision of care. The association of physical activity before and during pregnancy with birth outcomes needs evaluation using robust data. The lack of information among women of reproductive age about the benefits of the exercise during pregnancy and the low level of social support are two of the factors hindering engagement in prenatal exercise programs.

A knowledge of health advantages can lead to more favorable attitudes towards exercise during pregnancy among women, exercise professionals, and healthcare providers [5].

With the increasing amount of scientific evidence on the positive effects of prenatal physical activity, authors from different countries observe its insufficient level in pregnant women [32]. The gestational period is an opportunity to promote positive health behaviors [5,33]. Moreover, in many countries one can find guidelines supporting moderate-intensity physical activity during pregnancy, with specific frequency and duration/time indicated [5,33]. Also, higher intensity exercise programs, which can meet the expectations and needs of very active women before pregnancy, have become more and more popular recently [34]. Nowadays, sufficient evidence is available that shows various types and intensities of maternal exercise enhance proper fetal and child development, including their normal weight gain and metabolism [34,35]. According to researchers, prenatal exercise interventions reduced gestational weight gain and the risk of gestational diabetes for overweight and obese pregnant women, which reinforced the benefits of exercise during pregnancy [33]. Moreover, authors have found that prenatal exercise is safe and beneficial for fetuses.

Maternal exercise is associated with reduced odds of macrosomia and is not associated with neonatal complications or adverse childhood outcomes [3,36–41]. In a retrospective population study by Su et al., including all children born in Xiamen, China, in 2011–2018, the data revealed that 6982 (9.37%) of their mothers were obese and 8874 (12.07%) were overweight. Women from both these groups were more likely to develop PTB, completion of pregnancy by caesarean section, and macrosomia [42]. Similar results were obtained by Shahla et al., in a retrospective cohort study in Iran in 2008–2009, who concluded that an increased BMI level increased the risk of an unfavorable course of pregnancy, including premature delivery [43]. In our study, logistic regression showed that the risk of preterm labor increased with higher maternal BMI before pregnancy. An attempt was also made to assess how the pre-pregnancy BMI affects the birth weight of newborns and their Apgar score. The smallest group of participants (both in the group which had the full-term birth and PTB) were women underweight before pregnancy (4.6% of all women in the study). Interestingly, obese or overweight mothers accounted for as much as 30.7% of all studied women from both groups. These data show the scale of the problem of overweight and obesity in the Polish population. A similar distribution of data is presented in the study by Vince et al. [44], whose aim was to determine the relationship between maternal body mass index before pregnancy (pp-BMI) and the course of pregnancy in pregnant women in Croatia in 2017. Among 32,051 pregnant women, 5.3% were underweight, 65.5% had a normal BMI, 20.4% were overweight, and 8.8% were obese. Preterm deliveries occurred more frequently in underweight and obese women ($p < 0.001$) [44].

Importantly, the literature data indicate that prematurity is not directly related to high BMI (>30, obesity), but results from medical complications that usually accompany high BMI [45]. Our analysis shows that the mothers of children who had full term births were more likely to have normal weight or be underweight, while mothers who had preterm births were more likely to be underweight, overweight, or have obesity. In detailed analyses, we noted that that the problem of being underweight in the mother affected children born before 32 weeks of age to a greater extent, while overweight and obesity in the mother affected children born between 32–37 weeks of pregnancy to a greater extent.

One of the most important findings of our study is that pre pregnancy BMI affected the mode of the childbirth. Women who had normal pre-pregnancy BMI or were underweight had a lower risk of having a cesarean section (CS) compared to women with overweight or obesity. The last two decades have seen an increase in CS worldwide. In the middle and highly developed countries, almost half of the women gave birth by CS. Poland has one of the highest percentages of cesarean sections (42%) in Europe, where the average is 27% [46]. We are still looking for strategies to reduce CS and we should also consider education on the benefits of maintaining a healthy BMI as part of pre-conceptual care. Many authors obtained results that associated increasing BMI with increasing rates of adverse obstetric outcomes, including higher rates of CS [46–48].

There were changes in behavioral patterns during the COVID-19 pandemic that were associated with lockdowns and restrictions of access to certain resources. During the lockdown, trends of unfavorable changes were observed: decreased physical activity, increased sedentary time, increased snacking, decreased consumption of fresh food (especially fruit and fish), and increased consumption of sweets, cookies, and cakes. Yet, the opposite trends were also observed: increased home cooking and increased physical activity. All of these trends displayed associations with various individual characteristics [36–38]. Although our study was conducted before the COVID-19 pandemic, the results obtained allow for strategies to be developed in case social isolation becomes necessary. It is necessary to maintain positive role models among pregnant women as well as those planning to become pregnant, including offering them education or online exercises [49]. In line with Miranda et al. [32], our results also highlight the need for a multidisciplinary approach during prenatal care to reinforce the adoption of health-promoting behaviors during pregnancy.

The study findings align with recommendations from the American College of Obstetricians and Gynecologists (ACOG), which emphasize the positive impact of physical activity on pregnancy outcomes. Women who reported being physically active before and during pregnancy exhibited a significantly higher likelihood of achieving full-term births, accompanied by a noteworthy reduction in the incidence of very-premature and extremely premature births [50].

Additionally, the Chief Medical Officers' Physical Activity Guidelines in the UK support the notion that promoting physical activity is integral to overall health, with potential benefits extending to maternal and perinatal outcomes [51]. Importantly, our study identified a correlation between pre-pregnancy body mass index (BMI) and the mode of birth, with a higher BMI associated with an increased rate of cesarean sections. Moreover, pre-pregnancy BMI influenced the week of pregnancy completion, with inappropriate BMI contributing to a rise in the percentage of premature births.

5. Strengths and Limitations

The main strength of the study was that the data were collected in multi-centers in Poland, allowing for generalization of our conclusions to the Polish population. The relatively large number of study participants allowed for the subgroups analysis. Medical records used for the data collection were objective and reliable and could not be affected by the subjective assessment of mothers.

From this study we excluded women with multiple pregnancies, recognizing that this condition could limit their physical activity. On the one hand, this assumption provided us with greater group homogeneity and avoided misinterpretation of the data. Multiple pregnancies statistically lead to preterm birth more often and, in consequence, babies with lower birth weight due to their prematurity. These are also variables that can indirectly influence Apgar scores. In addition, multiple pregnancies are mostly terminated by CS [52]. Therefore, in analyses that include both singlet and multiple pregnancies, the impact of physical activity on labor and neonatal outcomes could be attenuated by the negative consequences of multiple pregnancies on these parameters. On the other hand, however, it would be valuable to analyze the outcomes of subgroup of women with multiple pregnancies, as well as women with pregnancy-related complications, such as shortening of the cervix or assisted conception.

In the context of our study, it is noteworthy to address the upper limit for recommended exercise levels during pregnancy. While our findings demonstrate the positive impact of self-perceived exercise before and during pregnancy on various birth outcomes, it is crucial to acknowledge that there exists a need for clear guidelines regarding the upper threshold of physical activity for expectant mothers. The current literature, including recommendations from reputable sources such as the American College of Obstetricians and Gynaecologists (ACOG), underscores the importance of regular physical activity during pregnancy [50]. However, the specific upper limit remains an area that requires precise delineation. Future research and healthcare guidelines should aim to establish evidence-based thresholds for exercise intensity, frequency, and duration to ensure the safety and well-being of both the pregnant woman and the developing fetus. Addressing this aspect is vital for providing comprehensive guidance to healthcare professionals and expectant mothers, fostering a balanced and health-promoting approach to prenatal physical activity.

One of the limitations of our study was that analysis did not include indications for caesarean section. However, it seems that the data obtained may be useful in the future to distinguish the analysis in only CSs performed due to lack of progress of labor, prolonged second period of labor, or threatened asphyxia. Moreover, for the determination of neonatal weight, centile charts for girls and boys were not used to determine percentile values; instead, only birth weight was used, which was then classified into specific birth weight categories. In future analyses, it would be extremely valuable to use a reference to centile charts for this variable.

Another limitation of the study was the lack of information on the type, intensity, duration, and frequency of physical activity undertaken and the length of time for which it was carried out. The data collected was based only on the subjective assessment of the exercise undertaken by the mothers. In future studies it would be valuable to use standardized tools, e.g., Pregnancy Physical Activity Questionnaire [53] or accelerometers to more precisely assess the level of physical activity. To determine the intensity of physical activity, it would be reasonable to use standardized fitness tests (e.g., to establish maximal exercise capacity through the maximal oxygen uptake and maximum heart rate values). Then, the use of heart rate monitors would allow for proper continuous monitoring of the intensity of physical activity [54]. It would also be useful to assess the impact of maternal exercise on the blood pressure values recorded in the pregnancy chart and the pattern of physical activity in the postpartum period (including the time of return to pre-pregnancy weight). These observations should be extended to the assessments of body mass composition and nutritional status. This, in turn, would allow for an analysis of how physical activity influences weight gain during pregnancy and thus how weight gain affects the birth outcomes.

According to the literature, an important issue in assessing the nutritional status of a child's mother is taking into account the quality of consumed products and identifying deficiencies in the diet. Particularly important is the deficit of elements such as zinc or iron, an inadequate concentration of which in the body may disturb the functioning of the immune system, thus increasing the risk of preterm labor [55]. In our study, most women declared supplementation with complex vitamin preparations. However, we were not able to assess whether or not, and to what extent, these women had vitamin and micro deficiency and macronutrients, and whether or not they were supplemented by appropriately selected preparations.

Since national minorities constitute a marginal part of Poland's population (around 2%), we did not ask the study participants about their ethnicity. However, due to the increasingly intense migration process in Europe, this issue is worth addressing in future research.

Despite the indicated weaknesses of our work, the obtained results may be useful in planning future, more complex studies aimed at improving a healthy lifestyle before and during pregnancy.

6. Conclusions

The study revealed that women who reported being physically active before and during pregnancy were more likely to have full-term birth and had a lower incidence of very premature and extremely premature births. Women who exercised during pregnancy more often gave birth to children with a normal body weight and were less likely to have children with low, very-low, or extremely low body weight. Pre-pregnancy BMI affects the method of pregnancy termination—in the group of women with a higher BMI there were more cesarean sections. Pre-pregnancy BMI also influenced the week of pregnancy termination, i.e., incorrect BMI contributed to an increase in the percentage of premature births.

Our findings indicate that promoting physical activity and weight management remains a priority in public health policy, and women of childbearing age should be encouraged to adopt or maintain an active and healthy lifestyle during pregnancy in order to avoid sedentary- and obesity-associated risks affecting birth and newborns' health.

Supplementary Materials: The following supporting information can be downloaded at: https://www.mdpi.com/article/10.3390/nu15234894/s1, Table S1: *t*-Student test; maternal exercise before pregnancy. Table S2. Logistic regression for the analyzed variables: group; the mother's pp weight; mother's pp-BMI; weight gain in pregnancy. Table S3. Likelihood ratio test for the analyzed variables: group; the weight of the mother at the time of pregnancy; mother's pp-BMI; weight gain in pregnancy. Table S4. Hosmer-Lemeshow test for the analyzed variables: group; pp mother's weight; Mother's pp-BMI; weight gain in pregnancy. Table S5. Model for the analyzed variables: group; the weight of the mother at the time of pregnancy; Mother's pp-BMI; weight gain in pregnancy. Table S6. Hosmer-Lemeshow division for the analyzed variables: group; the pre-pregnancy weight of the mother; Mother's pp-BMI; weight gain in pregnancy. Table S7. Exercise before pregnancy and gestational age at delivery [weeks]. Table S8. Exercise started during pregnancy and gestational age at delivery [weeks]. Table S9. Exercise started during pregnancy and newborn birth weight [g]. Table S10. Mode of the childbirth vs. pre-pregnancy BMI category. Table S11. Gestational age at delivery category [weeks] vs maternal pp-BMI.

Author Contributions: Conceptualization, A.W.S., A.S., R.S.-R. and J.W.; Formal analysis, A.W.S. and A.S.; Methodology, A.W.S., A.S. and J.W.; Project administration, A.W.S.; Writing—original draft A.W.S., A.S. and R.S.-R.; Writing—review and editing, A.W.S., A.S., R.S.-R. and J.W. All authors have read and agreed to the published version of the manuscript.

Funding: This research received no external funding.

Institutional Review Board Statement: The study was conducted in accordance with the Declaration of Helsinki and approved by the Independent Bioethics Committee for Scientific Research at the Medical University of Gdańsk. Decision of 15 September 2015, no. NKBB/393/2015 for studies involving humans.

Informed Consent Statement: Informed consent was obtained from all subjects involved in the study.

Data Availability Statement: Data are contained within the article and supplementary materials.

Conflicts of Interest: The authors declare no conflict of interest.

References

1. Bø, K.; Artal, R.; Barakat, R.; Brown, W.; Davies, G.A.L.; Dooley, M.; Evenson, K.R.; Haakstad, L.A.H.; Henriksson-Larsen, K.; Kayser, B.; et al. Exercise and pregnancy in recreational and elite athletes: 2016 evidence summary from the IOC expert group meeting, Lausanne. Part 1—Exercise in women planning pregnancy and those who are pregnant. *Br. J. Sports Med.* **2016**, *50*, 571–589. [CrossRef]
2. Bø, K.; Artal, R.; Barakat, R.; Brown, W.; Dooley, M.; Evenson, K.R.; Haakstad, L.A.H.; Larsen, K.; Kayser, B.; Kinnunen, T.I.; et al. Exercise and pregnancy in recreational and elite athletes: 2016 evidence summary from the IOC expert group meeting, Lausanne. Part 2—The effect of exercise on the fetus, labour and birth. *Br. J. Sports Med.* **2016**, *50*, 1297–1305. [CrossRef]
3. Davenport, M.H.; Meah, V.L.; Ruchat, S.M.; Davies, G.A.; Skow, R.J.; Barrowman, N.; Adamo, K.B.; Poitras, V.J.; Gray, C.E.; Jaramillo Garcia, A.; et al. Impact of prenatal exercise on neonatal and childhood outcomes: A systematic review and meta-analysis. *Br. J. Sports Med.* **2018**, *52*, 1386–1396. [CrossRef]
4. Davenport, M.H.; Ruchat, S.-M.; Sobierajski, F.; Poitras, V.J.; Gray, C.E.; Yoo, C.; Skow, R.J.; Garcia, A.J.; Barrowman, N.; Meah, V.L.; et al. Impact of prenatal exercise on maternal harms, labour and delivery outcomes: A systematic review and meta-analysis. *Br. J. Sports Med.* **2019**, *53*, 99–107. [CrossRef]
5. Szumilewicz, A.; Worska, A.; Santos-Rocha, R.; Oviedo-Caro, M.Á. Evidence-based and practice-oriented guidelines for exercising during pregnancy. In *Exercise and Physical Activity during Pregnancy and Postpartum: Evidence-Based Guidelines*; Springer: Berlin/Heidelberg, Germany, 2022; pp. 177–217.
6. Cai, C.; Ruchat, S.-M.; Sivak, A.; Davenport, M.H. Prenatal exercise and cardiorespiratory health and fitness: A meta-analysis. *Med. Sci. Sports Exerc.* **2020**, *52*, 1538–1548. [CrossRef]

7. Hopkins, S.A.; Cutfield, W.S. Exercise in pregnancy: Weighing up the long-term impact on the next generation. *Exerc. Sport Sci. Rev.* **2011**, *39*, 120–127. [CrossRef]
8. Catalano, P.M.; Shankar, K. Obesity and pregnancy: Mechanisms of short term and long term adverse consequences for mother and child. *BMJ* **2017**, *356*, j1. [CrossRef] [PubMed]
9. Kumari, A. Pregnancy outcome in women with morbid obesity. *Int. J. Gynecol. Obstet.* **2001**, *73*, 101–107. [CrossRef] [PubMed]
10. Sirimi, N.; Goulis, D.G. Obesity in pregnancy. *Hormones* **2010**, *9*, 299–306. [CrossRef] [PubMed]
11. Allahem, H.; Sampalli, S. Automated uterine contractions pattern detection framework to monitor pregnant women with a high risk of premature labour. *Inform. Med. Unlocked* **2020**, *20*, 100404. [CrossRef]
12. Ganer Herman, H.; Miremberg, H.; Dekalo, A.; Barda, G.; Bar, J.; Kovo, M. Preterm uterine contractions ultimately delivered at term: Safe but not out of danger. *Eur. J. Obstet. Gynecol. Reprod. Biol.* **2016**, *199*, 1–4. [CrossRef] [PubMed]
13. Batista, A.G.; Najdi, S.; Godinho, D.M.; Martins, C.; Serrano, F.C.; Ortigueira, M.D.; Rato, R.T. A multichannel time–frequency and multi-wavelet toolbox for uterine electromyography processing and visualisation. *Comput. Biol. Med.* **2016**, *76*, 178–191. [CrossRef] [PubMed]
14. Di Renzo, G.C.; Giardina, I.; Rosati, A.; Clerici, G.; Torricelli, M.; Petraglia, F.; the Italian Preterm Network Study Group. Maternal risk factors for preterm birth: A country-based population analysis. *Eur. J. Obstet. Gynecol. Reprod. Biol.* **2011**, *159*, 342–346. [CrossRef] [PubMed]
15. Vogel, J.P.; Chawanpaiboon, S.; Watananirun, K.; Lumbiganon, P.; Petzold, M.; Moller, A.-B.; Thinkhamrop, J.; Laopaiboon, M.; Seuc, A.H.; Hogan, D.; et al. Global, regional and national levels and trends of preterm birth rates for 1990 to 2014: Protocol for development of World Health Organization estimates. *Reprod. Health* **2016**, *13*, 76. [CrossRef]
16. World Health Organization. Available online: http://www.who.int/mediacentre/factsheets/fs363/en/ (accessed on 21 April 2022).
17. Blencowe, H.; Cousens, S.; Chou, D.; Oestergaard, M.; Say, L.; Moller, A.-B.; Kinney, M.; Lawn, J.; the Born Too Soon Preterm Birth Action Group. Born Too Soon: The global epidemiology of 15 million preterm births. *Reprod. Health* **2013**, *10* (Suppl. S1), S2. [CrossRef]
18. Wierzejska, R.; Jarosz, M. Niedożywienie i zaburzenia odżywiania u kobiet w wieku prokreacyjnym. *Postępy Nauk. Med.* **2012**, *12*, 965–970.
19. Vinturache, A.; Moledina, N.; McDonald, S.; Slater, D.; Tough, S. Pre-pregnancy Body Mass Index (BMI) and delivery outcomes in a Canadian population. *BMC Pregnancy Childbirth* **2014**, *14*, 422. [CrossRef]
20. Associations of the Pre-Pregnancy Body Mass Index and Gestational Weight Gain with Pregnancy Outcomes in Taiwanese Women | Asia Pacific Journal of Clinical Nutrition [Internet]. Available online: https://search.informit.or (accessed on 2 May 2022).
21. Lim, C.C.; Mahmood, T. Obesity in pregnancy. *Best Pract. Res. Clin. Obstet. Gynaecol.* **2015**, *29*, 309–319. [CrossRef]
22. von Elm, E.; Altman, D.G.; Egger, M.; Pocock, S.J.; Gøtzsche, P.C.; Vandenbroucke, J.P.; STROBE Initiative. The Strengthening the Reporting of Observational Studies in Epidemiology (STROBE) Statement: Guidelines for reporting observational studies. *Int. J. Surg.* **2014**, *12*, 1495–1499. [CrossRef]
23. DHHS. *Physical Activity Guidelines for Americans*, 2nd ed.; Department of Health and Human Services: Washington, DC, USA, 2018. Available online: https://health.gov/sites/default/files/2019-09/Physical_Activity_Guidelines_2nd_edition.pdf (accessed on 2 May 2022).
24. Weir, C.B.; Jan, A. *BMI Classification Percentile and Cut off Points*; StatPearls Publishing: Treasure Island, EL, USA, 2019.
25. Rasmussen, K.M.S.; Abrams, B.D.; Bodnar, L.M.; Butte, N.F.; Catalano, P.M.; Siega-Riz, A.M. Recommendations for weight gain during pregnancy in the context of the obesity epidemic. *Obstet. Gynecol.* **2010**, *116*, 1191–1195. [CrossRef]
26. Engle, W.A. Age terminology during the perinatal period. *Pediatrics* **2004**, *114*, 1362–1364.
27. Glass, H.C.; Costarino, A.T.; Stayer, S.A.; Brett, C.M.; Cladis, F.; Davis, P.J. Outcomes for extremely premature infants. Anesth Analg. *Obstet. Anesthesia Dig.* **2015**, *120*, 1337–1351.
28. UNICEF. Available online: https://data.unicef.org/topic/nutrition/low-birthweight/ (accessed on 2 May 2022).
29. American Academy of Pediatrics—Committee on Fetus and Newborn. Available online: https://www.acog.org/clinical/clinical-guidance/committee-opinion/articles/2015/10/the-apgar-score (accessed on 2 May 2022).
30. Santos, S.; Voerman, E.; Amiano, P.; Barros, H.; Beilin, L.J.; Bergström, A.; Charles, M.-A.; Chatzi, L.; Chevrier, C.; Chrousos, G.P.; et al. Impact of maternal body mass index and gestational weight gain on pregnancy complications: An individual participant data meta-analysis of European, North American and Australian cohorts. *BJOG Int. J. Obs. Gynaecol.* **2019**, *126*, 984–995. [CrossRef] [PubMed]
31. The International Weight Management in Pregnancy (i-WIP) Collaborative Group. Effect of diet and physical activity based interventions in pregnancy on gestational weight gain and pregnancy outcomes: Meta-analysis of individual participant data from randomised trials. *BMJ* **2017**, *358*, j3119.
32. Miranda, L.A.; de Moura, A.C.R.; Kasawara, K.T.; Surita, F.G.; Moreira, M.A.; Nascimento, S.L.D. Exercise and Physical Activity Levels and Associated Factors Among High-Risk Pregnant Women. *Rev. Bras. Hematol. Hemoter.* **2022**, *44*, 360–368. [CrossRef] [PubMed]
33. Szumilewicz, A.; Worska, A.; Rajkowska, N.; Santos-Rocha, R. Summary of guidelines for exercise in pregnancy–are they comprehensive enough for designing the contents of a prenatal exercise program? *Curr. Womens Health Rev.* **2015**, *11*, 3–12. [CrossRef]

34. Szumilewicz, A.; Santos-Rocha, R.; Worska, A.; Piernicka, M.; Yu, H.; Pajaujiene, S.; Shojaeian, N.-A.; Caro, M.A.O. How to HIIT while pregnant? The protocol characteristics and effects of high intensity interval training implemented during pregnancy: A systematic review. *Balt. J. Health Phys. Act.* **2022**, *14*, 1–16. [CrossRef]
35. Strom, C.J.; McDonald, S.M.; Remchak, M.-M.; Kew, K.A.; Rushing, B.R.; Houmard, J.A.; Tulis, D.A.; Pawlak, R.; Kelley, G.A.; Chasan-Taber, L.; et al. Maternal Aerobic Exercise, but Not Blood Docosahexaenoic Acid and Eicosapentaenoic Acid Concentrations, during Pregnancy Influence Infant Body Composition. *Int. J. Environ. Res. Public Health* **2022**, *19*, 8293. [CrossRef]
36. Deschasaux-Tanguy, M.; Druesne-Pecollo, N.; Esseddik, Y.; De Edelenyi, F.S.; Allès, B.; Andreeva, V.A.; Baudry, J.; Charreire, H.; Deschamps, V.; Egnell, M.; et al. Diet and physical activity during the coronavirus disease 2019 (COVID-19) lockdown (March–May 2020): Results from the French NutriNet-Santé cohort study. *Am. J. Clin. Nutr.* **2021**, *113*, 924–938. [CrossRef]
37. He, M.; Xian, Y.; Lv, X.; He, J.; Ren, Y. Changes in Body Weight, Physical Activity, and Lifestyle During the Semi-lockdown Period after the Outbreak of COVID-19 in China: An Online Survey. *Disaster Med. Public Health Prep.* **2021**, *15*, e23–e28. [CrossRef] [PubMed]
38. Knuppel, A. Diet, lifestyle, and livelihoods during coronavirus disease 2019 (COVID-19)–related lockdowns and the value of web-based nutrition studies. *Am. J. Clin. Nutr.* **2021**, *113*, 763–764. [CrossRef]
39. Magro-Malosso, E.R.; Saccone, G.; Di Mascio, D.; Di Tommaso, M.; Berghella, V. Exercise during pregnancy and risk of preterm birth in overweight and obese women: A systematic review and meta-analysis of randomized controlled trials. *Acta Obstet. Gynecol. Scand.* **2017**, *96*, 263–273. [CrossRef]
40. Muhammad, H.F.L.; Pramono, A.; Rahman, M.N. The safety and efficacy of supervised exercise on pregnant women with overweight/obesity: A systematic review and meta-analysis of randomized controlled trials. *Clin. Obes.* **2021**, *11*, e12428. [CrossRef]
41. Du, M.-C.; Ouyang, Y.-Q.; Nie, X.-F.; Huang, Y.; Redding, S.R. Effects of physical exercise during pregnancy on maternal and infant outcomes in overweight and obese pregnant women: A meta-analysis. *Birth* **2019**, *46*, 211–221. [CrossRef] [PubMed]
42. Su, W.-J.; Chen, Y.-L.; Huang, P.-Y.; Shi, X.-L.; Yan, F.-F.; Chen, Z.; Yan, B.; Song, H.-Q.; Lin, M.-Z.; Li, X.-J. Effects of Prepregnancy Body Mass Index, Weight Gain, and Gestational Diabetes Mellitus on Pregnancy Outcomes: A Population-Based Study in Xiamen, China, 2011–2018. *Ann. Nutr. Metab.* **2019**, *75*, 31–38. [CrossRef] [PubMed]
43. Yazdani, S.; Yosofniyapasha, Y.; Nasab, B.H.; Mojaveri, M.H.; Bouzari, Z. Effect of maternal body mass index on pregnancy outcome and newborn weight. *BMC Res. Notes.* **2012**, *5*, 34. [CrossRef] [PubMed]
44. Vince, K.; Brkić, M.; Poljičanin, T.; Matijević, R. Prevalence and impact of pre-pregnancy body mass index on pregnancy outcome: A cross-sectional study in Croatia. *J. Obstet. Gynaecol.* **2020**, *41*, 55–59. [CrossRef]
45. Aly, H.; Hammad, T.; Nada, A.; Mohamed, M.; Bathgate, S.; El-Mohandes, A. Maternal obesity, associated complications and risk of prematurity. *J. Perinatol.* **2010**, *30*, 447–451. [CrossRef]
46. Sys, D.; Baranowska, B.; Kajdy, A.; Tataj-Puzyna, U.; Gotlib, J.; Bączek, G.; Juszczakiewicz, P.; Rabijewski, M. Women's views and preferences regarding the mode of birth after cesarean section: Polish cross-sectional web-based survey. *Eur. J. Obstet. Gynecol. Reprod. Biol.* **2022**, *273*, 26–32. [CrossRef]
47. Bebeau, K.A.; Edenfield, A.L.; Hill, A.; Van Buren, E.; Finneran, M.M.; Meglin, M.F. Impact of pre-pregnancy obesity on cesarean delivery rates in nulliparous pregnant people undergoing induction of labor. *J. Matern. Neonatal Med.* **2022**, *35*, 9934–9939. [CrossRef]
48. Class, Q.A. Obesity and the increasing odds of cesarean delivery. *J. Psychosom. Obstet. Gynecol.* **2022**, *43*, 244–250. [CrossRef] [PubMed]
49. Yu, H.; Santos-Rocha, R.; Radzimiński, Ł.; Jastrzębski, Z.; Bonisławska, I.; Szwarc, A.; Szumilewicz, A. Effects of 8-Week Online, Supervised High-Intensity Interval Training on the Parameters Related to the Anaerobic Threshold, Body Weight, and Body Composition during Pregnancy: A Randomized Controlled Trial. *Nutrients* **2022**, *14*, 5279. [CrossRef] [PubMed]
50. American College of Obstetricians and Gynecologists. Physical Activity and Exercise during Pregnancy and the Postpartum Period [Internet]. 2020. Available online: https://www.acog.org/clinical/clinical-guidance/committee-opinion/articles/2020/04/physical-activity-and-exercise-during-pregnancy-and-the-postpartum-period (accessed on 25 September 2022).
51. Officers UCM. *UK Chief Medical Officers' Physical Activity Guidelines*; 2019. Available online: https://assets.publishing.service.gov.uk/media/5d839543ed915d52428dc134/uk-chief-medical-officers-physical-activity-guidelines.pdf (accessed on 25 September 2022).
52. Rezavand, N.; Veisi, F.; Malek-khosravi, S.; Zangeneh, M.; Kohzadi, M. Assessment of frequency of twin pregnancy and neonatal outcome in deliveries of Mo'tazedi Hospital, Kermanshah in 2004–2007. *J. Obstet. Gynecol. India* **2014**, *64*, 19–22. [CrossRef]
53. Chasan-Taber, L.; Schmidt, M.D.; Roberts, D.E.; Hosmer, D.; Markenson, G.; Freedson, P.S. Development and Validation of a Pregnancy Physical Activity Questionnaire. *Med. Sci. Sports Exerc.* **2004**, *36*, 1750–1760. [CrossRef] [PubMed]
54. Santos-Rocha, R.; Gutiérrez Corrales, I.; Szumilewicz, A.; Pajaujiene, S. Exercise testing and prescription in pregnancy. In *Santos-Exercise and Physical Activity During Pregnancy and Postpartum Evidence-Based Guidelines*, 2nd ed.; Rocha, R., Ed.; Springer Nature Switzerland AG: Cham, Switzerland, 2022; pp. 219–274.
55. Czerwińska, E. Czynniki wpływające na poród przedwczesny. *Ginekol i Perinatol Prakt.* **2018**, *3*, 52–57.

nutrients MDPI

Article

Maternal Body Mass Index Trends and Weight Gain in Singleton Pregnancies at the Time of Fetal Anatomic Survey: Changes in the Last Decade and New Trends in the Modern Era

Alexandra Ursache [1,2], Iuliana Elena Bujor [1,†], Alexandra Elena Cristofor [1,*], Denisa Oana Zelinschi [1,2], Dragos Nemescu [1,2,*] and Daniela Roxana Matasariu [1,2,†]

1 Department of Obstetrics and Gynecology, University of Medicine and Pharmacy 'Gr. T. Popa', 700115 Iasi, Romania; alexandra.ursache@umfiasi.ro (A.U.); iuliana-elena.bujor@d.umfiasi.ro (I.E.B.); zelinschi.denisa@email.umfiasi.ro (D.O.Z.); daniela.matasariu@umfiasi.ro (D.R.M.)
2 Department of Obstetrics and Gynecology, Cuza Voda Hospital, 700038 Iasi, Romania
* Correspondence: alexandra-elena_s_mihaila@d.umfiasi.ro (A.E.C.); dragos.nemescu@umfiasi.ro (D.N.)
† These authors contributed equally to this work.

Abstract: (1) Background: the worldwide impact of overweight and obesity is rising, increasingly resembling an epidemic (a price we have to pay for our new way of living). (2) Methods: our study aims to evaluate the temporal trends and patterns of singleton pregnant women's BMI (body mass index) in our region during a 12-year time frame between 2010 and 2021. (3) Results: We noticed a statistically significant difference between the BMIs of nulliparous and multiparous women and a significantly increased pregestational BMI in women with previous ART (assisted reproductive technology) procedures. Smoking pregnant women had a higher second trimester weight gain, regardless of parity. Women with folic acid supplementation alone had a higher BMI than those with folic acid and multivitamin intake. The weight of both nulliparous and multiparous women with chronic hypertension was statistically significantly higher in all three timeframes. Global weight gain did not reveal any statistically significant changes concerning women with pregestational diabetes, regardless of parity and the pregnancy trimester. (4) Conclusions: our article describes the trends in obesity and overweight in our middle-income country, in which this pathology is continuously growing, negatively influencing our reproductive-aged women and future generations.

Keywords: pregnancy; obesity; epidemiology; first trimester morphology; second trimester morphology; overweight

1. Introduction

Overweight and obesity have increased during the past few decades. The worldwide impact is rising, increasingly resembling an epidemic (a price we have to pay for our new way of living) [1,2]. Urbanization-related sedentariness associated with processed low-quality food negatively influences our health, resulting in a continuously increasing number of obese and overweight people. This has become a major public health issue, affecting not only the populations of developed countries but also those of low- and middle-income countries [3]. Our healthcare systems need to reshape the increasing pathologies associated with overweight and obesity [4]. In their retrospective study about women's healthcare utilization and costs, Morgan et al. revealed an increase of 23% in overweight pregnancies and 37% in obese pregnancies [5].

This condition has affected many women, and the curve still has an upward slope [6]. In some countries, the rates of obesity exceed 30%. This ascending trend has also become visible in Asian countries. In China, the rates have tripled since 2004 [3]. The rates of overweight and obesity among European women reached up to 44.7% in the last decade [2,7].

A national study in the United States revealed that almost 50% of pregnant women are either overweight or obese [8].

Overweight and obesity are defined using World Health Organization (WHO) criteria. BMI (body mass index) is calculated by dividing an individual's weight in kilograms by the square of their height in meters. After obtaining their BMI value, we can classify the individual as being underweight with a BMI under 18.5; normal weight with a BMI that ranges from 18.5 to 24.9; overweight with a BMI from 25 to 29.9; or obese with a BMI above 30. Obesity is also classified into three stages depending on the BMI value: class I (BMI = 30.0–34.9), class II (35.0–39.9), or class III (≥40.0) [9].

Nutritional disorders negatively impact both mothers' and children's outcomes [10]. Obesity and overweight are associated with almost all pregnancy complications, affecting women before conception, during pregnancy, and postpartum. In the pregestational period, both overweight and obesity cause fertility problems, miscarriages, chronic hypertension, type 2 diabetes, stroke, and heart problems. Women who start their pregnancy with a weight above normal and a BMI over 24.9 are more prone to placental (abnormal spiral arterial modification and placental hypertrophy), embryonic, and fetal growth pathologies. Overweight and obese women have an increased risk of birth complications, including cesarean delivery, instrumental delivery, induction of labor, obstructed labor, shoulder dystocia, hypertensive disorders, gestational diabetes, preterm births, thromboembolisms, stillbirths, infections, birth defects, large-for-gestational-age (LGA) fetuses, and macrosomia. They are also have an increased risk of postpartum complications, including hemorrhages, infections, and thromboembolisms [1,2,7,10–13]. The impact on the offspring is reflected in an increase in mortality and morbidity in fetuses and newborn children, and, as some studies depict, in long-term negative consequences in descendants that extend beyond the gestational period. As the literature reveals, children from obese mothers develop hypertensive disorders, diabetes, obesity, and cardiovascular dysfunctions [14] due to an inadequate intrauterine environment [15]. In the end, we cannot neglect or deny the economic implications of nutritional disorders, with both overweight and obesity indicating the prolonged need to address healthcare services [6,11]. These overwhelming complications of obesity do not improve by simply reducing weight gain during pregnancy due to pre-existing fat that is responsible for all the negative results stated above. Some studies have reported that the sources of all negative maternal and fetal outcomes are directly linked to the mother's weight before the pregnancy and less to weight gain during it [6].

The literature provides scarce data on weight trends in the obstetric population. In our country, only one study (conducted by Panaitescu et al.) has evaluated the prevalence of underweight, overweight, and obesity in the obstetric population during the first trimester of pregnancy between 11 and 13 weeks of gestation [7].

Our study aims to evaluate temporal trends and patterns in pregnant women's BMI during a 12-year timeframe. In addition to evaluating BMI trends in our population of pregnant women, we also examined BMI's particularities and variations depending on parity, smoking status, conceiving method, folic acid and multivitamin supplementation, chronic hypertension, and pregestational diabetes. The distribution of and variations in BMI in the Romanian obstetric population have not been reported until now.

2. Materials and Methods

We chose 3 stages at which to evaluate the weight of women: before pregnancy, in the first trimester of pregnancy (between 11 and 13 weeks of gestation), and in the second trimester at the moment of the morphological ultrasound (between 18 and 20 weeks of gestation).

We conducted a retrospective cohort study in which we included obstetrically monitored patients between 2010 and 2021. All the women included had singleton pregnancies. The BMIs before pregnancy were obtained by questioning the patients, and for the first and second trimesters of pregnancy by evaluating them. For the first trimester, we used the measurement of the embryo, a CRL (crown–rump length) between 45 and 85 mm (millimeter). For the second trimester, we evaluated our patients' weights and heights when the pregnancies had a gestational age between 18 and 24 weeks. We also analyzed patients' age, means of conception, smoking status, and other risk factors (folic acid or vitamin administration, chronic hypertension, or preexisting diabetes). We excluded all duplicate cases, each of our patients being registered in this study only once. The BMI categories were underweight ≤ 18.5; normal weight = 18.5–24.9; overweight = 25–29.9; and obesity = 30 or greater.

Statistical Analysis

We used the standard classification of BMI: underweight, normal weight, overweight, and obese. The statistics were carried out using SPSS application version 24.

Analysis of variance (ANOVA) was performed to test the differences in mean birth weight and mean gestational age, evaluating BMI variations and trends with the 6 above-mentioned categories (type of conception, smoking habits, parity, COVID-19 pandemic, and folic acid intake). A *p*-value of less than 0.05 was considered significant.

To identify the changes in weight trends, joinpoint regression was estimated for each parameter mentioned above using the Joinpoint Regression Program, Version 4.5.0.1 (Statistical Research and Applications Branch, National Cancer Institute, Rockville, MD, USA).

We used Astraia software version 1.27.1 for pregnancy evaluation and measurements.

3. Results

All the patients included in our study were Caucasian. After the exclusion of all duplicate cases, we totalized 8.579 patients (3.600 in the first trimester of pregnancy and 4.979 in the second trimester) (Figures 1 and 2).

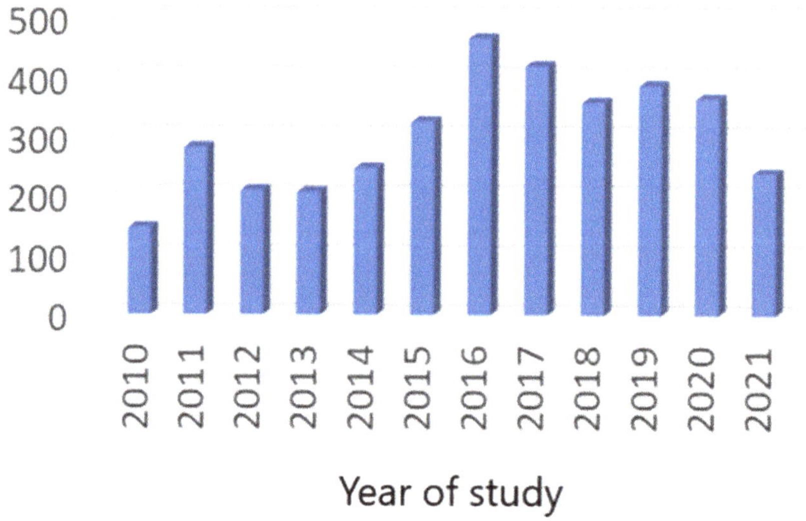

Figure 1. First trimester case distribution.

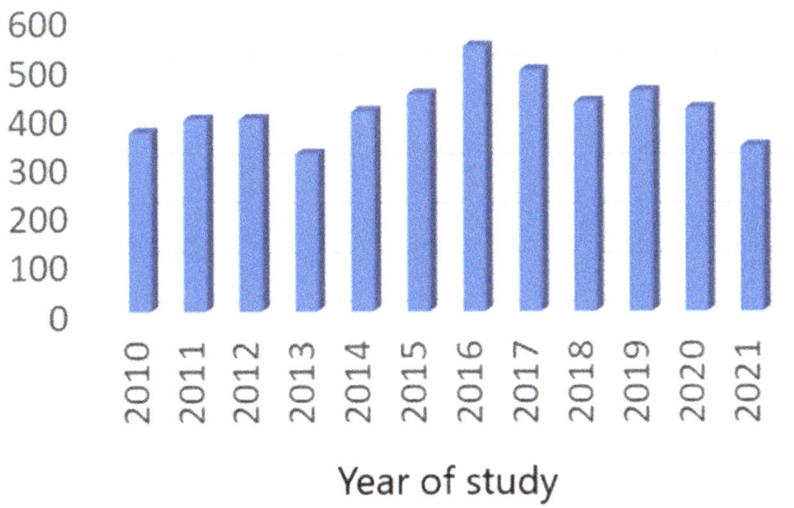

Figure 2. Second trimester case distribution.

We noticed a statistically significant difference between the BMIs of nulliparous and multiparous women. This difference was visible before pregnancy and continued throughout the entire gestational period. This aspect led us to separately evaluate multiparous and nulliparous women for each parameter.

3.1. Pregestational Results

When we analyzed BMI's nulliparous pregestational variance, we observed an unequivocal increasing tendency of overweight and obese cases in nulliparous patients throughout our study period. This tendency reached up to 30% in 2020 (Figure 3).

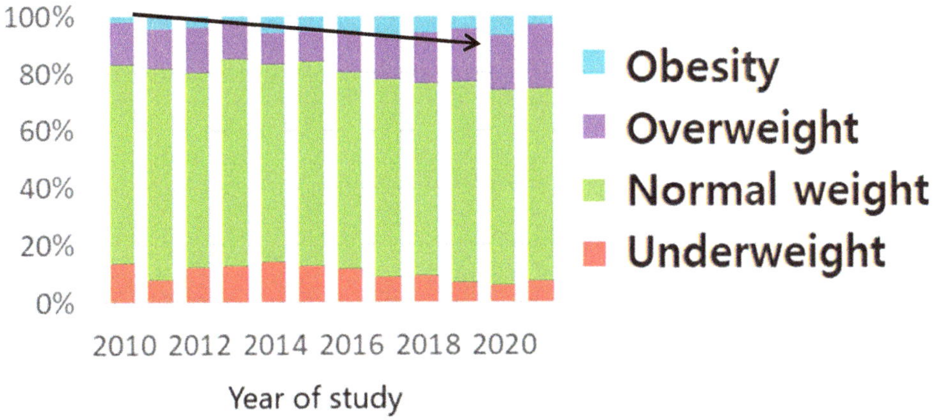

Figure 3. BMI pregestational distribution in nulliparous women (The arrow shows the increasing tendency of obesity as explained in the text).

This phenomenon was absent in multiparous women, with the pregestational BMI distribution being practically uniform (Figure 4).

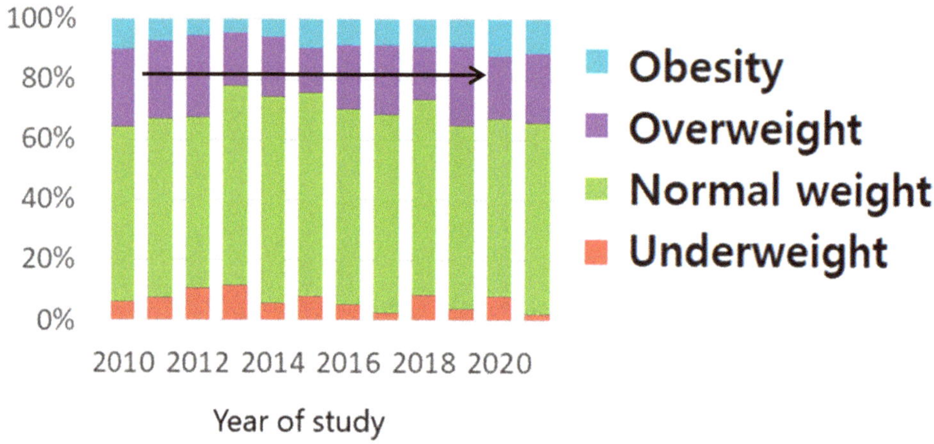

Figure 4. BMI pregestational distribution in multiparous women (The arrow shows the uniform distribution, as explained in the text).

3.2. First Trimester Results

We totalized 3.664 cases, but, when we excluded the duplicate ones, we obtained only 3.600 pregnant women who met the inclusion criteria. The mean age of our patients was 30.7 years (±4.8 years), 57.7% of them being nulliparous. When we analyzed the BMI class distribution, we noticed that approximately 29% of the pregnant women included in our study were either overweight (21.7%) or obese (7.7%) at the moment of the first trimester morphology scan. Of these cases, 65% had normal weight, and 5.7% were underweight (Table 1).

Table 1. First trimester pregnant women characteristics.

First Trimester Characteristics		
Mean age		30.69 ± 4.81
Gestational age		12.46 ± 0.65
CRL		61.92 ± 11.72
Nulliparous		57.7%
Folic acid	Without folic acid supplementation	20.3%
	Folic acid	47.6%
	Folic acid with multivitamins	32.1%
Chronic hypertension		1.9%
Diabetes		0.7%
Type of conception	Spontaneous	95.5%
	ART	4.3%
Smoking	Yes	8.7%
	No	86.7%
Initial BMI		22.93 ± 4.06
First trimester BMI		23.49 ± 4.08
BMI class	Underweight	5.7%
	Normal weight	65%
	Overweight	21.7%
	Obese	7.7%
Delta G% (weight gain)		2.57 ± 4.71

Despite the existence of differences between nulliparous and multiparous women in the pregestational period, as well as in the first and second trimesters of pregnancy, the weight gain in the first trimester was similar in both categories (Figure 5).

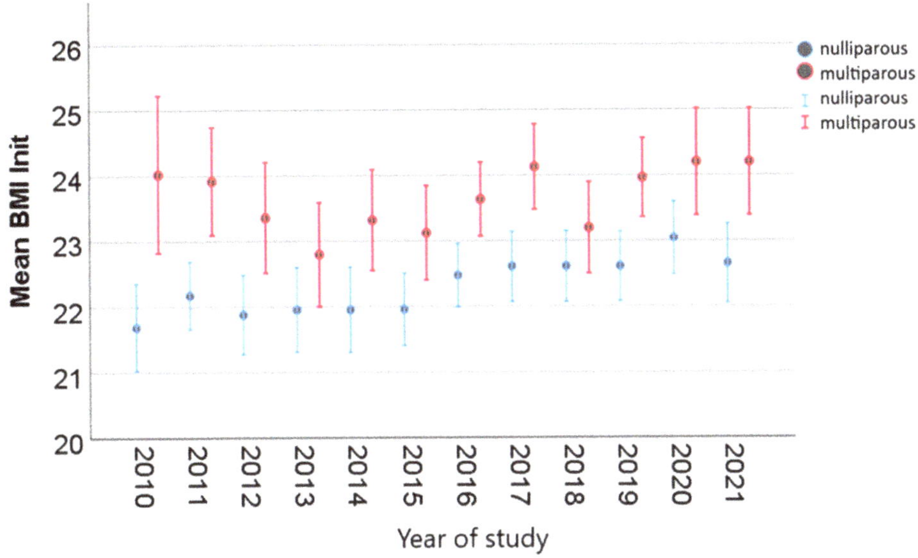

(**a**)

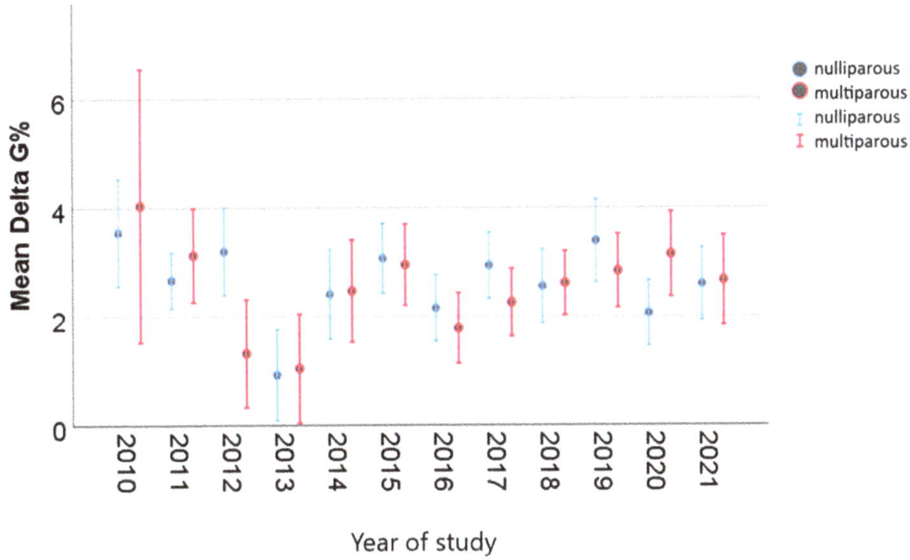

(**b**)

Figure 5. Weight gain (Delta G%) until the second morphological scan for both nulliparous and multiparous women ((**a**), initial BMI; (**b**) mean Delta G%, weight gain in the first trimester).

Analyzing the moment of the first trimester morphology scan in nulliparous women, we noticed an increase in the percentage of overweight and obese pregnant women, reaching up to 30% (Figures 3 and 5).

3.3. Second Trimester Results

For the second trimester, 4.979 pregnant women met the inclusion criteria. The mean age of our patients was 30.32 years old (±4.84). All of them had singleton pregnancies, 55.1% of them being nulliparous. All the other characteristics are depicted in Table 2. The evaluation was conducted between 18 and 24 weeks of gestation. Almost half of the pregnant women included in our study were overweight or obese (45.7%), with only 53.5% having a normal weight.

Table 2. Second trimester pregnant women's characteristics.

Second Trimester Pregnant Women's Characteristics		
Age		30.32 ± 4.84
Gestational age		22.09 ± 1.31
Nulliparous		55.1%
Folic acid	Without folic acid supplementation	20.6%
	Folic acid	45.3%
	Folic acid with multivitamins	34.1%
Chronic hypertension		1.9%
Diabetes		0.6%
Type of conception	Spontaneous	97.1%
	ART	2.9%
Smoking	Yes	8.9%
	No	86.9%
Initial BMI		22.96 ± 4.13
First trimester BMI		25.32 ± 4.16
BMI class	Underweight	0.8%
	Normal weight	53.5%
	Overweight	32.3%
	Obese	13.4%
Delta G% (weight gain)		10.7 ± 6.68

When analyzing nulliparous pregnant women during the second trimester of pregnancy, the same increasing tendency for overweight and obese becomes visible. BMI's distribution in multiparous pregnancies follows the tendency in the pregestational and first trimester time frames by remaining constant.

3.4. BMI Joinpoint Regression Analysis

We used joinpoint regression to obtain an objective evaluation of BMI.

We detected an annual 0.57 BMI increase in nulliparous women in the first trimester of pregnancy. This increase started in 2013 and reached a maximum mean value in 2020 (Figure 6). The BMI increased annually by 0.18 until 2013.

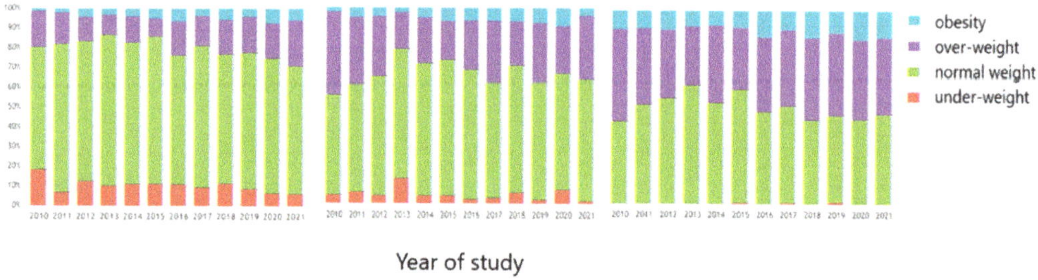

Figure 6. Multiparous weight trend from pregestational period until second trimester of pregnancy.

When analyzing the first trimester BMI tendency in multiparous women with the same joinpoint regression, we detected a significant annual 0.65 increase starting from 2013. The maximum value was reached in 2020 (Figure 7). During 2010–2013, the annual increase was 1.59 (Figure 8).

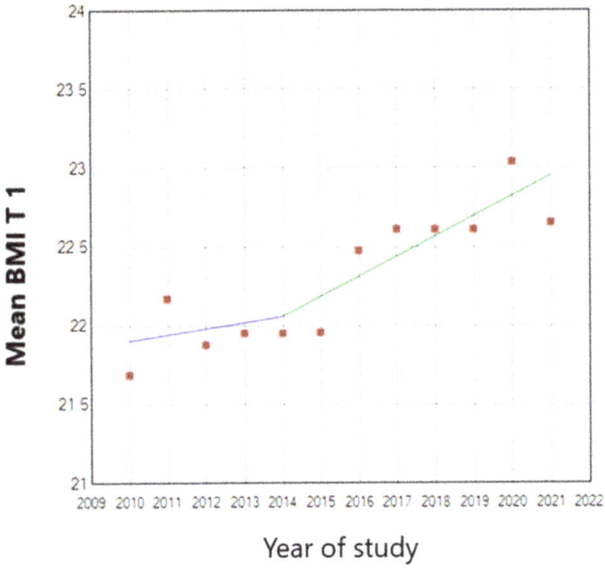

Figure 7. First trimester BMI trend in nulliparous women. (T 1—first trimester of pregnancy; the blue line represents the stationary tendency of the BMI until 2014 and the green line the ascendant tendency of the BMI).

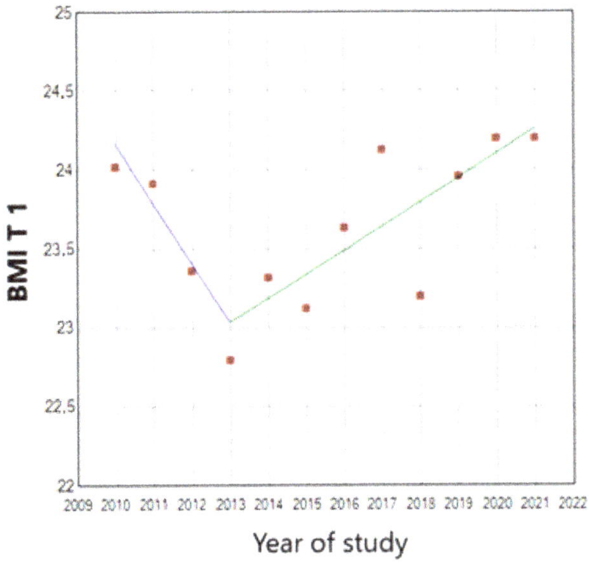

Figure 8. First trimester BMI trend in multiparous women (T 1—first trimester of pregnancy). (the blue line represents the descendent tendency of the BMI until 2014 and the green line the ascendant tendency of the BMI).

In the second trimester of pregnancy, both nulliparous and multiparous pregnant women encountered a continuous 0.46 and 0.42 annual BMI increase throughout the whole study period, respectively (Figure 9).

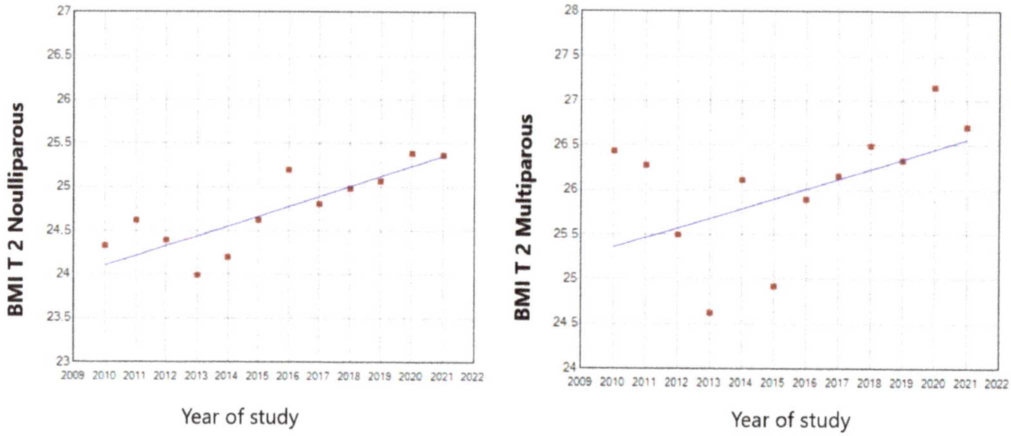

Figure 9. Second trimester BMI trends in nulliparous and multiparous pregnant women (T 2—second trimester of pregnancy).

3.5. BMI Variation with Other Parameters

3.5.1. Type of Conception

When evaluating pregestational BMI in nulliparous women depending on the type of conception, our results pointed out a significantly increased pregestational BMI in women with previous ART (assisted reproductive technology) procedures (IVF (in vitro fertilization) or ovarian stimulation) (Figure 10).

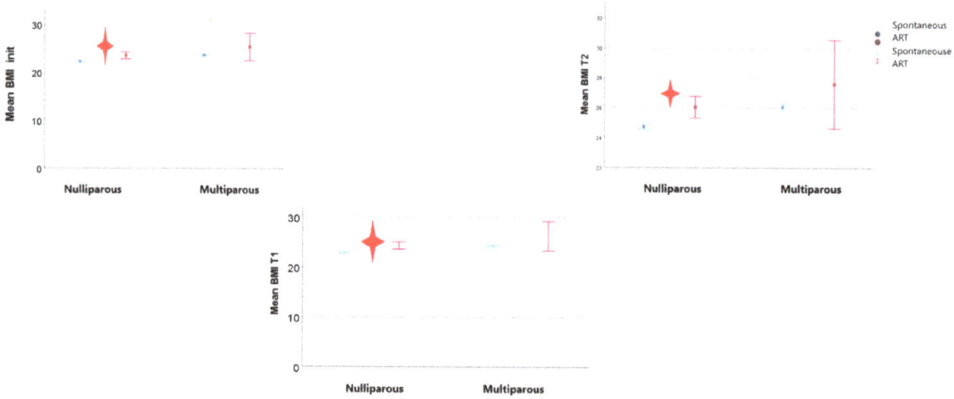

Figure 10. BMI trends depending on the type of conception (BMI_init—pregestational BMI; T1—first trimester of pregnancy; T2—second trimester of pregnancy; the red star indicated statistical significant results).

The tendency toward an increased BMI compared with patients with spontaneous conception was maintained throughout the first and the second trimesters of pregnancy. From a weight gain point of view, we detected no differences that concerned the type of conception or parity (Figure 11).

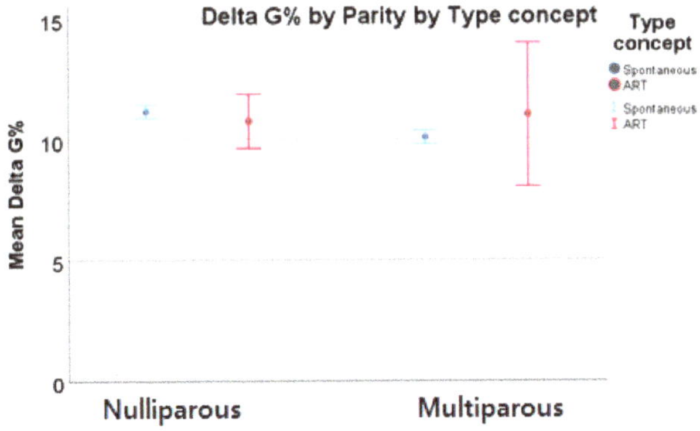

Figure 11. Weight gain depending on the type of conception.

3.5.2. Smoking Habits

The pregestational and first trimester BMIs of smoking women did not differ so much from that of non-smoking ones, regardless of parity. However, when we analyzed weight in the second trimester of pregnancy, we detected a significantly higher BMI mean value in smoking patients and in patients who quit smoking during pregnancy compared with non-smoking ones. Smoking pregnant women seemed to have higher second trimester weight gain, regardless of parity (Figure 12).

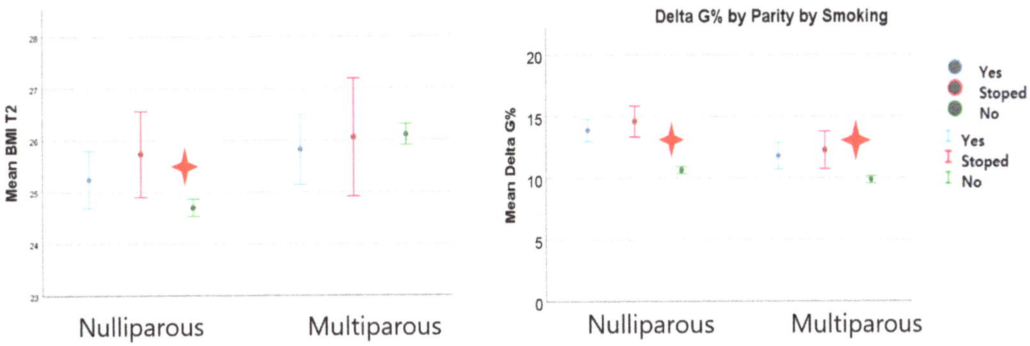

Figure 12. Second trimester BMI in smoker women and their weight gain the red star indicated statistical significant results).

3.5.3. Folic Acid Intake

We analyzed our cohort using folic acid intake, folic acid with multivitamin consumption, or diet supplementation with neither of these two as criteria. The results show no statistically significant pregestational or first or second trimester weight difference in nulliparous women. Instead, there was a statistically significant difference in BMI in the pregestational and first and second trimesters of pregnancy in multiparous women. The women with folic acid supplementation alone had a higher BMI than those with folic acid and multivitamin intake. Multiparous women without folic acid or vitamin consumption had a higher BMI than the other two categories (with folic acid and with vitamin intake), but the difference was not significant. The weight gain was statistically significant in nulliparous women with folic acid diet supplementation in the first trimester and in multiparous women with multivitamin intake during the second trimester until the morphology scan (Figure 13).

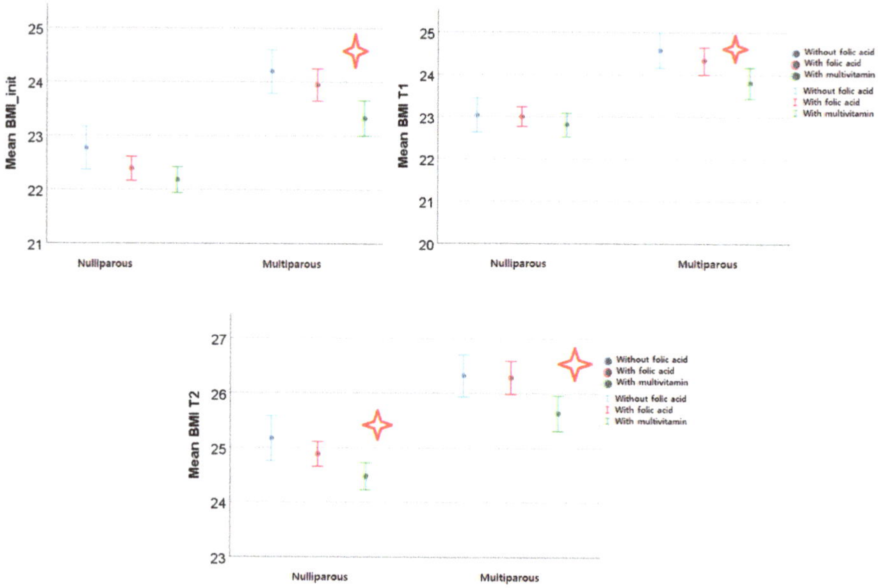

Figure 13. BMI trends depending on folic acid or multivitamin supplementation (BMI_init—pregestational BMI; T1—first trimester of pregnancy; and T2—second trimester of pregnancy; the red star indicated statistical significant results).

3.5.4. Chronic Hypertension

The weight of both nulliparous and multiparous women with chronic hypertension was statistically significantly higher in all three of the time frames in pregestational and the first and second trimesters of pregnancy. However, the weight gain until the second morphological evaluation was statistically significantly lower in women without chronic hypertension (Figure 14).

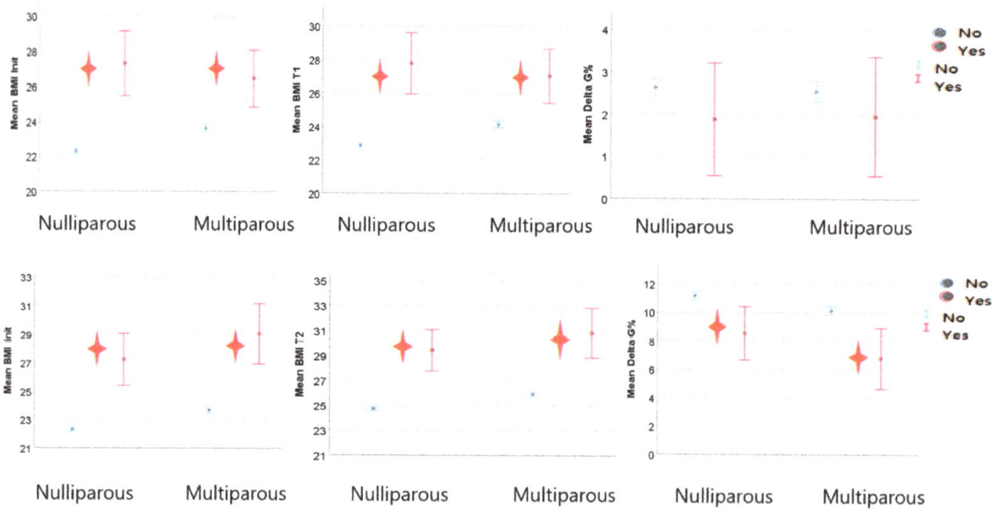

Figure 14. BMI trends in hypertensive women (the red star indicated statistical significant results).

3.5.5. Pregestational Diabetes

Multiparous diabetic women had statistically significantly higher BMIs than non-diabetic ones in the pre-pregnancy evaluation and the first trimester of pregnancy. The same observation was detected in the second trimester but for both diabetic nulliparous and multiparous pregnant women. The global weight gain did not reveal any statistically significant changes regardless of parity and the pregnancy trimester (Figure 15).

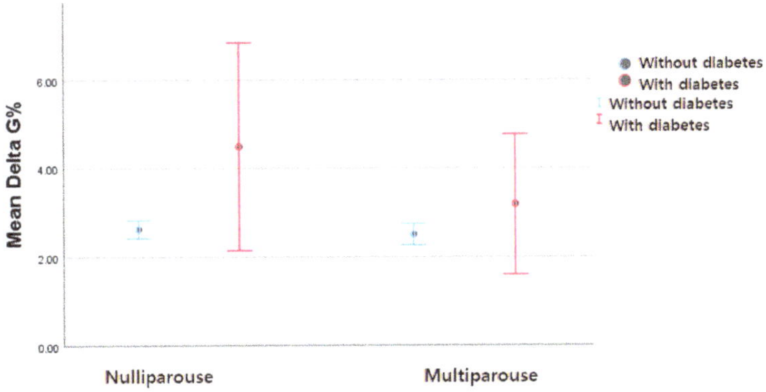

Figure 15. Global weight gain in women with chronic diabetes.

4. Discussion

This study allowed us to observe preconception and pregnancy BMI trends over 12 years and their variations depending on parity, the type of conception, smoking status, the COVID-19 pandemic, folic acid or multivitamin intake, chronic hypertension, and diabetes. The large time frame enabled us to obtain solid results and an accurate reflection of our eastern Romanian region. This is the first study conducted in our country that evaluates the BMI of women before pregnancy and during the first two trimesters. Another element that strengthens this study's value is the analysis of weight trends in women depending on smoking status, the conceiving method, folic acid and multivitamin supplementation, chronic hypertension, and pregestational diabetes.

Maternal nutrition in the pre-pregnancy period and during pregnancy plays an undebated essential role in the development of a fetus. Studies report negative consequences in both underweight and overweight/obesity cases. The intrauterine fetal environment needs to be optimal for the fetus to achieve its full growing and developing potential. Any disruption deeply marks its intrauterine and future childhood and adolescent development due to epigenetic factors. Therefore, we must take care of this to have healthy future generations. Nutritional problems deeply affect our contemporary society with their rising incidence, and it is very hard to implement effective measures to prevent them [1].

As stated in the literature, overweight and obesity have exhibited ascending curves in our women population, while the percentage of normal-BMI women has decreased over time [11,16–18]. The main factors involved in this increase are our new sedentary lifestyles, diet modifications characterized by an increased caloric intake of low-cost food, and shifts in our gut microbiomes [16].

Of our patients, 29% were overweight or obese at the moment of the first trimester morphology scan evaluation. The pre-pregnancy percentages were similar to those stated by Wang et al. in their 2021 United States study [19] but lower than the national estimates proposed by Hales et al. in 2020 for the first trimester of pregnancy [20]. However, the percentage increased until the second trimester morphological ultrasound, reaching 45.7%.

Our results are comparable to those stated by Panaitescu et al. in 2019, which evaluated BMI only in the first trimester of pregnancy, concerning the following parameters: maternal age, nulliparous proportion, and means of conception. The proportions of BMI classes are also similar. Parallel to our study, Panaitescu et al.'s results revealed the following first trimester BMI distribution: 6.76% of women were underweight, 66.37% were normal weight, and 26.82% were overweight and obese [7].

Regarding nulliparous women, similar results are depicted in studies from countries neighboring ours, such as Bulgaria and Turkey. The study carried out by Kamburova et al. in Bulgaria [21] states that 23.3% of women are overweight and obese. The percentage from Turkey is closer to ours, with 27.2% of women being obese and overweight in the first trimester of pregnancy [22]. Concerning the second trimester of pregnancy, the rates of overweight and obese women exceed 40%, as Fleming et al. in their study state to be the situation in most developing countries.

The peak for nulliparous women was reached in 2020, with a 30% increase compared with multiparous women, who exhibited a constant trend during the 12 years of study, but with a value of overweight and obesity that exceeded 30% [23,24]. As stated in Reynolds et al.'s [17] and McKeating et al.'s studies [23], multiparity is a risk factor for overweight and obesity. Our study's results also strengthen this idea. Studies have evaluated interpregnancy weight gain and maternal and fetal outcomes. The percentage of overweight and obese women was high and had a constant trend during the 12 years of our study. This reveals an important interpregnancy weight gain in our multiparous women. This increase in women's weight, which takes place from one pregnancy to another, has a negative influence on both mother and fetal outcomes. It is associated with pregnancy hypertensive disorders, diabetes, LGA fetuses, stillbirths, and C-section births [17,23–25] (McKeating). Our study also indicates that obese women are more prone to higher weight gain during pregnancy, in agreement with Rasmussen et al. [25].

We also detected a trend to postpone the first pregnancy, with the mean age for nulliparous women in our study being 30.69 $\pm$ 4.81. This tendency to postpone pregnancy is also visible in Panaitescu et al.'s study, strengthening the idea that this is a generalized phenomenon in our country [7].

Our study might underestimate the proportion of overweight and obesity in women who fail in spontaneous conception because this systemic inflammatory pathology is frequently associated with infertility, miscarriage, and congenital malformations [26,27]. We only included women who succeeded in conceiving via ovarian stimulation or IVF in our study.

When analyzing overweight and obesity depending on the other variables in our study, the results regarding smoking women were consistent with those of McKeating et al. They found no difference between smoking and non-smoking women concerning the percentage of overweight and obesity in the pre-pregnancy and first trimester time frames. However, in the second trimester, we observed increased weight gain, with higher proportions of overweight and obese pregnant women in smokers and those who quit smoking during pregnancy.

As stated in our study, Akter et al. found an increase in the percentage of overweight people during the pandemic mainly due to a sedentary lifestyle [28]. This aspect was also sustained by Restrepo et al. in their United States study [29].

Mlodzik-Czyzewska et al.'s case control study underlines that low folate intake and low serum folate values are associated with overweight and obesity [30]. This trend is also visible in our study, especially in multiparous women, such that multiparous women without any supplementation had higher BMI values than those with vitamin or folic acid supplementation. Many studies reveal the weight gain protector effect of a mother's folic acid intake on their children [31]. These results underline the importance of folic acid supplementation, either alone or in association with a multivitamin, in the pregestational period in women who desire to conceive. Supplementation with folic acid has two major benefits for both the mother and the child concerning its protective weight gain effect, the counterbalancing of which extends throughout generations.

Being overweight and obese before pregnancy implies a multitude of well-known complications. A wide range of such complications, such as preeclampsia, admission to the neonatal intensive care unit, fetal growth pathology, premature birth, C-section delivery, and superimposed preeclampsia, negatively influence a woman with chronic hypertension throughout her pregnancy's evolution. As stated in the literature, chronic hypertensive disorder is directly associated with overweight and obesity [32]. Our study reinforces these aspects. Our chronic hypertensive cohort of women had higher BMIs than the rest. However, the interesting aspect that we noticed was that the weight gain until the second morphological evaluation was statistically significantly lower in women without chronic hypertension.

The literature proves a direct relationship between the increase in obesity rates and pre-pregnancy diabetes [33]. These two pathologies are highly interconnected. This is sustained by our results, which obtained a higher BMI in diabetic women compared with non-diabetic ones and a statistically significantly increased BMI in multiparous women. However, the weight gain during pregnancy until the second morphological scan was not statistically significantly higher in women with chronic diabetes than in those without.

The assessment of pre-pregnancy BMI becomes very important when considering that the major impact on maternal and fetal outcomes is consistent with overweight and obesity before pregnancy, and weight gain during pregnancy has a reduced influence [34]. Dietary and other interventions aiming to improve maternal and fetal outcomes ought to concentrate on the pre-pregnancy period to obtain a significant result, underlining the importance of our study, which evaluated women's pre-pregnancy BMIs. This also adds value to our study, which succeeded in revealing women's BMI class distribution before and during pregnancy.

Another important aspect is that the BMI class distribution in the population varies with race, ethnicity, maternal age, and a country's economic status. The population in our study was homogenous. All the women included were Caucasian. The proportion of pre-pregnancy overweight and obese women was far smaller than the 46% described by Fisher et al. in their United States study (Fisher). Moreover, of the three times that BMI was evaluated in our study, the pre-pregnancy value was assessed by interviewing the patient the first time only, and the second two values were obtained via a direct evaluation of each pregnant woman by healthcare professionals in a limited timeframe. Another of our study's strengths resides in the 12-year period we took into consideration.

One of the limitations of our study is that it was exclusive to women who could not conceive, so the rate of pre-pregnancy overweight and obesity was underestimated. Furthermore, our study was limited to only one center in the private sector.

5. Conclusions

Obesity is, and will remain for a long time, one of the major burdens of the world's healthcare systems. It has gained prevalence over time as an epidemic. The health complications and overall impact on maternal and fetal outcomes surpass a specific moment in time, extending to future generations due to epigenetics.

Our article describes the trends of obesity and overweight in our middle-income country, in which this pathology is undergoing continuous growth, negatively influencing our reproductive-aged women and future generations.

Overweight and obese patients require expensive individualized health management.

We need to make a sustained effort to stop this trend and succeed in improving the health of our people.

Author Contributions: Conceptualization, D.R.M. and A.U.; methodology, A.E.C.; software, D.N.; validation, A.E.C., D.O.Z. and D.N.; formal analysis, D.N.; investigation, D.O.Z.; resources, D.N.; data curation, D.R.M.; writing—original draft preparation, A.U.; writing—review and editing, D.R.M.; visualization, I.E.B.; supervision, A.U.; project administration, D.R.M.; funding acquisition, A.E.C. All authors have read and agreed to the published version of the manuscript.

Funding: This research received no external funding.

Institutional Review Board Statement: This study was conducted following the Declaration of Helsinki and approved by the Ethics Committee of the "Cuza Voda" University Hospital (10426/24 August 2021).

Informed Consent Statement: Written informed consent was obtained from the patients to publish this paper.

Data Availability Statement: Data are contained within the article.

Conflicts of Interest: The authors declare no conflict of interest.

References

1. Ratnasiri, A.W.G.; Lee, H.C.; Lakshminrusimha, S.; Parry, S.S.; Arief, V.N.; DeLacy, I.H.; Yang, J.S.; DiLibero, R.J.; Logan, J.; Basford, K.E. Trends in maternal prepregnancy body mass index (BMI) and its association with birth and maternal outcomes in California, 2007-2016: A retrospective cohort study. *PLoS ONE* **2019**, *14*, e0222458. [CrossRef] [PubMed]
2. Paljk, I.; Verdenik, I.; Blickstein, I.; Tul, N. Maternal BMI and weight gain in singleton pregnancies: Has something changed in the last decade? *J. Matern. Fetal Neonatal Med.* **2021**, *34*, 7–11. [CrossRef]
3. Martin, B.; Sacks, D.A. The global burden of hyperglycemia in pregnancy—Trends from studies in the last decade. *Diabetes Res. Clin. Pract.* **2018**, *145*, 17–19. [CrossRef]
4. Morais, S.S.; Ide, M.; Morgan, A.M.; Surita, F.G. A novel body mass index reference range—An observational study. *Clinics* **2017**, *72*, 698–707. [CrossRef] [PubMed]
5. Morgan, K.L.; Rahman, M.A.; Macey, S.; Atkinson, M.D.; Hill, R.A.; Khanom, A.; Paranjothy, S.; Husain, M.J.; Brophy, S.T. Obesity in pregnancy: A retrospective prevalence-based study on health service utilisation and costs on the NHS. *BMJ Open* **2014**, *4*, e003983. [CrossRef] [PubMed]
6. Poston, L. Obesity in pregnancy; Where are we, where should we go? *Midwifery* **2017**, *49*, 4–6. [CrossRef]
7. Panaitescu, A.M.; Rotaru, D.; Ban, I.; Peltecu, G.; Zagrean, A.M. The prevalence of underweight, overweight and obesity in a Romanian population in the first trimester of pregnancy—Clinical implications. *Acta Endocrinol. (Buchar.)* **2019**, *15*, 323–332. [CrossRef]
8. Branum, A.M.; Kirmeyer, S.E.; Gregory, E.C. Prepregnancy body mass index by maternal characteristics and state: Data from the birth certificate, 2014. *Natl. Vital Stat. Rep.* **2016**, *65*, 1–11.
9. World Health Organization. Obesity: Preventing and managing the global epidemic. Report of a WHO consultation. *World Health Organ. Tech. Rep. Ser.* **2000**, *894*, 1–253.
10. Maxwell, C.; Gaudet, L.; Cassir, G.; Nowik, C.; McLeod, N.L.; Jacob, C.É.; Walker, M. Guideline No. 391-Pregnancy and Maternal Obesity Part 1: Pre-conception and Prenatal Care. *J. Obstet. Gynaecol. Can.* **2019**, *41*, 1623–1640. [CrossRef]
11. Deputy, N.P.; Dub, B.; Sharma, A.J. Prevalence and Trends in Prepregnancy Normal Weight—48 States, New York City, and District of Columbia, 2011–2015. *MMWR Morb. Mortal. Wkly. Rep.* **2018**, *66*, 1402–1407. [CrossRef] [PubMed]
12. Horta, B.L.; Barros, F.C.; Lima, N.P.; Assunção, M.C.F.; Santos, I.S.; Domingues, M.R.; Victora, C.G.; Pelotas Cohorts Study Group. Maternal anthropometry: Trends and inequalities in four population-based birth cohorts in Pelotas, Brazil, 1982–2015. *Int. J. Epidemiol.* **2019**, *48*, i26–i36. [CrossRef] [PubMed]
13. Scott-Pillai, R.; Spence, D.; Cardwell, C.; Hunter, A.; Holmes, V. The impact of body mass index on maternal and neonatal outcomes: A retrospective study in a UK obstetric population, 2004–2011. *BJOG* **2013**, *120*, 932–939. [CrossRef] [PubMed]
14. Godfrey, K.M.; Costello, P.M.; Lillycrop, K.A. The developmental environment, epigenetic biomarkers and long-term health. *J. Dev. Orig. Health Dis.* **2015**, *6*, 399–406. [CrossRef]
15. Poston, L.; Harthoorn, L.F.; Van Der Beek, E.M.; Contributors to the ILSI Europe Workshop. Obesity in pregnancy: Implications for the mother and lifelong health of the child. A consensus statement. *Pediatr. Res.* **2011**, *69*, 175–180. [CrossRef]
16. Ng, M.; Fleming, T.; Robinson, M.; Thomson, B.; Graetz, N.; Margono, C.; Mullany, E.C.; Biryukov, S.; Abbafati, C.; Abera, S.F.; et al. Global, regional, and national prevalence of overweight and obesity in children and adults during 1980–2013: A systematic analysis for the Global Burden of Disease Study 2013. *Lancet* **2014**, *384*, 766–781. [CrossRef]
17. Reynolds, C.M.E.; Egan, B.; McMahon, L.; O'Malley, E.G.; Sheehan, S.R.; Turner, M.J. Maternal obesity trends in a large Irish university hospital. *Eur. J. Obstet. Gynecol. Reprod. Biol.* **2019**, *238*, 95–99. [CrossRef]
18. Fisher, S.C.; Kim, S.Y.; Sharma, A.J.; Rochat, R.; Morrow, B. Is obesity still increasing among pregnant women? Prepregnancy obesity trends in 20 states, 2003–2009. *Prev. Med.* **2013**, *56*, 372–378. [CrossRef]
19. Wang, M.C.; Freaney, P.M.; Perak, A.M.; Greenland, P.; Lloyd-Jones, D.M.; Grobman, W.A.; Khan, S.S. Trends in Prepregnancy Obesity and Association with Adverse Pregnancy Outcomes in the United States, 2013 to 2018. *J. Am. Heart Assoc.* **2021**, *10*, e020717. [CrossRef]
20. Hales, C.M.; Carroll, M.D.; Fryar, C.D.; Ogden, C.L. Prevalence of obesity and severe obesity among adults: United States, 2017–2018. *NCHS Data Brief* **2020**, *360*, 1–8.
21. Kamburova, M.S.; Hristova, P.A.; Georgieva, S.L.; Khan, A. Adverse effects of maternal age, weight and smoking during pregnancy in Pleven, Bulgaria. *South Eastern Eur. J. Public Health (SEEJPH)* **2015**, *4*, 39–48. [CrossRef]

22. Daşıkan, Z. Weight Gain in Pregnancy: Do Pregnant Women Receive Correct Weight Gain Recommendation in Prenatal Care? *Turk. Klin. Jinekoloji Obstet.* **2015**, *25*, 32–38. [CrossRef]
23. McKeating, A.; Maguire, P.J.; Daly, N.; Farren, M.; McMahon, L.; Turner, M.J. Trends in maternal obesity in a large university hospital 2009–2013. *Acta Obstet. Gynecol. Scand.* **2015**, *94*, 969–975. [CrossRef] [PubMed]
24. Oteng-Ntim, E.; Mononen, S.; Sawicki, O.; Seed, P.T.; Bick, D.; Poston, L. Interpregnancy weight change and adverse pregnancy outcomes: A systematic review and meta-analysis. *BMJ Open* **2018**, *8*, e018778. [CrossRef]
25. Rasmussen, K.M.; Yaktine, A.L. *Weight Gain during Pregnancy: Reexamining the Guidelines Institute of Medicine and National Research Council Committee to Reexamine IOM Pregnancy Weight Guidelines*; National Academies Press: Washington, DC, USA, 2009. [CrossRef]
26. Catalano, P.M.; Shankar, K. Obesity and pregnancy: Mechanisms of short term and long term adverse consequences for mother and child. *BMJ* **2017**, *356*, j1. [CrossRef]
27. Langley-Evans, S.C.; Pearce, J.; Ellis, S. Overweight, obesity and excessive weight gain in pregnancy as risk factors for adverse pregnancy outcomes: A narrative review. *J. Hum. Nutr. Diet.* **2022**, *35*, 250–264. [CrossRef]
28. Akter, T.; Zeba, Z.; Hosen, I.; Al-Mamun, F.; Mamun, M.A. Impact of the COVID-19 pandemic on BMI: Its changes in relation to socio-demographic and physical activity patterns based on a short period. *PLoS ONE* **2022**, *17*, e0266024. [CrossRef]
29. Restrepo, B.J. Obesity Prevalence Among U.S. Adults During the COVID-19 Pandemic. *Am. J. Prev. Med.* **2022**, *63*, 102–106. [CrossRef]
30. Mlodzik-Czyzewska, M.A.; Malinowska, A.M.; Chmurzynska, A. Low folate intake and serum levels are associated with higher body mass index and abdominal fat accumulation: A case control study. *Nutr. J.* **2020**, *19*, 53. [CrossRef]
31. Wang, G.; DiBari, J.; Bind, E.; Steffens, A.M.; Mukherjee, J.; Azuine, R.E.; Singh, G.K.; Hong, X.; Ji, Y.; Ji, H.; et al. Association Between Maternal Exposure to Lead, Maternal Folate Status, and Intergenerational Risk of Childhood Overweight and Obesity. *JAMA Netw. Open* **2019**, *2*, e1912343. [CrossRef]
32. Badon, S.E.; Dublin, S.; Nance, N.; Hedderson, M.M.; Neugebauer, R.; Easterling, T.; Cheetham, T.C.; Chen, L.; Holt, V.L.; Avalos, L.A. Gestational weight gain and adverse pregnancy outcomes by pre-pregnancy BMI category in women with chronic hypertension: A cohort study. *Pregnancy Hypertens.* **2021**, *23*, 27–33. [CrossRef] [PubMed]
33. Fadl, H.E.; Simmons, D. Trends in diabetes in pregnancy in Sweden 1998–2012using. *BMJ Open Diabetes Res. Care* **2016**, *4*, e000221. [CrossRef] [PubMed]
34. Zhang, J.; Zhang, R.; Chi, J.; Li, Y.; Bai, W. Pre-pregnancy body mass index has greater influence on newborn weight and perinatal outcome than weight control during pregnancy in obese women. *Arch. Public Health* **2023**, *81*, 5. [CrossRef] [PubMed]

nutrients

MDPI

Article

Preconception Maternal Mentoring for Improved Fetal Growth among Indonesian Women: Results from a Cluster Randomized Controlled Trial

Hamam Hadi [1,2,*], Siti Nurunniyah [3], Joel Gittelsohn [4], Ratih Devi Alfiana [3], Fatimatasari [3], Emma C. Lewis [4] and Detty Nurdiati [5]

1 Alma Ata Graduate School of Public Health, The University of Alma Ata, Yogyakarta 55183, Indonesia
2 Alma Ata Center for Healthy Life and Foods (ACHEAF), The University of Alma Ata, Yogyakarta 55183, Indonesia
3 Department of Midwifery, Faculty of Health Sciences, The University of Alma Ata, Yogyakarta 55183, Indonesia; nurunniyah.siti@almaata.ac.id (S.N.); ratihdevi@almaata.ac.id (R.D.A.); fatimatasari@almaata.ac.id (F.)
4 Human Nutrition, Department of International Health, Johns Hopkins University Bloomberg School of Public Health, Baltimore, MD 21205, USA; jgittel1@jhu.edu (J.G.); elewis40@jhu.edu (E.C.L.)
5 Department of Obstetrics & Gynecology, Faculty of Medicine, Public Health, and Nursing, Universitas Gadjah Mada, Yogyakarta 55281, Indonesia; dnurdiati@yahoo.com
* Correspondence: hhadi@almaata.ac.id; Tel.: +62-274-434-2288; Fax: +62-274-434-2269

Abstract: The prevalence of stunting in young children is associated with poor growth during the prenatal and early postnatal periods. A maternal mentoring program was developed for Indonesian women to improve birth outcomes. A cluster-randomized controlled trial (CRCT) was conducted in three sub-districts of the Special Region of Yogyakarta, Indonesia. A total of 384 eligible participants were randomly allocated to either an intervention (received the maternal mentoring program and standard care; n = 189) or control (received standard care only; n = 195) group. The maternal mentoring program provided preconception health education; health monitoring; and text message reminders for preconception women. Fetal growth was measured between gestational weeks 27 and 30 using the estimated fetal weight generated from ultrasonographic measurements. Birth weight was measured within 24 h of birth. A structured questionnaire captured women's demographics, pregnancy readiness, and body mass indexes (BMIs). After adjustment, fetal weight was 14% (95% CI: 5.1–23.0) higher in the intervention group than in the control group, and the average weight-for-length Z-score at birth was 0.16 (95% CI: 0.04–0.30) higher in the intervention group than in the control group. The maternal mentoring program was associated with improved fetal growth and birth weight in this population and should be considered for scale-up to other settings, nationally and globally.

Keywords: maternal mentoring; preconception; fetal growth; maternal and child health; Indonesia

1. Introduction

Maternal and child health is a pressing health challenge worldwide. Restricted linear growth in particular presents major public health implications for under-resourced communities in low- and middle-income countries (LMICs) [1–3]. In Indonesia, the maternal mortality rate (MMR) and infant mortality rate (IMR) have been on the decline but remain relatively higher than the 2015 Millennium Development Goals target of only 102 deaths per 100,000 live births [4–6]. In addition, impaired growth and development of children is especially concerning in developing countries, where the prevalence of stunting and wasting in children under 2 years of age is 29.1% and 6.3%, respectively [7]. In Indonesia, 21.6% of children are stunted, and 7.7% are wasted, surpassing the average among all developing countries [8].

Stunting can result from inadequate fetal growth, which is typically characterized by having a birth weight that does not match the gestational age at birth (referred to as 'Small for Gestational Age (SGA)'). SGA babies born at term have a 2.43-times greater risk of stunting and a 2.52-times greater risk of wasting compared with normal-weight babies, and not surprisingly, those born preterm are at even greater risk (a 4.51-times greater risk of stunting and a 4.19-times greater risk of wasting) [9]. There are no data regarding the current prevalence of SGA in Indonesia, but it is estimated that approximately 6% of babies are born with a low birth weight (LBW) among those whose weights are recorded. Across all developing countries, estimates are higher, reaching nearly 27% of all live births being considered SGA [10]. Importantly, exclusive breastfeeding has been found to play a significant role in protecting young children from stunting in under-resourced populations [11], but the prevalence of exclusive breastfeeding remains low in these settings [12,13].

Moreover, despite intervention approaches aimed at ensuring pregnant women receive adequate early prenatal care, many settings where birth outcomes are poor have not seen substantial improvements [14]. Thus, based on the literature and our understanding from previous formative research conducted in Indonesia, we believe that interventions to improve birth outcomes should begin at an earlier stage, prior to conception [14,15], during which healthcare providers may have greater opportunities to intervene and successfully improve outcomes for both the mother and baby.

Preconception health services, including maternal mentoring programs, typically involve a series of interventions aimed at identifying and modifying behaviors pertaining to biomedical and social risks associated with maternal and child health before, during, and after pregnancy [16,17]. Several studies conducted in other settings show that preconception health services can improve childbirth and pregnancy outcomes, thus reducing the likelihood of maternal and infant mortality [18,19]. Likewise, it is well documented that poor preconception health is associated with poor pregnancy outcomes [20,21].

Many women in under-resourced settings are not well equipped to adopt certain health-related behaviors prior to becoming pregnant. Relatedly, potential risks associated with poor pregnancy outcomes are more likely to arise in women who are unaware of these risks or their consequences and are often unprepared for pregnancy. Therefore, when made readily accessible, preconception health services can serve as a protective factor by providing pregnant women with adequate health services before their babies enter crucial stages of development [22].

To date, no preconception interventions have been developed and tested in Indonesia. Given the current state of maternal and child outcomes in this setting, there is a strong need for interventions that target preconception in Indonesian women. The present study sought to examine the impact of a maternal mentoring program provided to Indonesian women during preconception and pregnancy on fetal growth and birth weight [23].

2. Materials and Methods

The present study was conducted under the Community Alma Ata Partnership through the Updated Research and Education (CAPTURE) project. Detailed methods of this study have been reported elsewhere [24,25]. A cluster-randomized controlled trial (CRCT) design was used consisting of preconception women residing in either the Sedayu Subdistrict, Pajangan Subdistrict, or Pleret Subdistrict of the Special Region of Yogyakarta, Indonesia. Recruitment was conducted using national marriage registration data. Members of the research team met with preconception women and explained the research process, as well as the potential benefits and disadvantages of participating. If willing and able to participate, women were then asked to sign an informed consent form. The inclusion criteria included: (1) being a woman of childbearing age (but not currently pregnant) and currently married; (2) planning to remain in the research area for at least the next two years; and (3) giving informed consent. Women were excluded from this study if they (1) became pregnant at the beginning of this study; (2) anticipated moving in the next two years; or

(3) planned to delay pregnancy. Of the total 1281 women recruited, 384 met the inclusion criteria and were willing to move forward with participation. The data were collected from this final sample via the CAPTURE data system from October 2018 to February 2021.

A total of 384 women were recruited within 122 identified clusters, and each was randomly allocated to either the intervention group (*n* = 189) or the control group (*n* = 195). Among them, 152 women in the intervention group and 158 in the control group became pregnant during the study period. We followed these pregnant women, and by February 2021, there were 113 newborns in the intervention group and 119 newborns in the control group who had their weights and lengths measured. Due to the COVID-19 pandemic, we did encounter some challenges in following the remaining women from our initial sample. Data were obtained using a questionnaire conducted at two time points: pre-test and post-test. Pre-tests occurred during the period before pregnancy, while post-tests occurred three weeks later. Clusters were randomly allocated to the treatment group using computer-generated random allocation [26]. Clusters 1–61 were assigned to the intervention group, and clusters 62–122 were assigned to the control group. Thus, the intervention and control groups each consisted of 61 clusters.

The mentors consisted of undergraduate students enrolled in the program areas of midwifery, nutrition, nursing, pharmacy, and hospital administration, and who had prior involvement in maternal and child health surveillance activities conducted under the CAPTURE project.

The maternal mentoring program delivered to the intervention group involved the following sequential components: (1) preconception health education delivered once during an initial home visit via face-to-face counseling in addition to providing a supplemental educational booklet; (2) monthly monitoring of pregnancy status via WhatsApp (WA) or basic Short Messaging Service (SMS), where women were asked to respond to the text prompt, "Have you experienced signs or symptoms of pregnancy such as late menstruation, nausea, vomiting, or others?"; and (3) once women reported experiencing signs of pregnancy, they were sent a text reminder to book their first antenatal care (ANC) visit immediately. Follow-up messages were sent every other day and included reminders to comply with routine provider visits and recommended iron supplementation. The control group received standard care based on current nationally recommended procedures for women of childbearing age.

The CAPTURE team trained mentors to ensure that they were competent in their role as preconception health counselors during the initial home visit phase of the program. In addition, a standardized preconception education booklet and worksheet were used to ensure intervention quality and validity [27].

Fetal weight between weeks 27 to 30 was estimated using ultrasonography (USG) examination conducted by trained obstetricians. Each pregnant woman in the study sample was scheduled to visit an approved obstetrician once she entered the 27th week of gestation. Birth weight and birth length were measured within 24 h of the newborn's birth by a trained midwife or nurse in the health clinic or hospital in which the delivery took place. Weight was measured using a digital weighing scale (SECA 876, Hannover, Germany) to the nearest 100 g, while length was measured using SECA measuring tapes to the nearest millimeter. A weight-for-length Z-score, length-for-age Z-score, and weight-for-age Z-score were generated using Stata 15 [28] for each newborn.

All data were then analyzed using Stata 15, which involved constructing a frequency distribution to determine participant characteristics, as well as bivariate and multivariable analyses. The average difference test between treatment groups was performed using chi-square and independent t-tests. Multilevel mixed-effects linear regression was used to explore the effect of the intervention on fetal growth and infant birthweight, with the factors of cluster, age, parity, level of education, employment status, income, and maternal body mass index (BMI) controlled for.

3. Results

There were no significant differences detected in socioeconomic or demographic characteristics between the intervention and control groups (Table 1). The majority of participants were of a healthy reproductive age, were nulliparous, had less than 12 years of education, were employed, had an income equal to or below the regional minimum wage, and reported having spent less than six months preparing for pregnancy.

Table 1. Participant characteristics at baseline.

Variable	Intervention Group Total (n = 189) (%)	Control Group Total (n = 195) (%)	* p-Value
Age			
<20	6 (3.2)	15 (7.7)	0.15
20–35	176 (93.1)	174 (89.2)	
>35	7 (3.7)	6 (3.1)	
Parity			
Nulliparous	182 (96.2)	190 (97.4)	0.52
Multiparous	7 (3.8)	5 (2.6)	
Education level			
≤12 years	153 (81)	166 (85.1)	0.28
>12 years	36 (19)	29 (14.9)	
Employment status			
Yes	140 (74.1)	139 (71.3)	0.54
No	49 (25.9)	56 (28.7)	
Income			
≤Regional income	143 (75.7)	142 (72.8)	0.53
>Regional income	46 (24.3)	53 (27.2)	
Time for pregnancy preparation			
≤6 months	153 (81)	167 (85.6)	0.22
>6 months	36 (19)	28 (14.4)	
Maternal body mass index			
<18.5	28 (14.8)	35 (17.9)	0.06
18.5–24.5	117 (61.9)	133 (68.2)	
>24.5	44 (23.3)	27 (13.8)	

* p-value from the chi-squared/Fisher's exact test.

3.1. The Effect of Maternal Mentoring on Fetal Growth

The estimated fetal weight (EFW) at 27–30 weeks of gestational age was 245.5 g higher ($p < 0.001$) in the intervention group compared with the control group (Table 2). Likewise, the percentile of EFW was 17.7 points higher ($p < 0.001$) in the intervention group compared with the control group (Table 2). The birth weight of babies was found to be 78.8 g higher ($p < 0.05$) in the intervention group than in the control group (Table 2). Both WLZ and WAZ were significantly higher ($p < 0.05$) in the intervention group than in the control group (Table 2). No impact was seen in terms of birth length.

Table 2. Fetal and newborn anthropometric characteristics.

	Study Groups		
Fetal Anthropometric Characteristics	**Intervention, *n* = 113**	**Control, *n* = 119**	*** *p*-Value**
Estimated fetal weight/EFW (g), mean (SD)	1415.8 (443.3)	1170.3 (226.8)	<0.001
Percentile of EFW, mean (SD)	57.7 (34.5)	40.0 (26.6)	<0.001
	Intervention, *n* = 129	Control, *n* = 123	
Newborn birth weight (g), mean (SD)	3117.8 (277.5)	3039.0 (264.7)	<0.05
WLZ score, mean (SD)	−0.3 (0.7)	−0.5 (0.7)	<0.05
WAZ score, mean (SD)	−0.4 (0.6)	−0.5 (0.6)	<0.05
Newborn length (cm), mean (SD)	49.2 (1.2)	49.1 (1.1)	>0.05
LAZ score, mean (SD)	−0.2 (0.7)	−0.2 (0.6)	>0.05

EBW was estimated using USG measurements. EBW percentile was calculated based on intergrowth. WLZ score was calculated based on intergrowth standard. WAZ score was calculated based on intergrowth standard. * *p*-value was obtained from independent *t*-test.

3.2. The Effect of Maternal Mentoring on Estimated Fetal Weight

Further analyses using cluster-adjusted multilevel mixed-effects linear regression were performed to examine the effect of maternal mentoring on the EFW percentile. In addition to adjusting for clusters, variables including maternal age, maternal education, maternal employment status, maternal monthly income, and maternal BMI were also adjusted for. Based on this, we determined that the EFW percentile was 14 points higher (95% CI: 5.1–23.0) in the intervention group than in the control group (Table 3).

Table 3. Effect of maternal mentoring on percentile of estimated fetal weight.

EFW Percentile	**Cluster-Adjusted Multilevel Mixed-Effects Linear Regression**		
	Coefficient	**SE**	**(95% CI)**
Study group			
Intervention	14.0	4.6	5.1–23.0
Control	-	-	-
Age (years)			
<20	4.4	7.9	−11.2–20.0
20–35	-	-	-
>35	−6.2	12.9	−31.5–19.1
Maternal education			
≤12 years	−13.7	5.5	−24.5–(−3.0)
>12 years	-	-	-
Employment status			
Employed	-	-	-
Unemployed	−4.47	4.4	−13.2–4.2
Maternal monthly income			
<national wage	-	-	-
≥national wage	−5.74	4.8	−15.0–3.6
Maternal body mass index			
Underweight	−4.4	5.5	−15.3–6.4
Normal	-	-	-
Overweight	−10.5	5.4	−21.3–0.15

Regression coefficients, SE, and 95% CI were generated from multilevel mixed-effects linear regression adjusting for cluster, age, maternal education, employment status, maternal monthly income, and BMI (*n* cluster = 106).

3.3. The Effect of Maternal Mentoring on Newborn Birth Weight

After adjusting the multivariate models, we found a significant difference in birth weight between the intervention and control groups (Table 4). Accordingly, the mean newborn birth weight was 65.7 g higher (95% CI: 1.9–129.5) in the intervention group than in the control group adjusted for cluster, maternal age, maternal education, socioeconomic status, and maternal preconception BMI (Table 4).

Table 4. Effect of maternal mentoring on newborn birth weight.

Newborn Birth Weight	Cluster-Adjusted Multilevel Mixed-Effects Linear Regression		
	Coefficient	SE	(95% CI)
Study group			
Intervention	65.7	32.52	1.9–129.5
Control	-	-	-
Age (years)			
<20	−12.7	63.9	−137.8–112.5
20–35	−32.6	116.6	−261.1–195.9
>35			
Maternal education			
≤12 years	−52.3	42.0	−134.6–30.1
>12 years	-	-	-
Employment status			
Employed	39.2	35.6	−30.7–108.9
Unemployed	-	-	-
Maternal monthly income			
<national wage	-	-	-
≥national wage	−27.6	38.5	−103.1–47.8
Maternal body mass index			
Underweight	57.4	42.9	−26.8–141.6
Normal	-	-	-
Overweight	−8.8	44.7	−96.5–78.9

Regression coefficients, SE, and 95% CI were generated from multilevel mixed-effects linear regression adjusting for cluster, age, maternal education, employment status, maternal monthly income, and BMI (*n* cluster = 106).

3.4. The Effect of Maternal Mentoring on Newborn Weight-for-Length Z-Score

After adjusting the multivariate models, we found a significant difference in birth weight, but not in birth length, between the intervention and control groups (Table 4). Accordingly, the mean weight-for-length Z-score was 0.16 points higher (95% CI: 0.01–0.30) in the intervention group than in the control group adjusted for cluster, maternal age, maternal education, socioeconomic status, and maternal preconception BMI (Table 5).

Table 5. Effect of maternal mentoring on newborn weight-for-length Z-score.

Weight-for-Length Z-Score	Cluster-Adjusted Multilevel Mixed-Effects Linear Regression		
	Coefficient	SE	(95% CI)
Study group			
Intervention	0.162	0.08	0.04–0.3
Control	-	-	-
Maternal age (years)			
<20	4.4	7.9	−11.2–20.0
20–35	-	-	-
>35	−6.2	12.9	−31.6–19.1
Maternal education			
≤12 years	−13.7	5.45	−24.5–(−3.0)
>12 years	-	-	-

Table 5. *Cont.*

Weight-for-Length Z-Score	Cluster-Adjusted Multilevel Mixed-Effects Linear Regression		
	Coefficient	SE	(95% CI)
Maternal employment status			
Employed	−4.5	4.44	−13.2–4.2
Unemployed	-	-	-
Maternal monthly income			
<national minimum wage	-	-	-
≥national minimum wage	−5.7	4.76	−15.09–3.59
Maternal body mass index			
Underweight	0.11	5.53	−0.10–0.3
Normal	-	-	-
Overweight	−0.22	−5.46	0.08–0.4

Regression coefficients, SE, and 95% CI were generated from multilevel mixed-effects linear regression adjusting for cluster, age, maternal education, employment status, maternal monthly income, and BMI.

3.5. The Effect of Maternal Mentoring on Newborn Birth Length

After adjusting the multivariate models, we could not find a significant difference in birth length between the intervention and control groups (Table 6). Using the same statistical modeling, we could not find a significant difference in newborn length-for-age Z-score and newborn weight-for-age Z-score (not shown).

Table 6. Effect of maternal mentoring on newborn birth length.

Newborn Birth Length	Cluster-Adjusted Multilevel Mixed-Effects Linear Regression		
	Coefficient	SE	(95% CI)
Study group			
Intervention	0.08	0.14	−0.19–0.35
Control	-	-	-
Maternal age (years)			
<20	−0.26	0.27	−0.79–0.26
20–35	-	-	-
>35	−0.24	0.49	−1.2–0.72
Maternal education			
≤12 years	−0.15	0.18	−24.5–(−3.0)
>12 years	-	-	-
Maternal employment status			
Employed	−4.5	4.44	−0.50–0.20
Unemployed	-	-	-
Maternal monthly income			
<national minimum wage	-	-	-
≥national minimum wage	0.21	0.15	−0.09–0.50
Maternal body mass index			
Underweight	0.06	0.18	−0.29–0.41
Normal	-	-	-
Overweight	−0.15	0.19	−0.51–0.22

Regression coefficients, SE, 95% CI were generated from multilevel mixed-effects linear regression adjusting for cluster, age, maternal education, employment status, maternal monthly income, and BMI.

4. Discussion

The preconception maternal mentoring program described herein is the only program of its kind to be delivered as an intervention in Indonesian women with an overall goal of improving maternal and child health [25]. In the present analysis, we found that receiving the maternal mentoring program during preconception and pregnancy significantly improved fetal growth and birth weight for newborns. We also found that the newborn weight-for-length Z-score (WLZ), but not the length-for-age Z-score (LAZ), was significantly higher for women who received the program compared with those who only received standard care.

A number of previous preconception interventions have been conducted to examine their impacts on maternal knowledge [18,29,30], maternal self-efficacy [31,32], maternal risk behaviors [29,30,32–35], and various birth outcomes [29,36]. Preconception nutritional supplementation in particular has been shown to improve newborn birth length [37] which is the strongest predictor of linear growth status and stunting in the first two years of life [38].

Although one study showed that preconception education and counseling did not significantly reduce low birth weight, the intervention materials used in the study were only delivered to women at one time point during the preconception stage [36]. Therefore, we posit that the effect of the materials was not strong enough in this instance to elicit a change in women's risk behaviors. In addition, the study did not provide women with adequate information about complying with routine provider visits and recommended iron supplementation before and during pregnancy.

Herein, we reported that the maternal mentoring program in our study led to greater reported readiness for pregnancy (i.e., women felt more prepared for pregnancy, had more time for motherhood, had time to discuss their pregnancy with their partner, were more likely to consume recommended iron and folic acid supplementation, were more likely to maintain a healthy diet, were more likely to not smoke, were more likely to avoid over-the-counter and herbal drugs, were more likely to have health care insurance, were more able to manage stress, and were more likely to seek early detection of STDs) [24]. Preconception maternal mentoring improved the timing of first ANC visits, and women who received preconception maternal mentoring were three times more likely to have an earlier ANC visit than those who did not receive this mentoring [25]. This latter finding may help to explain, in part, the effect of the maternal mentoring program on improved fetal growth and birth weight in this study given that early ANC has been associated with improved birth outcomes.

We believe our intervention is unique from previous studies focused on providing maternal mentoring programs in other settings, as our intervention included a comprehensive package of educational materials and multiple time points for delivery from preconception to post-delivery. Meanwhile, many previous studies have only consisted of one single educational or counseling session [30,31,33,35,36], or have consisted of more than one session but without support for accessing routine provider visits or recommended iron supplementation before and during pregnancy [30,31,33].

In the present study, each woman in the intervention group received basic education during preconception, as well as monthly WhatsApp/SMS messages until pregnancy, and other message reminders every other day to comply with routine provider visits and recommended iron supplementation during pregnancy until delivery. This approach is comprehensive and could be considered a strength of our study. In addition, as many women have access to mobile devices, this approach is also likely to be feasible among the broader population of women in this setting and should be considered by healthcare providers and the national government given the ease and low cost of sending automated messages.

Importantly, a previous study found that monthly nutritional education delivered during the third trimester led to 60% higher weight gain, 20% higher birth weight, and 94% lower LBW for newborns [39]. Similarly, guided nutritional counseling delivered during pregnancy through home visits led to a 0.95kg higher average gestational weight gain and 0.26 kg higher average birth weight in one previous intervention [40]. Moreover, nutritional education for pregnant women has been shown to result in improved newborn birth weight, especially when spouses are involved in the education. In one particular study, newborn birth weight was 0.40 kg higher for the newborns of couples where both partners received nutritional education compared with only the woman [41]. Each of these nutritional education sessions was delivered at least three times during either a home visit or counseling. Therefore, it is possible that the intensity and frequency of nutritional education and counseling sessions play an important role in the success of behavioral change interventions aiming to improve birth outcomes.

Additionally, there is a lack of evidence to show that maternal mentoring significantly impacts newborn birth length. In our study, the newborn length-for-age Z-score was not found to be different between the intervention and control groups. However, one multi-country randomized controlled trial conducted in rural and semi-rural settings demonstrated that the newborn birth length-for-age Z-score was 0.19 points higher for women who received nutritional supplementation at least 3 months prior to conception compared with women who did not receive any nutritional intervention [37]. This higher LAZ, in turn, led to a significantly lower prevalence of stunting at six months and twenty-four months of age among the children whose mothers had received preconception nutritional intervention [38]. In the case of our study, it is possible that having greater health knowledge among those women who received maternal mentoring led to better eating practices prior to conception; however, we did not collect data on nutrient intake prior to conception. A takeaway from a multi-country study in relation to ours is that nutritional intervention approaches seemed to more strongly impact the newborn LAZ in settings with a higher prevalence of malnutrition [37].

Given that inadequate fetal growth is strongly associated with stunting in developing countries, including Indonesia, the present study provides strong support for implementing maternal mentoring in addition to standard care for preconception and pregnant women in this setting. It is important to note that this study sample was obtained from women in Yogyakarta, who mostly have mobile devices, and may not be representative of all women across rural and urban regions of Indonesia; therefore, future research should explore the impact of such programs in broader populations in order to successfully reach the national goals for reduced stunting and wasting among children.

5. Conclusions

To our knowledge, this is the first intervention of its kind to investigate the impact of preconception maternal mentoring on fetal growth and birth weight outcomes in Indonesia, where child stunting and wasting remain common. Our findings demonstrate that a comprehensive maternal mentoring program provided in addition to standard care procedures may be feasible and effective for improving fetal growth and increasing birth weight, especially among a particularly under-resourced population of women. Future efforts are needed on behalf of researchers, healthcare providers, and policymakers to determine how maternal mentoring programs such as the one described herein can be adapted and scaled to improve outcomes for both mothers and children across Indonesia and worldwide.

Author Contributions: H.H. was involved in the research initiation, research design, data analysis, and writing of this manuscript. S.N. was involved in the research preparation, data collection, management, data analysis, and manuscript preparation. F. and R.D.A. were involved in the data collection and manuscript preparation. J.G., E.C.L. and D.N. were involved in writing and reviewing this manuscript. All authors have read and agreed to the published version of the manuscript.

Funding: The University of Alma Ata as well as the Ministry of Education and Culture, Research and Technology, and Higher Education, the Republic of Indonesia No: 108/E/KPT/2023, 27 July 2023, contributed to this manuscript's preparation.

Institutional Review Board Statement: This study received ethical approval from the Medical and Health Research Ethics Commission of Gadjah Mada University under approval number KE/FK1289/EC/2018.

Informed Consent Statement: Informed consent was obtained from all subjects involved in this study.

Data Availability Statement: The authors are very pleased to share the research data used in this manuscript.

Acknowledgments: The University of Alma Ata supported this work. The first author would also like to acknowledge the financial support from the Ministry of Education and Culture, Research and Technology, and Higher Education, the Republic of Indonesia, through the grant of World Class Professor No: 108/E/KPT/2023, 27 July 2023. We also acknowledge the contribution of Yhona Paratmanitya and other faculty members and students of the Faculty of Health Sciences, the University of Alma Ata, who were involved in the CAPTURE Project. We also acknowledge the contribution of the Directorate of Human Resources, Directorate General of Higher Education Research and Technology, Ministry of Education, Culture Research and Technology, Indonesia.

Conflicts of Interest: The authors declare no conflict of interest.

References

1. World Health Organization. *Global Nutrition Targets 2025: Policy Brief Series WHO/NMH/NHD/14.4*; World Health Organization: Geneva, Switzerland, 2014.
2. UNICEF. *Tracking Progress on Child and Maternal Nutrition: A Survival and Development Priority*; UNICEF: Geneva, Switzerland, 2009.
3. The World Bank Group. *The World Bank Annual Report 2017: End Extreme Poverty, Boost Shared Prosperity*; World Bank: Washington, DC, USA, 2017.
4. Ministry of Health Indonesia. *Basic Health Research 2018*; Ministry of Health Indonesia: Batam, Indonesia, 2018.
5. Statistics Indonesia; National Population and Family Planning Board; Ministry of Health. *Indonesia Demographic and Health Survey 2012*; Ministry of Health Indonesia: Batam, Indonesia, 2013.
6. World Health Organization (WHO). *WHO Recommendations on Antenatal Care for A Positive Pregnancy Experience*; World Health Organization: Geneva, Switzerland, 2016; Volume 6.
7. Ssentongo, P.; Ssentongo, A.E.; Ba, D.M.; Ericson, J.E.; Na, M.; Gao, X.; Fronterre, C.; Chinchilli, V.M.; Schiff, S.J. Global, regional and national epidemiology and prevalence of child stunting, wasting and underweight in low- and middle-income countries, 2006–2018. *Sci. Rep.* **2021**, *11*, 1–12. [CrossRef]
8. Kemenkes. *Hasil Survei Status Gizi Indonesia (SSGI) 2022*; Kemenkes: 2023; pp. 1–7. Available online: https://ayosehat.kemkes.go.id/pub/files/files46531._MATERI_KABKPK_SOS_SSGI.pdf (accessed on 27 October 2023).
9. Christian, P.; Lee, S.E.; Angel, M.D.; Adair, L.S.; Arifeen, S.E.; Ashorn, P.; Barros, F.C.; Fall, C.H.; Fawzi, W.W.; Hao, W.; et al. Risk of childhood undernutrition related to small-for-gestational age and preterm birth in low- and middle-income countries. *Int. J. Epidemiol.* **2013**, *42*, 1340–1355. [CrossRef] [PubMed]
10. Black, R.E. Global Prevalence of Small for Gestational Age Births. *Nestle Nutr. Inst. Workshop Ser.* **2015**, *81*, 1–7. [PubMed]
11. Hadi, H.; Fatimatasari, F.; Irwanti, W.; Kusuma, C.; Alfiana, R.D.; Asshiddiqi, M.I.N.; Nugroho, S.; Lewis, E.C.; Gittelsohn, J. Exclusive breastfeeding protects young children from stunting in a low-income population: A study from eastern indonesia. *Nutrients* **2021**, *13*, 4264. [CrossRef]
12. UNICEF/WHO. Global Breastfeeding Scorecard 2022: Protecting Breastfeeding Through Further Investments and Policy Actions. Glob Breastfeed Collect [Internet]. 2022; pp. 1–6. Available online: https://www.who.int/publications/i/item/WHO-HEP-NFS-22.6 (accessed on 14 February 2023).
13. Victora, C.G.; Bahl, R.; Barros, A.J.D.; Franca, G.V.A.; Horton, S.; Krasevec, J.; Murch, S.; Sankar, M.J.; Walker, N.; Rollins, N.C.; et al. Breastfeeding in the 21st century: Epidemiology, mechanisms, and lifelong effect. *Lancet* **2016**, *387*, 475–790. [CrossRef]
14. Is early prenatal care too late? From the march of dimes birth defects foundation. *Contemp. Ob. Gyn.* **2002**, *47*.
15. Is early prenatal care too late? *Emerg. Med.* **2002**, *47*. Available online: https://www.contemporaryobgyn.net/view/march-dimes-updates-early-prenatal-care-too-late (accessed on 27 October 2023).
16. Dean, S.V.; Imam, A.M.; Lassi, Z.S.; Bhutta, Z.A. *Systematic Review of Preconception Risks and Interventions*; Aga Khan University: Karachi, Pakistan, 2012. Available online: https://media.tghn.org/articles/Preconception_Report.pdf (accessed on 27 October 2023).
17. Robbins, C.L.; Zapata, L.B.; Farr, S.L.; Kroelinger, C.D.; Morrow, B.; Ahluwalia, I.; D'Angelo, D.V.; Barradas, D.; Cox, S.; Goodman, D.; et al. Core state preconception health indicators—Pregnancy risk assessment monitoring system and behavioral risk factor surveillance system, 2009. *Morb. Mortal. Wkly. Rep. Surveill. Summ.* **2009**, *63*, 1–62.
18. Withanage, N.N.; Botfield, J.R.; Srinivasan, S.; Black, K.I.; Mazza, D. Effectiveness of preconception interventions in primary care: A systematic review. *Br. J. Gen. Pract.* **2022**, *72*, E865–E872. [CrossRef]
19. Hussein, N.; Kai, J.; Qureshi, N. The effects of preconception interventions on improving reproductive health and pregnancy outcomes in primary care: A systematic review. *Eur. J. Gen. Pract.* **2016**, *22*, 42–52. [CrossRef]
20. Das, R.N.; Devi, R.S.; Kim, J. Mothers' lifestyle characteristics impact on her neonates' low birth weight. *Int. J. Women's Health Reprod. Sci.* **2014**, *2*, 229–235.
21. Genuis, S.J.; Genuis, R.A. Preconception Care: A New Standard of Care within Maternal Health Services. *Biomed Res. Int.* **2016**, *2016*, 6150976. [CrossRef] [PubMed]
22. Ricks, N.; Comer, L.; Liu, F.; DeGrande, H.; Adeniran, O. Substance use and preconception care: A review of the literature. *Int. J. Women's Health Reprod. Sci.* **2017**, *5*, 3–10. [CrossRef]

23. Lassi, Z.S.; Mansoor, T.; Salam, R.A.; Das, J.K.; Bhutta, Z.A. Essential pre-pregnancy and pregnancy interventions for improved maternal, newborn and child health. *Reprod. Health* **2014**, *11* (Suppl. S1), S2. [CrossRef]
24. Nurunniyah, S.; Julia, M.; Hadi, H.; Nurdiati, D.S.; Lewis, E.C. The effect of a Maternal Mentoring Programme on Pregnancy Readiness among Indonesian Women: Results of a Cluster Randomised Control Trial. *Afr. J. Nurs. Midwifery* **2022**, *24*, 16. [CrossRef]
25. Paratmanitya, Y.; Helmyati, S.; Nurdiati, D.S.; Lewis, E.C.; Gittelsohn, J.; Hadi, H. The effect of a maternal mentoring program on the timing of first antenatal care visit among pregnant women in Bantul, Indonesia: Results of a cluster randomized trial. *Health Promot. Perspect.* **2021**, *11*, 307. [CrossRef]
26. Kim, J.; Shin, W. How to do random allocation (randomization). *Clin. Orthop. Surg.* **2014**, *6*, 103–109. [CrossRef]
27. Nurunniyah, S.; Nurdiati, D.S.; Julia, M.; Hadi, H. Development process of the preconception education booklet. *Int. J. Res. Med. Sci.* **2021**, *9*, 1864. [CrossRef]
28. 28. StataCorp LP. *Stata Statistical Software: Release 15*; Stata Corp LLC.: College Station, TX, USA, 2017.
29. Elsinga, J.; de Jong-Potjer, L.C.; van der Pal-de Bruin, K.M.; le Cessie, S.; Assendelft, W.J.J.; Buitendijk, S.E. The Effect of Preconception Counselling on Lifestyle and Other Behaviour Before and During Pregnancy. *Women's Health Issues* **2008**, *18* (Suppl. S6), S117–S125. [CrossRef]
30. Schwarz, E.B.; Sobota, M.; Gonzales, R.; Gerbert, B. Computerized counseling for folate knowledge and use: A randomized controlled trial. *Am. J. Prev. Med.* **2008**, *35*, 568–571. [CrossRef]
31. Bastani, F.; Hashemi, S.; Bastani, N.; Haghani, H. Impact of preconception health education on health locus of control and self-efficacy in women. *East. Mediterr. Health J.* **2010**, *16*, 396–401. [CrossRef] [PubMed]
32. Hillemeier, M.M.; Downs, D.S.; Feinberg, M.E.; Weisman, C.S.; Chuang, C.H.; Parrott, R.; Velott, D.; Francis, L.A.; Baker, S.A.; Dyer, A.M.; et al. Improving Women's Preconceptional Health. Findings from a Randomized Trial of the Strong Healthy Women Intervention in the Central Pennsylvania Women's Health Study. *Women's Health Issues* **2008**, *18* (Suppl. S6), S87–S96. [CrossRef] [PubMed]
33. Robbins, J.M.; Cleves, M.A.; Collins, H.B.; Andrews, N.; Smith, L.N.; Hobbs, C.A. Randomized trial of a physician-based intervention to increase the use of folic acid supplements among women. *Am. J. Obstet. Gynecol.* **2005**, *192*, 1126–1132. [CrossRef] [PubMed]
34. Floyd, R.L.; Sobell, M.; Velasquez, M.M.; Ingersoll, K.; Nettleman, M.; Sobell, L.; Mullen, P.D.; Ceperich, S.; von Sternberg, K.; Bolton, B.; et al. Preventing alcohol-exposed pregnancies: A randomized controlled trial. *Am. J. Prev. Med.* **2007**, *32*, 1–10. [CrossRef]
35. Cena, E.R.; Joy, A.B.; Heneman, K.; Espinosa-Hall, G.; Garcia, L.; Schneider, C.; Swanson, P.C.W.; Hudes, M.; Zidenberg-Cherr, S. Learner-centered nutrition education improves folate intake and food-related behaviors in nonpregnant, low-income women of childbearing age. *J. Am. Diet. Assoc.* **2008**, *108*, 1627–1635. [CrossRef]
36. Lumley, J.; Donohue, L. Aiming to increase birth weight: A randomised trial of pre-pregnancy information, advice and counselling in inner-urban Melbourne. *BMC Public Health* **2006**, *6*, 299. [CrossRef]
37. Hambidge, K.M.; Westcott, J.E.; Garcés, A.; Figueroa, L.; Goudar, S.S.; Dhaded, S.M.; Pasha, O.; Ali, S.A.; Tshefu, A.; Lokangaka, A.; et al. A multicountry randomized controlled trial of comprehensive maternal nutrition supplementation initiated before conception: The Women First trial. *Am. J. Clin. Nutr.* **2019**, *109*, 457–469. [CrossRef]
38. Hambidge, K.M.; Westcott, J.E.; Garcés, A.; Figueroa, L.; Goudar, S.S.; Dhaded, S.M.; Pasha, O.; Ali, S.A.; Tshefu, A.; Lokangaka, A.; et al. Birth length is the strongest predictor of linear growth status and stunting in the first 2 years of life after a preconception maternal nutrition intervention: The children of the Women First trial. *Am. J. Clin. Nutr.* **2022**, *116*, 86–96. [CrossRef]
39. Jahan, K.; Roy, S.K.; Mihrshahi, S.; Sultana, N.; Khatoon, S.; Roy, H.; Datta, L.R.; Roy, A.; Jahan, S.; Khatun, W.; et al. Short-term nutrition education reduces low birthweight and improves pregnancy outcomes among urban poor women in Bangladesh. *Food Nutr. Bull.* **2014**, *35*, 414–421. [CrossRef]
40. Demilew, Y.M.; Alene, G.D.; Belachew, T. Effect of guided counseling on dietary practices of pregnant women in West Gojjam Zone, Ethiopia. *PLoS ONE* **2020**, *15*, e0233429. [CrossRef]
41. Tsegaye, D.; Tamiru, D.; Belachew, T. Effect of a theory-based nutrition education intervention during pregnancy through male partner involvement on newborns' birth weights in Southwest Ethiopia. A three-arm community based Quasi-Experimental study. *PLoS ONE* **2023**, *18*, e0280545. [CrossRef] [PubMed]

nutrients

MDPI

Review

The Effects of Prenatal Iron Supplementation on Offspring Neurodevelopment in Upper Middle- or High-Income Countries: A Systematic Review

Najma A. Moumin [1,2], Emily Shepherd [1,3], Kai Liu [3,4], Maria Makrides [1,2], Jacqueline F. Gould [1,2], Tim J. Green [1,5] and Luke E. Grzeskowiak [1,6,*]

1 Women and Kids, South Australian Health and Medical Research Institute, Adelaide, SA 5000, Australia; najma.moumin@sahmri.com (N.A.M.); emily.shepherd@sahmri.com (E.S.); maria.makrides@sahmri.com (M.M.); jacqueline.gould@sahmri.com (J.F.G.); tgreen@flinders.edu.au (T.J.G.)
2 Discipline of Pediatrics, Adelaide Medical School, The University of Adelaide, Adelaide, SA 5005, Australia
3 Discipline of Obstetrics and Gynecology, Adelaide Medical School, The University of Adelaide, Adelaide, SA 5005, Australia; kai.liu@adelaide.edu.au
4 Lifelong Health, South Australian Health and Medical Research Institute, Adelaide, SA 5000, Australia
5 College of Nursing and Allied Health, Caring Futures Institute, Flinders University, Adelaide, SA 5042, Australia
6 College of Medicine and Public Health, Flinders Health and Medical Research Institute, Flinders University, Adelaide, SA 5042, Australia
* Correspondence: luke.grzeskowiak@flinders.edu.au

Abstract: Iron supplementation is commonly recommended for the prevention and treatment of maternal iron deficiency (ID) or iron deficiency anemia (IDA). However, the impacts of prophylactic of therapeutic prenatal iron supplementation on child neurodevelopment in upper middle-income (UMI) and high-income countries (HICs), where broad nutritional deficiencies are less common, are unclear. To investigate this, we conducted a systematic review, searching four databases (Medline, CINAHL, EMBASE, Cochrane Library) through 1 May 2023. Randomized controlled trials (RCTs) assessing oral or intravenous iron supplementation in pregnant women reporting on child neurodevelopment (primary outcome: age-standardized cognitive scores) were eligible. We included three RCTs (five publications) from two HICs (Spain and Australia) (N = 935 children; N = 1397 mothers). Due to clinical heterogeneity of the RCTs, meta-analyses were not appropriate; findings were narratively synthesized. In non-anemic pregnant women, prenatal iron for prevention of IDA resulted in little to no difference in cognition at 40 days postpartum (1 RCT, 503 infants; very low certainty evidence). Similarly, the effect on the intelligence quotient at four years was very uncertain (2 RCTs, 509 children, very low certainty evidence). No RCTs for treatment of ID assessed offspring cognition. The effects on secondary outcomes related to language and motor development, or other measures of cognitive function, were unclear, except for one prevention-focused RCT (302 children), which reported possible harm for children's behavioral and emotional functioning at four years. There is no evidence from UMI countries and insufficient evidence from HICs to support or refute benefits or harms of prophylactic or therapeutic prenatal iron supplementation on child neurodevelopment.

Keywords: iron supplementation; neurodevelopment; pregnancy; prenatal

1. Introduction

Iron requirements increase substantially during pregnancy to facilitate maternal blood volume expansion and fetal iron transfer, placing women at risk of iron deficiency (ID) with or without anemia [1,2]. A 2019 Lancet Global Health report noted that approximately 36% of pregnant women (15–49 years) are anemic, and ID is responsible for one quarter to one half of all cases worldwide [2]. Although low- and middle-income countries (LMICs) are disproportionately affected, the prevalence of iron deficiency anemia (IDA) among pregnant women is as high as 15% in some high-income countries (HICs) [2]; 28 to 85% of European women have been estimated to be ID in the third trimester of pregnancy, the peak of fetal iron transfer [3].

Oral iron supplementation is recognized as a first-line therapy to correct maternal ID and IDA [4–10]; however, routine supplementation to prevent ID is not recommended in most HICs [4–6,9,11] due to limited evidence of clinical benefits for maternal and child health outcomes. Despite this, prenatal multivitamins containing up to 60 mg of elemental iron are commonly consumed by women, irrespective of iron status [12]. The implications for child neurodevelopment are unknown. Evidence surrounding the optimal oral dose for treating IDA is also unclear, with recommendations varying from 40 to 200 mg of elemental iron between countries [13–16].

Observational studies have long reported associations between maternal ID and poor cognitive outcomes in children [17–19]. However, recent evidence from a large Dutch cohort study (N = 2479 mother–child dyads) has also linked high maternal iron status in early pregnancy with both a lower IQ and a smaller brain size in children at six and ten years, respectively [20]. In the study, although one third of women with high serum ferritin in early pregnancy reported prenatal multivitamin use, it is unclear what dose of iron, if any, these contained [20]. Previous systematic reviews and meta-analyses evaluating prenatal iron supplementation and childhood neurodevelopment were unable to draw definitive conclusions, including due to the limited number of studies at the time and a focus on prophylactic iron supplementation (rather than all forms of treatment) [21,22]. They were also strongly influenced by data from LMICs [21], and as such, their findings were unlikely to be generalizable to high-resource settings, where nutritional deficiencies are less prevalent. A contemporary evaluation of the impacts of prenatal iron supplementation for the prevention and/or treatment of IDA on child neurodevelopment in UMI and HICs is therefore necessary, especially given the ubiquity of iron-containing prenatal supplements in these settings.

2. Materials and Methods

This systematic review was prepared in accordance with the Preferred Reporting Items for Systematic Reviews and Meta-Analyses (PRISMA) checklist [23] (Table S1) and was registered with the International Prospective Register of Systematic Reviews [24] (CRD42023429580).

2.1. Data Sources and Search Strategy

We consulted an experienced research librarian to develop the search strategy using combinations of controlled vocabulary (such as MeSH) and free text words (Table S2). We then performed comprehensive searches across four main databases (Medline, CINAHL, EMBASE, Cochrane Library) through 1 May 2023. Additional manual searches on Google Scholar for recent RCTs were also completed. No date or language restrictions were applied; however, because of logistical constraints, for non-English papers, only those with an available English full-text translation were retrieved.

2.2. Eligiblity Criteria and Study Selection

We included RCTs (individual or cluster-randomized) where the intervention occurred in pregnant women living in upper middle-income (UMI) or HICs as defined by the World Bank gross national income per capita at the time of the study [25]. RCTs were eligible if: (1) women received oral or intravenous (IV) iron in pregnancy; (2) the comparator group received placebo or no intervention, iron via a different dose or for a different duration, or iron with a co-intervention where the quantities of other nutrients were equal across treatment groups; and (3) offspring neurodevelopmental outcomes were reported. Our primary outcome was the global cognition or intelligence quotient (IQ), where a psychometric test provided an age-standardized score (mean = 100, standard deviation (SD) = 15). Secondary outcomes included other measures of neurodevelopment, such as other aspects of cognitive functioning, language, motor skills, academic abilities, and emotional and behavioral functioning. Studies were excluded if they were quasi-randomized, cross-over and non-RCTs, cohort studies, case-control studies, cross-sectional studies, case series, and case reports. Conference abstracts were excluded.

Retrieved publications were uploaded into Covidence [26] for duplicate removal and screening. Two independent reviewers (NAM and TJG) completed title and abstract screening. The same reviewers assessed full-text articles for inclusion.

2.3. Data Extraction and Quality Appraisal

Data were extracted using a standardized form, piloted by NAM and KL, and reviewed by ES. NAM and KL completed data extraction independently; any discrepancies were resolved through discussion with JFG. Where outcome data were missing or data conversions were needed, we contacted study authors.

The quality appraisal of included RCTs was conducted independently by NAM and KL using established guidelines from the Cochrane Handbook for Systematic Reviews of Interventions [27]. The certainty of the evidence was appraised following the Grading of Recommendations, Assessment, Development and Evaluation (GRADE) approach [28] for our primary outcome.

2.4. Data Synthesis

Due to expected variations in assessment tools, we planned to perform random-effects meta-analyses using Review Manager, Version 5.4 [29] to calculate standardized mean differences with 95% confidence intervals (CI) for primary and secondary outcomes according to child age at assessment: $\leq$12 months, 1–3 years, and 4–8 years.

We planned to conduct subgroup analyses according to participant (maternal iron and hemoglobin status) and treatment (timing, dose, and duration) characteristics. Sensitivity analyses excluding studies with a high risk of bias were also planned.

3. Results

3.1. Search Results and Trial Characteristics

Our initial search identified 4509 articles, 880 of which were duplicates. After screening 3629 articles, 58 were assessed in full for inclusion, and five (relating to three RCTs) were included in this review (Figure 1). Of those excluded, 32 reported on studies conducted in LMICs, 20 did not include the population of interest (one animal and 19 child supplementation RCTs), and one RCT was reported as a conference abstract only. A list of the excluded studies is provided in Table S3.

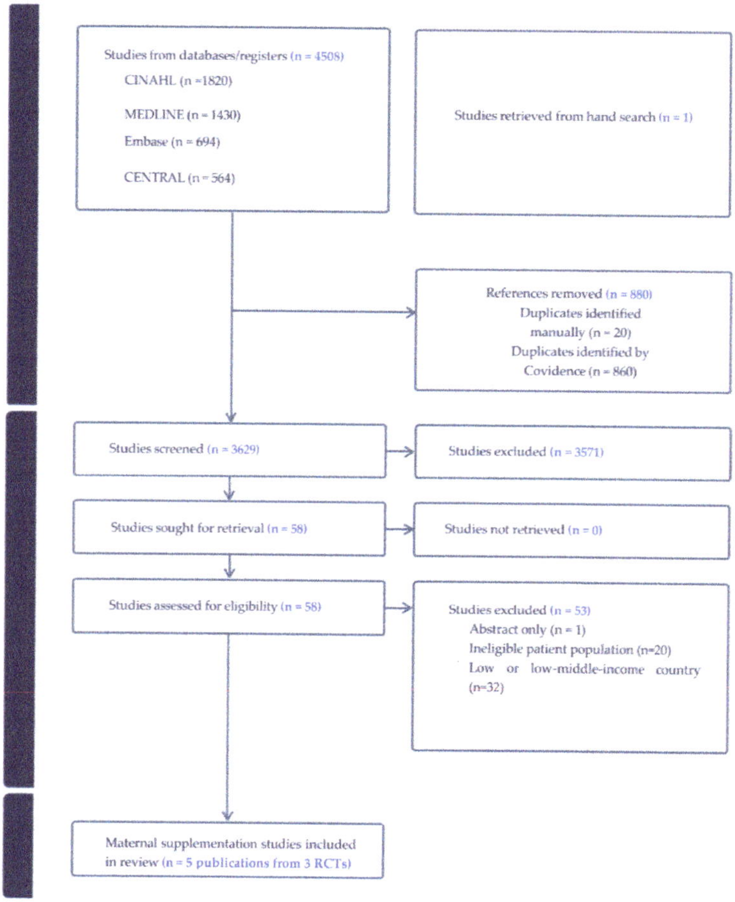

Figure 1. Study flow diagram.

3.2. Study Characteristics

A summary of the included RCTs is provided in Table 1. Five publications reported findings from three prenatal iron supplementation RCTs in two high-income countries, Australia [30–32] and Spain [33,34]. Additional data were sought from the authors of two RCTs [30,33,34], and both provided the information requested.

Table 1. Characteristics of included RCTs.

Citation		Population Enrolled, Location	Sample Size Enrolled	Intervention Arms (Type, Dose, Frequency)	Duration of Intervention	Outcome, Instrument Used, Age Assessed	Children Assessed
Prevention of IDA							
AMBIT RCT	Zhou 2006 [32]	Non anaemic (Hb > 110 g/L) pregnant women with unknown iron status at 20 wks gestation, Australia	n = 216 intervention, n = 214 placebo	*Intervention*: 20 mg oral iron, once daily *Control*: Placebo, once daily	20 wks gestation until delivery	4 years: IQ, behavior using SBIS and SDQ	4 years [32] *Intervention*: IQ (n = 153), behavior (n = 151) *Control*: IQ (n = 149), behavior (n = 149)
	Parsons 2008 [31]					6–8 years: behavior using SDQ and STS for children	6–8 years [31] *Intervention*: parent-rated SDQ (n = 132), teacher-rated SDQ (n = 112), parent-rated STS (n = 132) *Control*: parent-rated SDQ (n = 132), teacher-rated SDQ (n = 113), parent-rated STS (n = 132)

Table 1. *Cont.*

Citation		Population Enrolled, Location	Sample Size Enrolled	Intervention Arms (Type, Dose, Frequency)	Duration of Intervention	Outcome, Instrument Used, Age Assessed	Children Assessed
ECLIPSES RCT	Iglesias-Vazquez 2022 [33]	Non anaemic (Hb > 110 g/L) pregnant women with unknown iron status, ≤12 wks gestation, Spain	Stratum 1 (Hb 110–130 g/L): n = 268 intervention, n = 261 control	*Stratum 1* *Intervention*: 80 mg oral iron, daily *Control*: 40 mg oral iron, daily	12 wks gestation until delivery	40 days: cognitive, motor, and language development using Bayley-III 4 years: IQ using WPPSI-IV and NEPSY-II	40 days [33] *Intervention*: Stratum 1 (n = 161), Stratum 2 (n = 93) *Control*: Stratum 1 (n = 167) Stratum 2 (n = 82)
	Iglesias-Vazquez 2023 [34]		Stratum 2 (Hb > 130 g/L): n = 132 intervention, n = 130 control	*Stratum 2* *Intervention*: 40 mg oral iron, daily *Control*: 20 mg oral iron, daily			4 years [34] *Intervention*: Stratum 1 (n = 92), Stratum 2 (n = 55) *Control*: Stratum 1 (n = 90) Stratum 2 (n = 51)
Treatment of ID							
IV Iron RCT	Froessler 2023 [30]	ID (SF < 15 µg/mL or SF < 50 µg/mL and TSAT < 20% with elevated CRP) pregnant women in the second or third trimester, Australia	n = 139 intervention, n = 165 control	*Intervention*: 1000 mg IV FCM, single dose *Control*: 500 mg IV FCM, single dose	Once	12 months: communication, gross motor, fine motor, problem solving, personal–social development using ASQ	12 months [30] *Intervention*: ASQ (n = 53) *Control*: ASQ (n = 75–77)

Abbreviations: ASQ: Ages and Stages Questionnaire; Bayley-III: Bayley Scales of Infant Development version 3; CRP: c-reactive protein; FCM: ferric carboxymaltose; Hb: haemoglobin; ID: iron deficiency; IDA: iron deficiency anaemia; IQ: intelligence quotient; IV: intravenous; NEPSY-II: Neuropsychological Assessment second edition; RCT: randomized controlled trial; SBIS: Stanford–Binet Intelligence Scale; SDQ: Strengths and Difficulties Questionnaire; SF: serum ferritin; STS: Short Temperament Scale; TSAT: transferrin saturation; wks: weeks; WPPSI-IV: Wechsler Preschool and Primary Scale of Intelligence version 4.

Two of the RCTs [31–34] supplemented non-anemic women (hemoglobin > 110 g/L) with oral iron from their first or second trimester until delivery for the prevention of IDA; however, there were differences in their comparators. In the AMBIT RCT (Refs. [31,32]), women received 20 mg of oral iron or placebo. In comparison, in the ECLIPSES RCT [33,34], women with normal hemoglobin (110–130 g/L) were randomized to either 80 or 40 mg iron daily (Stratum 1) and those with high hemoglobin (>130 g/L) to either 40 or 20 mg iron daily (Stratum 2). The third RCT (IV Iron RCT) compared two doses (500 or 1000 mg) of IV ferric carboxymaltose (FCM) for treating ID defined as serum ferritin (SF) < 15 µg/mL or SF < 50 µg/mL and transferrin saturation <20% with elevated c-reactive protein in the second or third trimester [30].

Child neurodevelopment was reported as a secondary outcome in the three RCTs and only one was adequately powered to assess this outcome [32]. Measures of neurodevelopment varied between RCTs, as did the instruments used and the ages of the children at assessment (see Table 1). Some assessments were administered by psychologists or research assistants, whilst others were parent- or teacher-completed questionnaires. Evaluated outcomes included various measures of cognitive, language, and motor development, and emotional and behavioral functioning.

3.3. Risk of Bias

Table 2 provides a summary of the risk of bias for the included RCTs (with further details in Table S4). All were at high risk of attrition bias due to incomplete outcome data > 20% [27]. All had an unclear or high risk of reporting bias due to lack of clear outcome pre-specification.

Table 2. Risk of bias.

Author, Year		Selection Bias (Random Sequence Generation)	Selection Bias (Allocation Concealment)	Performance Bias (Blinding of Participants and Personnel)	Detection Bias (Blinding of Outcome Assessment)	Attrition Bias (Incomplete Outcome Data)	Reporting Bias (Selective Outcome Reporting)	Other Bias
Prevention of IDA								
AMBIT RCT	Zhou 2006 [32]	Low risk	Low risk	Low risk	Low risk	High risk	Unclear risk	Low risk
	Parsons 2008 [31]			High risk	High risk			

Table 2. *Cont.*

Author, Year		Selection Bias (Random Sequence Generation)	Selection Bias (Allocation Concealment)	Performance Bias (Blinding of Participants and Personnel)	Detection Bias (Blinding of Outcome Assessment)	Attrition Bias (Incomplete Outcome Data)	Reporting Bias (Selective Outcome Reporting)	Other Bias
ECLIPSES RCT	Iglesias-Vazquez 2022 [33]	Low risk	Low risk	Low risk	Low risk	High risk	Low risk	High risk [a]
	Iglesias-Vazquez 2023 [34]						Unclear risk	High risk [b]
Treatment of ID								
IV Iron RCT	Froessler 2022 [30]	Low risk	Low risk	Low risk	Low risk	High risk	High risk	Low risk

Abbreviations: ID: iron deficiency; IDA: iron deficiency anaemia; RCT: randomized controlled trial. [a] Intent to treat analyses requested but were not available. Results are per-protocol. [b] Intent to treat analyses requested and provided.

3.4. Effect of Prenatal Iron Supplementation on Primary Outcome: Age-Standardized Cognitive Score or Intelligence Quotient

Only one prevention RCT (ECLIPSES) measured cognition in infancy using the Bayley-III at ~40 days post-partum [33]. Very low certainty evidence suggested that higher- versus lower-dose prenatal iron did not benefit or harm cognitive development in infants < 12 months (80 mg versus 40 mg oral iron: MD −0.98, 95% CI −2.87, 0.91, 328 infants; 40 mg versus 20 mg oral iron: MD 2.00, 95% CI −0.69, 4.69, 175 infants) (Table 3).

Table 3. Summary of results: primary outcomes.

Primary Outcome	Number of Participants (RCTs)	MD (95% CI)	Quality of Evidence (GRADE)
Oral iron for prevention of IDA			
Global cognition infants at 40 days (Bayley-III)			
Baseline Hb 110–130 g/L			
80 mg versus 40 mg oral iron	328 (1 RCT) [33]	−0.98 (−2.87, 0.91)	⊕○○○ [a,b] Very Low
Baseline Hb > 130 g/L			
40 mg versus 20 mg oral iron	175 (1 RCT) [33]	2.00 (−0.69, 4.69)	⊕○○○ [a,b] Very Low
Intelligence quotient 4 years (SBIS or WPPSI-IV)			
Baseline Hb 110–130 g/L			
80 mg versus 40 mg oral iron	182 (1 RCT) [34]	0.57 (−3.00, 4.14)	⊕○○○ [a,c] Very low
Baseline Hb > 130 g/L			
40 mg versus 20 mg oral iron	106 (1 RCT) [34]	0.77 (−3.30, 4.84)	⊕○○○ [a,c] Very low
Baseline Hb > 110 g/L			
20 mg oral iron versus placebo	302 (1 RCT) [32]	0.00 (−2.48, 2.48)	⊕○○○ [a,d] Very Low

Note: GRADE Working Group grades of evidence. Very low certainty: we have very little confidence in the effect estimate: the true effect is likely to be substantially different from the estimate of effect. Abbreviations: Bayley-III: Bayley Scales of Infant Development version 3; CI: confidence interval; GRADE: Grading of Recommendations, Assessment, Development and Evaluation; g/L: gram per liter; Hb: haemoglobin; IDA: iron deficiency anaemia; MD: mean difference; RCT: randomized controlled trial; SBIS: Stanford–Binet Intelligence Scale; WPPSI-IV: Wechsler Preschool and Primary Scale of Intelligence version 4. [a] Downgraded 1 level for imprecision: wide confidence interval crossing line of no effect including potentially harmful or beneficial effect. [b] Downgraded 2 levels for risk of bias: attrition ~40% and per-protocol analysis. [c] Downgraded 2 levels for risk of bias: attrition ~60% and unclear risk of selective outcome reporting. [d] Downgraded 2 levels for risk of bias: attrition ~30% and unclear risk of selective outcome reporting.

Both prevention RCTs (AMBIT [32] and ECLIPSES [34]) measured offspring IQ at four years using the Stanford–Binet Intelligence Scale (SBIS) and the Wechsler Preschool and Primary Scale of Intelligence Version 4 (WPPSI-IV), respectively. Very low-certainty evidence suggested that neither higher versus lower dose iron (80 mg versus 40 mg oral iron: MD 0.57; 95% CI −3.00, 4.14, 182 children; 40 mg vs. 20 mg oral iron: MD 0.77, 95% CI −3.30, 4.84, 106 children) nor iron versus placebo (MD 0.00, 95% CI −2.48, 2.48, 302 children) improved or diminished IQ at four years (Table 3).

There was no age-standardized assessment of child cognition in the RCT evaluating the treatment of ID.

3.5. *Effect of Prenatal Iron Supplementation on Secondary Outcomes*

3.5.1. Language: Prevention of IDA

There were no clear differences in language or subscales of language (expressive and receptive language) scores (Bayley-III) at 40 days between children born to women receiving higher versus lower doses of iron in both strata of the ECLIPSES RCT. The proportion of infants showing signs of developmental delays (score < 85) was similar between the groups.

At the four-year follow-up of the AMBIT RCT, there were no clear differences in the verbal reasoning scores (SBIS) of children born to women receiving iron or placebo. Similarly, in the ECLIPSES RCT four-year follow-up, there were no clear differences between the treatment groups in both strata in any subscales of IQ related to language (verbal comprehension index, vocabulary acquisition index, non-verbal index) (WPPSI-IV) in intention-to-treat analyses (unpublished data) (Table S5). However, per-protocol analyses reported significant differences in subscales of the IQ test according to maternal serum ferritin status at entry [34]. Children whose mothers received 80 mg of iron but entered pregnancy with serum ferritin > 65 μg/L had lower verbal comprehension index and vocabulary acquisition index scores; there were no differences between intervention and control children of women with low (<15 μg/L) or normal (15–65 μg/L) serum ferritin in early pregnancy in either stratum.

3.5.2. Language: Treatment of ID

There were no clear differences in communication scores between children of women treated for ID with 1000 versus 500 mg of IV FCM (Ages and Stages Questionnaire (ASQ)) at 12 months (Table S5).

3.5.3. Motor Development: Prevention of IDA

There were no clear differences in motor or subscales of motor development (Bayley-III) at 40 days between children born to women receiving higher versus lower iron doses from both strata in the ECLIPSES RCT. The proportion of infants showing signs of developmental delays (score < 85 for main scale or <7 for subscales) was also similar between the groups.

3.5.4. Motor Development: Treatment of ID

Likewise, there were no clear differences between children born to mothers receiving higher versus lower doses of iron in gross or fine motor scores at 12 months (ASQ) in the IV Iron RCT.

3.5.5. Child Emotional and Behavioral Functioning: Prevention of IDA

Both RCTs assessing behavior in older children measured aspects of behavior related to emotion. In the AMBIT RCT follow-up, there were no clear differences in the total behavioral difficulties mean score or any sub-domains (Strengths and Difficulties Questionnaire (SDQ)) between the children born to women receiving iron versus placebo at the four or six to eight year follow up [31,32]. However, more children born to women who received iron had a total difficulties score $\geq$ 17 (indicating abnormal behavior) at four years of age. Although this effect was not present at six to eight years of age, abnormal scores for teacher-rated peer problems were higher in the iron versus placebo group (RR 3.70, 95%

CI 1.06, 12.91). There were no clear differences between the groups in the mean scores for child temperament measured (Short Temperament Scale for Children (STS)) at the six to eight-year follow-up or the percentage of children with difficult temperament (>1 SD above the mean).

In the four-year follow-up of the ECLIPSES RCT, there were no differences in emotion recognition (Developmental Neuropsychological Assessment (NEPSY-II)) in either stratum in intent-to-treat analyses (unpublished data). However, reported per-protocol analyses stratified by the maternal serum ferritin status at RCT entry showed higher emotion recognition scores in children of women supplemented with 80 mg iron who entered pregnancy with normal hemoglobin of 110–130 g/L and serum ferritin < 15 μg/L compared with children of women supplemented with 40 mg iron [34]. Conversely, children of women supplemented with 40 mg iron who entered pregnancy with high hemoglobin > 130 g/L and serum ferritin > 65 μg/L scored lower on emotion recognition than children of women supplemented with 20 mg.

3.5.6. Child Emotional and Behavioral Functioning: Treatment of ID

There were no clear differences between children born to women who received higher versus lower doses of iron in personal–social development scores (ASQ) at 12 months in the IV Iron RCT (unpublished data).

3.5.7. Other Cognitive Outcomes: Prevention of IDA

Other outcomes relating to memory, processing speed, and visual and quantitative reasoning were assessed in the AMBIT RCT and ECLIPSES RCT at the four-year follow-up [32,34]. Neither RCT showed any clear differences between groups for these outcomes (Table S5).

4. Discussion

We screened 3629 articles and ultimately included three RCTs with 935 children from two HICs, Spain and Australia. No RCTs from UMI countries were identified. Meta-analyses were not possible due to the small number of clinically heterogeneous RCTs. The quality of evidence was very low, and all three RCTs had a high risk of bias in the incomplete outcome domain. Considering the two RCTs focused on the prevention of IDA, prenatal iron supplementation versus placebo, and higher versus lower doses of iron showed no clear evidence of benefit or harm on age-standardized cognitive scores or IQ. Across the three RCTs (assessing the prevention of IDA and treatment of ID), there were similarly little to no effects on language, motor development, child emotional and behavioral functioning, or other aspects of cognition related to memory, processing speed, and visual or quantitative reasoning.

Child cognitive outcomes are among many clinical outcomes necessary to consider when balancing the risks and benefits of iron supplementation in pregnancy. A 2015 Cochrane review evaluated the impact of preventive oral iron on several maternal and neonatal health outcomes including maternal ID, anemia, death, infection during pregnancy, low birthweight, preterm birth, neonatal death, and congenital anomalies. Apart from hematological improvements for the mother at term, beneficial effects on other clinical outcomes were equivocal [7]. In LMICs, where the prevalence of IDA is high, the World Health Organization recommends that pregnant women take 30–60 mg of oral iron from early pregnancy until delivery [10]. However, in HICs, prophylactic iron use in pregnancy is not routinely recommended, due to the potential risks of iron overload [35–37]. In these settings, tailored recommendations based on the women's iron status may be preferable [37].

Lending support for caution with routine supplementation, evidence from the two prevention-focused RCTs in our review suggests potential harms to childhood emotional and behavioral functioning [31,32] and subscales of intelligence related to language and memory [34] at four years. Care is required with the interpretation of these findings due to RCT limitations. Despite receiving 20 mg of oral iron from 20 weeks' gestation through delivery and reporting a high compliance of 86%, one third of intervention women were ID at delivery in the AMBIT RCT [32], raising questions about adherence and whether this potentially influenced the magnitude of effect. Furthermore, sub-group analyses according to maternal ferritin in the ECLIPSES RCT were adjusted for maternal iron status late in pregnancy after women already received the intervention, potentially introducing bias into the causal pathway [34]. Thus, the impact of prophylactic prenatal iron on child neurodevelopment in high-resource settings remains uncertain.

Similarly, there was insufficient evidence to determine the impact of different doses of iron for the treatment of established ID on child neurodevelopment. The IV Iron RCT was powered on the proportion of participants who required a repeat iron infusion to determine the superiority of one dose over another for correcting ID [30]. Although both groups received the same dose (500 mg IV FCM) for the repeat infusion, women in the 500 mg group were over two times more likely to require a repeat infusion compared with women in the 1000 mg group (RR 2.05, 95% CI 1.45–2.91; $p < 0.001$) [30], which may have masked any potential differences in ASQ scores attributable to the different doses of iron. The lack of studies comparing long-term neurodevelopmental outcomes with IV or oral iron is also notable, particularly given the rapid increase in use (and cost) of IV iron in this population, and the lack of evidence supporting improvement in maternal or infant clinical outcomes [8,38].

All five publications reviewed had a high risk of bias in the incomplete outcome reporting domain due to significant loss to follow-up (30–66%). Furthermore, only one publication included a sample size calculation and was adequately powered to detect an effect on IQ [32]. The remainder either did not report a sample size estimate for the outcomes measured or were powered on a different primary outcome altogether [30,33,34]. Although intent-to-treat analyses were requested for both follow-up studies from the ECLIPSES RCT [33,34], data were only provided for the four-year follow-up (unpublished). While the Bayley-III assessment at 40 days may be useful for assessing signs of major disabilities, cognitive abilities are not well-developed or measurable at this age and results of this outcome may not be generalizable. Finally, both parents and teachers who completed outcome assessments were unblinded in the follow-up at six to eight years in the AMBIT RCT [31].

To our knowledge, this is the first systematic review assessing the effects of prenatal iron supplementation on child neurodevelopment in HICs in the context of the prevention of IDA and treatment of ID. Our review includes two new RCTs that were not included in previous systematic reviews and meta-analyses [21,22]. We planned to examine the effect of baseline hemoglobin and iron status, dose, duration, and the timing of iron supplementation in pregnancy on offspring neurodevelopment; however, this was not possible due to a lack of data. The included RCTs were clinically heterogenous, precluding meta-analysis, and making it difficult to draw definitive conclusions. Despite uncertainty in the findings, the possibility of harm to children born to iron-replete women who received further supplementation highlights the urgent need for adequately powered RCTs to determine the safety of routine supplement use in high-resource settings.

5. Conclusions

Very low-certainty evidence suggests that prenatal iron compared with a placebo or a high versus low dose for the prevention of IDA may not confer harm or benefit on child neurodevelopment in high-resource settings. The effect on cognition is unknown and the certainty of evidence for other aspects of neurodevelopment is very low for higher versus lower doses of prenatal iron for the treatment of ID. High-quality well-powered RCTs are required to determine the impacts of routine iron supplementation for preventing ID and of different doses of iron for treatment of ID on child neurodevelopmental outcomes in both UMI and HICs.

Supplementary Materials: The following supporting information can be downloaded at: https://www.mdpi.com/article/10.3390/nu16152499/s1: Table S1: Prisma checklist; Table S2: Search terms; Table S3: Excluded studies; Table S4: Risk of bias rationale; Table S5: Secondary outcomes.

Author Contributions: N.A.M., T.J.G., L.E.G. and M.M. conceived of the study; N.A.M., T.J.G., E.S., J.F.G. and L.E.G. developed the research protocol; N.A.M., E.S., J.F.G. and L.E.G. developed the search terms with support from an experienced research librarian; N.A.M. and T.J.G. completed title and abstract screening and full-text screening; N.A.M., K.L. and E.S. developed the data extraction template; N.A.M. and K.L. completed data extraction and study appraisal; E.S., J.F.G. and L.E.G., provided input into data synthesis; N.A.M. completed the qualitative summary; J.F.G. and L.E.G. provided input on the interpretation of findings; N.A.M. wrote the first draft of the manuscript; all authors provided critical input and approved the final manuscript. All authors have read and agreed to the published version of the manuscript.

Funding: M.M. and E.S. are supported by Australian National Health and Medical Research Council (NHMRC) Investigator Grants APP2016756 and ID2007800, respectively. L.E.G. receives salary support from a Channel 7 Children's Research Foundation Fellowship (CRF-210323).

Institutional Review Board Statement: Data from published studies were used in this review and ethics approval was not required.

Acknowledgments: We thank the RCT authors who provided us with the additional data we requested.

Conflicts of Interest: The authors declare no conflict of interest.

References

1. Saloojee, H.; Pettifor, J.M. Iron deficiency and impaired child development. *BMJ* **2001**, *323*, 1377. [CrossRef] [PubMed]
2. Stevens, G.A.; Paciorek, C.J.; Flores-Urrutia, M.C.; Borghi, E.; Namaste, S.; Wirth, J.P.; Suchdev, P.S.; Ezzati, M.; Rohner, F.; Flaxman, S.R.; et al. National, regional, and global estimates of anaemia by severity in women and children for 2000–19: A pooled analysis of population-representative data. *Lancet Glob. Health* **2022**, *10*, e627–e639. [CrossRef] [PubMed]
3. Milman, N.; Taylor, C.L.; Merkel, J.; Brannon, P.M. Iron status in pregnant women and women of reproductive age in Europe. *Am. J. Clin. Nutr.* **2017**, *106*, 1655S–1662S. [CrossRef]
4. Frayne, J.; Pinchon, D. Anaemia in pregnancy. *Aust. J. Gen. Pract.* **2019**, *48*, 125–129. [CrossRef]
5. National Institutes of Health. Iron: Fact Sheet for Health Professionals. Available online: https://ods.od.nih.gov/factsheets/Iron-HealthProfessional/#en64 (accessed on 30 October 2023).
6. Pavord, S.; Myers, B.; Robinson, S.; Allard, S.; Strong, J.; Oppenheimer, C.; British Committee for Standards in Haematology. UK guidelines on the management of iron deficiency in pregnancy. *Br. J. Haematol.* **2012**, *156*, 588–600. [CrossRef] [PubMed]
7. Pena-Rosas, J.P.; De-Regil, L.M.; Garcia-Casal, M.N.; Dowswell, T. Daily oral iron supplementation during pregnancy. *Cochrane Database Syst. Rev.* **2015**, *2015*, CD004736. [CrossRef] [PubMed]
8. Qassim, A.; Grivell, R.M.; Henry, A.; Kidson-Gerber, G.; Shand, A.; Grzeskowiak, L.E. Intravenous or oral iron for treating iron deficiency anaemia during pregnancy: Systematic review and meta-analysis. *Med. J. Aust.* **2019**, *211*, 367–373. [CrossRef]
9. Health New Zealand. Te Whatu Ora. In *Iron in Pregnancy and Post-Partum*; Health New Zealand: Auckland, New Zealand, 2022.
10. The World Health Organization. *Essential Nutrition Actions: Improving Maternal, Newborn, Infant and Young Child Health and Nutrition*; The World Health Organization: Geneva, Switzerland, 2013.
11. Bresson, J.L.; Burlingame, B.; Dean, T.; Fairweather-Tait, S.; Heinonen, M.; Hirsch-Ernst, K.I.; Mangelsdorf, I.; McArdle, H.; Naska, A.; Neuhauser-Berthold, M. Scientific opinion on dietary reference values for iron. *EFSA J.* **2015**, *13*, 1–115.
12. Commissioned by Elevit Executed by Researchify. The Pregnancy Nutrition Survey by Elevit: Survey of 1000+ Australians Aged 18–54. Available online: https://www.bayer.com.au/en/modern-diets-may-be-leaving-aussie-women-nutritionally-under-prepared-for-pregnancy (accessed on 31 October 2023).
13. Malinowski, A.K.; Murji, A. Iron deficiency and iron deficiency anemia in pregnancy. *CMAJ* **2021**, *193*, E1137–E1138. [CrossRef]
14. National Blood Authority. *Patient Blood Management Guideline: Module 5—Obstetrics and Maternity*; National Health and Medical Research Council: Canberra, Australia, 2015.
15. Pavord, S.; Daru, J.; Prasannan, N.; Robinson, S.; Stanworth, S.; Girling, J.; Committee, B.S.H. UK guidelines on the management of iron deficiency in pregnancy. *Br. J. Haematol.* **2020**, *188*, 819–830. [CrossRef]
16. Siu, A.L. Screening for Iron Deficiency Anemia and Iron Supplementation in Pregnant Women to Improve Maternal Health and Birth Outcomes: U.S. Preventive Services Task Force Recommendation Statement. *Ann. Intern. Med.* **2015**, *163*, 529–536. [CrossRef]
17. Geng, F.; Mai, X.; Zhan, J.; Xu, L.; Zhao, Z.; Georgieff, M.; Shao, J.; Lozoff, B. Impact of Fetal-Neonatal Iron Deficiency on Recognition Memory at 2 Months of Age. *J. Pediatr.* **2015**, *167*, 1226–1232. [CrossRef] [PubMed]
18. McCarthy, E.K.; Murray, D.M.; Hourihane, J.O.B.; Kenny, L.C.; Irvine, A.D.; Kiely, M.E. Behavioral consequences at 5 y of neonatal iron deficiency in a low-risk maternal–infant cohort. *Am. J. Clin. Nutr.* **2021**, *113*, 1032–1041. [CrossRef] [PubMed]
19. Tamura, T.; Goldenberg, R.L.; Hou, J.; Johnston, K.E.; Cliver, S.P.; Ramey, S.L.; Nelson, K.G. Cord serum ferritin concentrations and mental and psychomotor development of children at five years of age. *J. Pediatr.* **2002**, *140*, 165–170. [CrossRef] [PubMed]

20. Sammallahti, S.; Tiemeier, H.; Reiss, I.K.M.; Muckenthaler, M.U.; El Marroun, H.; Vermeulen, M. Maternal early-pregnancy ferritin and offspring neurodevelopment: A prospective cohort study from gestation to school age. *Paediatr. Perinat. Epidemiol.* **2022**, *36*, 425–434. [CrossRef] [PubMed]
21. Jayasinghe, C.; Polson, R.; van Woerden, H.C.; Wilson, P. The effect of universal maternal antenatal iron supplementation on neurodevelopment in offspring: A systematic review and meta-analysis. *BMC Pediatr.* **2018**, *18*, 150. [CrossRef] [PubMed]
22. Szajewska, H.; Ruszczynski, M.; Chmielewska, A. Effects of iron supplementation in nonanemic pregnant women, infants, and young children on the mental performance and psychomotor development of children: A systematic review of randomized controlled trials. *Am. J. Clin. Nutr.* **2010**, *91*, 1684–1690. [CrossRef] [PubMed]
23. Page, M.J.; McKenzie, J.E.; Bossuyt, P.M.; Boutron, I.; Hoffmann, T.C.; Mulrow, C.D.; Shamseer, L.; Tetzlaff, J.M.; Akl, E.A.; Brennan, S.E.; et al. The PRISMA 2020 statement: An updated guideline for reporting systematic reviews. *PLoS Med.* **2021**, *18*, e1003583. [CrossRef] [PubMed]
24. PROSPERO. International Prospective Registry of Systematic Reviews. Available online: https://www.crd.york.ac.uk/prospero/ (accessed on 25 July 2024).
25. The World Bank. World Bank Country and Lending Groups: Country Classification. Available online: https://datahelpdesk.worldbank.org/knowledgebase/articles/906519-world-bank-country-and-lending-groups (accessed on 25 July 2024).
26. *Covidence Systematic Review Software*; Veritas Health Innovation: Melbourne, Australia, 2023.
27. Higgins, J.P.; Thomas, J.; Chandler, J.; Cumpston, M.; Li, T.; Page, M.J. *Cochrane Handbook for Systematic Reviews of Interventions*, version 6.3 (updated February 2022); Cochrane: London, UK, 2022.
28. Schünemann, H.J.B.J.; Guyatt, G.; Oxman, A. *Handbook for Grading the Quality of Evidence and the Strength of Recommendations Using the GRADE Approach*, Updated October 2013; The GRADE Working Group, 2013.
29. The Cochrane Collaboration. *Review Manager (RevMan) [Computer Program]*; Version 5.4; Cochrane: London, UK, 2020.
30. Froessler, B.; Schubert, K.O.; Palm, P.; Church, R.; Aboustate, N.; Kelly, T.L.; Dekker, G.A.; Hodyl, N.A. Testing equivalence of two doses of intravenous iron to treat iron deficiency in pregnancy: A randomised controlled trial. *BJOG Int. J. Obstet. Gynaecol.* **2023**, *130*, 15–23. [CrossRef]
31. Parsons, A.G.; Zhou, S.J.; Spurrier, N.J.; Makrides, M. Effect of iron supplementation during pregnancy on the behaviour of children at early school age: Long-term follow-up of a randomised controlled trial. *Br. J. Nutr.* **2008**, *99*, 1133–1139. [CrossRef]
32. Zhou, S.J.; Gibson, R.A.; Crowther, C.A.; Baghurst, P.; Makrides, M. Effect of iron supplementation during pregnancy on the intelligence quotient and behavior of children at 4 y of age: Long-term follow-up of a randomized controlled trial. *Am. J. Clin. Nutr.* **2006**, *83*, 1112–1117. [CrossRef] [PubMed]
33. Iglesias-Vazquez, L.; Hernandez-Martinez, C.; Voltas, N.; Canals, J.; Coronel, P.; Gimeno, M.; Arija, V. Adapting prenatal iron supplementation to maternal needs results in optimal child neurodevelopment: A follow-up of the ECLIPSES Study. *BMC Pregnancy Childbirth* **2022**, *22*, 710. [CrossRef] [PubMed]
34. Iglesias-Vazquez, L.; Voltas, N.; Hernandez-Martinez, C.; Canals, J.; Coronel, P.; Gimeno, M.; Basora, J.; Arija, V. Importance of Maternal Iron Status on the Improvement of Cognitive Function in Children After Prenatal Iron Supplementation. *Am. J. Prev. Med.* **2023**, *65*, 395–405. [CrossRef] [PubMed]
35. Dewey, K.G.; Oaks, B.M. U-shaped curve for risk associated with maternal hemoglobin, iron status, or iron supplementation. *Am. J. Clin. Nutr.* **2017**, *106*, 1694S–1702S. [CrossRef] [PubMed]
36. Hansen, R.; Sejer, E.P.F.; Holm, C.; Schroll, J.B. Iron supplements in pregnant women with normal iron status: A systematic review and meta-analysis. *Acta Obstet. Gynecol. Scand.* **2023**, *102*, 1147–1158. [CrossRef] [PubMed]
37. Milman, N. Iron in Pregnancy—How Do We Secure an Appropriate Iron Status in the Mother and Child? *Ann. Nutr. Metab.* **2011**, *59*, 50–54. [CrossRef]
38. Shand, A.W.; Nassar, N. Rapid increase in intravenous iron therapy for women of reproductive age in Australia. *Med. J. Aust.* **2021**, *214*, 285–285.e1. [CrossRef]

nutrients

MDPI

Review

Maternal Fiber Intake and Perinatal Depression and Anxiety

Neda Ebrahimi [1,*], Tiffany Turner [2], Faith Gallant [3], Abinaa Chandrakumar [1], Roshni Kohli [1], Rebecca Lester [1], Victoria Forte [1] and Kieran Cooley [1,4,5,6]

[1] Department of Research and Clinical Epidemiology, Canadian College of Naturopathic Medicine, Toronto, ON M2K 1E2, Canada; kcooley@ccnm.edu (K.C.)
[2] Department of Research and Clinical Epidemiology, Canadian College of Naturopathic Medicine, Vancouver, BC V3L 5N8, Canada
[3] NCCO Rehabilitation, Toronto, ON M4J 3S2, Canada; faithgallant.7@gmail.com
[4] School of Public Health, University of Technology Sydney, Sydney, Ultimo 2007, Australia
[5] National Centre for Naturopathic Medicine, Southern Cross University, Lismore 2480, Australia
[6] Department of Human Biology, University of Toronto, Toronto, ON M5S 3J6, Canada
* Correspondence: nebrahimi@ccnm.edu

Abstract: (1) Background: Dietary fiber can significantly alter gut microbiota composition. The role of the gut microbiome in the Gut–Brain Axis and modulation of neuropsychiatric disease is increasingly recognized. The role of antenatal diet, particularly fiber intake, in mitigating maternal mental health disorders remains unexplored. The objective of this review is to investigate the association between maternal fiber intake and perinatal depression and anxiety (PDA). (2) Methods: A literature review of PubMed and Google Scholar was conducted using appropriate keyword/MeSH terms for pregnancy, diet, fiber, and mental health. Observational and clinical trials published between 2015 and 2021 were included and data pertaining to dietary patterns (DP), food intake, mental health, and demographic data were extracted. The top three fiber-containing food groups (FG) per study were identified using a sum rank scoring system of fiber per 100 g and fiber per serving size. The consumption of these top three fiber FGs was then ranked for each dietary pattern/group. Mental health outcomes for each study were simplified into three categories of improved, no change, and worsened. The relationship between top three fiber FGs consumed within each DP and mental health outcomes was analyzed using Spearman's correlation. (3) Results: Thirteen of fifty-two studies met the inclusion criteria. Ten (76.9%) studies assessed DPs (seven examined depression only, two examined depression and anxiety, and one examined anxiety only). Seven (53.9%) studies reported at least one significant positive relationship between mental health outcomes and DPs while three reported at least one negative outcome. Three (23.1%) studies compared intake of different food groups between depressed and non-depressed groups. In studies of DPs, the average consumption ranking of the top three fiber FGs bore a significant inverse association with mental health outcomes [$r = -0.419$ (95%CI: -0.672–-0.078)] $p = 0.015$. In studies comparing the intake of different FGs between depressed and non-depressed groups, the consumption of top-ranking fiber foods was higher in the non-depressed groups, but significantly higher in four of the ten high fiber FGs. (4) Conclusions: This study reframes findings from previously published studies of maternal diet and mental health outcomes to focus on fiber intake specifically, using a fiber ranking system. A significant correlation between lower intake of fiber and poorer mental health outcomes warrants further investigation in future studies.

Keywords: dietary fiber; perinatal mental health; maternal diet; maternal depression; maternal anxiety

1. Introduction

1.1. Perinatal Depression and Anxiety (PDA)

Postpartum depression and anxiety are common disabling health issues prevalent worldwide. The global prevalence of postpartum depression (PPD) is over 17% among postpartum women [1]. In Canada, postpartum anxiety (PPA) and PPD occur in 23%

of new mothers [2]. A study conducted by Bowen et al. reported that 27% of pregnant Canadian mothers have major depression [3]. A 2018 Canadian Survey on Maternal Health found a prevalence rate of 17.9% and 13.8% in depression and anxiety symptoms within the 13 months postpartum, respectively [4]. A meta-analysis of 30 countries reported a 4.2% prevalence rate of clinically diagnosed depression and anxiety in the 24 weeks postpartum [5]. PPD has been shown to impair secure attachment patterns and imposes serious adverse effects on the physical and mental health of the mother–infant dyad [6,7]. Of specific note, a meta-analysis of 122 studies from the United Sated, Europe, Asia, Australia, and New Zealand found that PDD impacted the care a mother was able to provide for her children. It is anticipated that this could originate from early physical separation or a lack of material emotional availability. Authors noted that the quality of the mother–infant relationship had an impact on infant development, further affecting the relationship, causing a positive feedback loop [7]. In addition to impacting the mother–infant dyad, PDD has serious impacts on the well-being and quality of life of the mother. For instance, maternal mental health disorders continue to increase the risk of maternal suicide in Western countries including Canada [8]. Additionally, individuals with PPD have been found to be more likely to consult general practitioners, pediatricians, or mental health professionals for non-routine care, demonstrating the impact PDD can have on their overall health [7]. While treatment options for PPD include pharmacotherapy and psychotherapy, safety concerns and limited access to these treatment options pose barriers to implementation [9]. To address these barriers and consider patient preferences for treatments that align with their views on antidepressant use and breastfeeding [10,11], non-pharmacological approaches for PPD appear to be warranted.

1.2. Gut Microbiome and Mental Health

There is now a growing body of evidence supporting the connection between mental health and the gut microbiome, owing to the bidirectional communication pathways between the intestines and the brain (Gut–Brain Axis (GBA)). The GBA communication is mediated by several players including the immune system, neuroendocrine, hypothalamic–pituitary–adrenal (HPA) axis, short-chain fatty acids (SCFA), and autonomic, enteric, central nervous systems [12]. Gut health, decided by the microbial profile and their metabolic byproducts, known as the gut microbiome, is continuously modified by many environmental factors, such as diet, stress, smoking, drug use, etc. These factors can cause perturbance of the microbiome, leading to a more pathologic profile; this shift, referred to as microbial dysbiosis, is associated with a continuously expanding list of inflammatory and non-communicable diseases including several neuropsychiatric disorders [13]. Furthermore, microbial dysbiosis contributes to the permeability of the intestinal mucosa (leaky gut), causing an upregulated immune response resulting in chronic neuroinflammation over time [14]. Increased inflammatory biomarkers including inflammatory cytokines have indeed been found in patients with major depression and generalized anxiety disorder (GAD). Inflammatory cytokines can cross the blood–brain barrier and interact with pathophysiological processes involved in depression, including neurotransmitter metabolism, neuroendocrine function, and neural plasticity [15]. Recent studies have shown interesting trends in specific microbial species over others in patients suffering from major depressive disorder (MDD) and GAD [16]. In a retrospective study, Jiang et al. found a correlation between increased levels of family *Enterobacteriaceae* and *genus Alistipes*, but reduced levels of genus *Faecalibacterium* in major depressive disorder [17]. In a prospective study, Jiang et al. found that participants with GAD had significantly decreased microbial richness and diversity, a reduced number of bacteria that produce short-chain fatty acids, and overgrowth of the bacterial genera *Escherichia*, *Shigella*, *Fusobacterium*, and *Ruminococcus gnavus* species [18].

1.3. Diet, Microbiome and Mental Health

The relationship between diet and risk of depression and anxiety disorders has been investigated in numerous studies of non-pregnant adults. Healthy eating patterns containing fruits, vegetables, meats, fish, grains, and dairy products are shown to be associated with a lower likelihood of depression and anxiety [19,20].

Many features of a 'healthy' diet attributed to positive mental health outcomes may include the higher content of antioxidants, phytochemicals, vitamins, and minerals. Additionally, the greater consumption of whole fruits, grains, and greens, naturally exposes individuals to a greater amount of dietary fiber, which is a key modifier of the microbial profile. What remains unknown, however, is the direct impact of dietary fiber on the microbiome, the GBA, and mental health outcomes.

Dietary fiber is defined as plant-derived carbohydrates and includes non-starch polysaccharides, resistant oligosaccharides, lignin, and resistant starch [21]. Fiber has been recognized worldwide as an important staple of a healthy diet, yet most countries report inadequate fiber intake [22]. Fibers can be categorized as soluble and insoluble. Soluble fibers can dissolve in water and form a gel-like substance; they lower blood cholesterol and stabilize blood sugar levels. Insoluble fibers add bulk to the stool, aid in the prevention of constipation and maintenance of digestive health. Studies have revealed an interconnection between fiber and alteration of the gut microbiome and intestinal barrier. Microbiota actively metabolize fiber in the cecum and large intestine, where it remains unaltered by intestinal enzymes [21,23]. The byproducts of fiber fermentation by microbiota are short-chain fatty acids (SCFA), of which acetate, propionate, and butyrate are the most studied [21].

Various sources of fiber have been shown to change the strains of the gut bacteria [21]. A reduction in soluble fiber is linked to an alteration of microbial metabolites such as loss of phylum Bacteroidetes and an increase in class Clostridia and phylum Proteobacteria species [18].

Dysbiosis is marked by an increase in proinflammatory bacteria. A reduction in anti-inflammatory bacteria has been observed in MDD, particularly an increase in the phyla Bacteroidetes/Firmicutes ratio [15]. The increase in Bacteroidetes has been associated with depression-related intestinal inflammation [16]. In a clinical study, an increase in dietary fiber/prebiotics along with postbiotics like SCFA, increased the abundance of beneficial bacteria; while another study has shown Bifidobacterium strains possess anti-inflammatory effects by modulating tryptophan metabolism and 5-hydroxytryptamine (5-HT) synthesis [13]. These findings suggest that targeting intestinal microbiota as a measure to prevent and manage mental disorders should be further explored [17].

1.4. Microbiome in Pregnancy

The gestational period is associated with marked changes in the maternal gut and vaginal microbiome. The changes in microbiome composition occur throughout pregnancy and are most pronounced in the third trimester. Increases in genera *Akkermansia*, *Bifidobacterium*, and phylum Firmicutes are seen in parallel to the increased need for energy storage. Increases in proinflammatory bacterial phyla, such as Proteobacteria and Actinobacteria, are thought to have protective effects on the mother and the fetus [24]. In late pregnancy, there is an overall reduction in the gut microbiota, characterized by a decrease in the number of phyla Firmicutes and an increase in Proteobacteria, Actinobacteria, and genus *Streptococcus* [25]. Vertical transmission of bacteria from mother to infant is particularly important in establishing the infant gut microbiome and the development and maturation of their immune system. In the days after birth, the skin, mouth, and intestine of infants delivered vaginally will be populated by micro-organisms from the mother's vaginal area, feces, breast milk, mouth, and skin. Initially after birth, the intestinal microbiota of the newborn is dominated by family *Enterobacteriaceae* and genus *Staphylococcus* but is later replaced by genus *Bifidobacterium* and some lactic acid bacteria [25]. The gut microbiota interacts with gut immune cells, establishing tolerance and dictating the development of inflammatory and autoimmune disorders. The first 1000 days of life is a critical period in the establishment of an infant/child's microbiome and their subsequent long-term health outcomes. Thus, the health of the maternal microbiome during pregnancy and postpartum has a long-reaching impact, beyond maternal well-being [25]. As such, diet, particularly fiber, may play a crucial role to the health of the microbiome and consequently the health of mother and infant.

1.5. Gestational Diet, Microbiome, and PDA

Many studies have focused on maternal nutrition, pregnancy, and neonatal outcomes [26]. Few, however, have prioritized mental health outcomes. Commonly studied dietary patterns include the fertility diet, low carbohydrate diet, Western-type diet, Mediterranean diet, and Dietary Approaches to Stop Hypertension (DASH). A "health-conscious" dietary pattern, consisting of vegetables, fruits, nuts, pulses, fish and seafood, olive oil, and dairy products is protective against postpartum depressive symptoms. Another study exhibited that "traditional", and "health-conscious" dietary patterns had a protective effect on anxiety symptoms. The relationship between maternal fiber intake and symptoms of depression and anxiety has not been investigated [22,23].

1.6. Study Objective

The objective of this review and evidence synthesis is to understand if a relationship between maternal fiber intake and mental health outcomes is present. Given the knowledge gap on the role of fiber specifically, in diet and PDA studies, we aim to re-examine published literature in the last 7 years to decipher the contribution of fiber, on mental health outcomes of pregnant women. This timeline was chosen so that the information collected was relevant to the most current changes/updates to dietary guidelines, fiber fortification of foods (snacks specifically), and general dietary trends subject to fads, information, and recommendations that affect dietary intake in different cohorts [27]. Our aim is to close the knowledge gap in the current literature and provide a new perspective on dietary studies in maternal mental health.

2. Materials and Methods

A literature review of PubMed and Google Scholar was conducted using keyword/MeSH terms: [diet, nutrition, dietary pattern, diet quality, fiber, prebiotic, oligosaccharides, complex carbs, prebiotics, symbiotic, fructooligosaccharides, inulin, oligofructose, galactooligosaccharide, xylooligosaccharides, vegetables, fruits, whole grains, legumes, fiber/fibre supplements, vegetarian] AND [mental health, anxiety, depression, mental illness, well-being, mood, stress, psychiatric disorders, psychological status, dysthymia, baby blues] AND [antenatal, pregnancy, postpartum, perinatal, peripartum, maternal, gestational age, lactation, breastfeeding].

Observational and clinical trials published since 2015 in pregnant and/or postpartum cohorts were included. Reviews, meta-analyses, studies prior to 2015, animal studies and studies of other mental health disorders were excluded. Article titles and abstracts were screened by three independent reviewers. Studies meeting inclusion criteria were reviewed, and variables related to diet, fiber intake, mental health outcomes, and demographic data were extracted.

The food items for each food group (FG) (i.e., grains, fruits, vegetables, nuts, etc.) in a study were extracted and evaluated for fiber content. Fiber content for every 100 g serving and typical serving size (TSS) of that food item was derived from food databases (i.e., United States Department of Agriculture (USDA), Canada Food and Nutrient Dataset (CFND), etc.). A fiber score (FS) was calculated by multiplying the fiber content per 100 g serving by the TSS; established cut points for % of recommended daily values were used as guides for FS (e.g., <5% of recommended daily value is considered 'a little') [28]. The FS and fiber per 100 g of all food item within a FG were averaged to calculate the FS and fiber/100 g for the given FG.

The FGs were then ranked according to highest FS and the highest fiber content per 100 g serving; the ranks were then summed to create a final fiber rank (FFR) per food group. Lower FFR corresponds to a higher fiber content. The three top-ranking FGs (i.e., FGs with the lowest FFR) for each dietary pattern in each study were identified and the relationship to mental health outcomes observed were reanalyzed using correlational statistics.

To our knowledge, comprehensive methods or resources to extrapolate fiber content for synthesis have not been established and up to 75% of dietary studies fail to capture fiber intake at all [29,30]. The next sections describe our process using hypothetical examples to estimate crude fiber exposure in each study.

In studies that did not make their food item lists available, the first and last and/or corresponding authors of studies were contacted to provide the list of foods, or the Food Frequency Questionnaires used in their studies to assess the diet in their cohorts. After three unsuccessful attempts, our reviewers used multiple government and industry websites to determine the most popular/typical food items within each food group. To identify what is most consumed from each food group in each country a combination of published literature, government websites, and a search of online popular supermarket brands were used. While the former sources were scarce and non-existent for most, identifying and searching popular brands proved to be exceedingly cumbersome and required sampling from several different popular stores and brands to come up with an estimated fiber and serving size for a given FG. Once this was compiled for each food group, we proceeded to calculate FFRs for each food group.

To account for the vast variation in serving sizes, we also ranked food groups by their fiber per 100 g serving. The sum rank of both (FS and fiber/100 g) were used to ultimately decide which 3 FGs had the highest fiber content. The following sections demonstrate this using hypothetical examples.

2.1. Determining Typical Serving Size (TSS)

As serving sizes vary by country, food and cuisine types, and personal preference, we defined typical serving size (TSS) as the medium size, volume, or quantity of any given food.

Example 1. (Orange) *On the United States Department of Agriculture (USDA) website https://fdc.nal.usda.gov (accessed on 11 October 2023) the TSS for "Orange, all commercial varieties, raw", is listed as 96 g, 131 g, and 184 g for one small, medium, and large orange, respectively, and 190 g for one cup of sectioned oranges. For our FS calculations we chose the medium size. Our assumption is that when eating an orange, the typical person peels and eats a medium size orange.*

Example 2. (Pineapple) *For "Pineapple, raw, traditional varieties", one pineapple weighs about 1 kg, 1 slice = 84 g, 1 cup diced = 174.4, and 1/2 cup diced = 85 g. To determine the FS, we used 3/4 cup = 129 g as the 'typical' serving size. This is considered the in-between serving size between a full cup and 1/2 cup. The assumption is that when eating pineapples, the typical person will consume just under 1 cup of cubed pineapple.*

Example 3. (Beans) *"Boiled, black, mature beans" are reported to weigh 91 g, 127 g, and 182 g for 1/2 cup, 3/4 cup, and 1 cup on the Canadian Nutrient File database (CNFD) https://food-nutrition.canada.ca/cnf-fce/?lang=eng (accessed on 11 October 2023). For calculating FS, we used the 127 g = 175 mL or 3/4 cup as the TSS of edible beans.*

Example 4. (Prepared Dishes) *In bean-based dishes or rice-based dishes (i.e., curry, seafood fried rice, chili, etc.), we examined common recipes listed on the USDA, CNFD, and/or popular restaurant websites that had published nutritional information by serving size. For example, the most common serving size reported for chili is 1 cup. Thus, we used 1 cup as the TSS which is reported to weigh 236–267 g on USDA website for different chili dishes https://fdc.nal.usda.gov/fdc-app.html#/ (accessed on 11 October 2023). We used the average of this range to determine FS for chili (and other prepared dishes in a similar manner).*

2.2. Calculating Fiber Scores (FS)

For any given FG, the average fiber per 100 g serving (edible portion, no refuse) and the TSS of all food items in that FG, were inputted. For example, if a study included pineapples, bananas, and oranges in their fruits FG, the fiber/TSS is calculated by multiplying the fiber/100 g serving by the TSS for that fruit.

Fiber scores (FS) are then assigned based on fiber/TSS values. The FS is a nominal value between 1 and 4. Less than 1 g of fiber/SS is a score of 1 and is defined as 'very low', 1 to <2 g corresponds to a FS of 2 and is defined as 'low', 2 to <5 g correspond to a score of 3 and is defined as 'moderate', and anything containing 5 g or more corresponds to a score of 4 and is defined as 'very high'. In the absence of standard definitions for high, medium, and low fiber, the FS definition and values were arbitrarily chosen by the authors, but consistent with typical dietary definitions (See Table 1).

Table 1. Defining fiber scores.

Fiber/Serving Size (grams)	Definition	Fiber Score
<1 g	Very Low	1
1 to <2 g	Low	2
2 to <5 g	Moderate	3
5+ g	Very High	4

Table 2 demonstrates how FS for the 'Fruits Food Group' in a hypothetical study would be calculated using fruit items: pineapples, bananas, and oranges. The FS for the FG fruits in this example is determined by averaging the fiber/TSS of all included fruits. In this example, an average fiber/TSS of 2.36 corresponds to a FS = 3 (Table 1) and is defined as moderate level of fiber content.

Table 2. Example of FS calculation for the food group fruits.

Food Group Items	Fiber/100 g	TSS (g)	Fiber/TSS	Fiber Score
Pineapple	1.4 g	129 g	1.8 g	2
Banana	1.7 g	118 g	2.01 g	3
Orange	2.5 g	131 g	3.27 g	3
Fruits Food Group			2.36 g	3

2.3. Calculating Final Fiber Ranks (FFR)

After calculating FS for each of the FGs in a study, we then ranked the FGs according to fiber content per 100 g as well as fiber score. The sum of both ranks was used to create a final fiber rank (FFR) for the given FGs. The top-ranking fiber FGs (i.e., lowest FFR) were then used for our analysis. Table 3 demonstrates the ranking process. In Table 3, the highest fiber ranking FGs are: (1) legumes, (2) nuts, and (3) fruits and (4) cereals/grains. The fruits and cereals/grains tied in 3rd place. After ranking FGs according to FFR and identifying the highest fiber ranking FGs (i.e., FGs with the lowest FFR), we analyzed their consumption within each dietary pattern in the study.

Table 3. Deriving final fiber ranks (FFR) for each food group.

FGs	Fiber/100 g	Fiber/100 g Rank	FS	FS Rank	Sum of Ranks	FFR
Fruits	1.87	4	3	2	6	3
Legumes	3.5	1	4	1	2	1
Nuts	3	2	2	3	5	2
Cereals and Grains	2.7	3	2	3	6	3

2.4. *Consumption Ranking of Highest Fiber FGs in Each DP*

Table 4 shows a hypothetical study, in which 7 FGs are sorted from most to least consumed in each of the three identified dietary patterns. The consumption ranking of the highest fiber containing FGs, legumes (FFR = 1) and nuts (FFR = 2), are analyzed within each DP. In this example, legume consumption is ranked 5th, 1st, and 7th in DP-1, DP-2, and DP-3, respectively; whereas nut consumption is ranked as 7th, 3rd, and 5th in the same DPs.

Table 4. Consumption of highest fiber ranking FGs in each dietary pattern.

Consumption Ranking	% Consumption Ranking	Dietary Pattern-1	Dietary Pattern-2	Dietary Pattern 3
1	14.2	Seafood	Legumes *	Soda
2	28.6	Fruits	Fruits	Cereals and Grains
3	42.9	Meats and Poultry	Nuts *	Fruits
4	57.1	Sodas	Seafood	Seafood
5	71.4	Legumes *	Cereals and Grains	Nuts *
6	85.7	Cereals and Grains	Meats and Poultry	Meats and Poultry
7	100	Nuts *	Sodas	Legumes *

* Highest fiber containing FGs. (Legumes FFR = 1; nuts FFR = 2).

Given that different number of FGs are analyzed in each study, we express the consumption ranking as percentage ranks. In this example 7 FG are included, so the percent consumption rank for legumes is 71.4%, 14.2%, and 100% in DPs-1, DP-2, and DP-3, respectively; and for nuts, 100%, 42.9%, and 71.4% in the same order DPs. Hence, only DP-2 has the highest consumption for the highest fiber FGs in this example.

2.5. *Simplifying Mental Health Outcomes*

We then examined the association between reported mental health outcomes in relation to the consumption ranking and percent consumption ranking of the highest fiber FGs within the DPs.

To do this, we simplified reported statistically significant outcomes for anxiety and depression in each study as 'same' (Score = 0), 'improved' (Score = +1), and 'worse' (Score = −1) for each DP. For studies where asynchronous findings were reported for anxiety and depression, the net score was used to represent the overall mental health score. For example, if one outcome worsened and the other improved, the net effect is treated as zero (i.e., no change), and if one worsened while the other did not change, the net effect would be scored a '−1' (worse), and if one improved and the other did not change, the net score for mental health would be '+1' (improved).

2.6. *Statistical Analysis*

Given the ordinal nature of the outcome variable (mental health Score: 1, 0, −1), we used Spearman's correlation to evaluate the relationship between consumption rank and percent consumption rank of the top 3 fiber FGs and the simplified mental health outcomes within each DP. The 95% confidence intervals, Spearman's rho, and two-tailed significances were reported for each relationship.

3. Results

A total of 53 studies were identified in the initial database searches. After duplication removal, fifty-one studies were screened of which twenty-eight were omitted (fifteen studies were published prior to 2015, four reviews, four missing maternal mental health outcomes, four focused on dietary quality/behavior/diversity, and one non-pregnant cohort). A total of twenty-three studies appeared eligible for full text review, of which ten were later excluded due to significant challenges in identifying food groups/items (six), wrong direction of association (one), comparing specific food groups only (one), and extreme poverty/food insecurity (two) at the country of study (Figure 1). Thirteen studies were included for the final analysis [31–43].

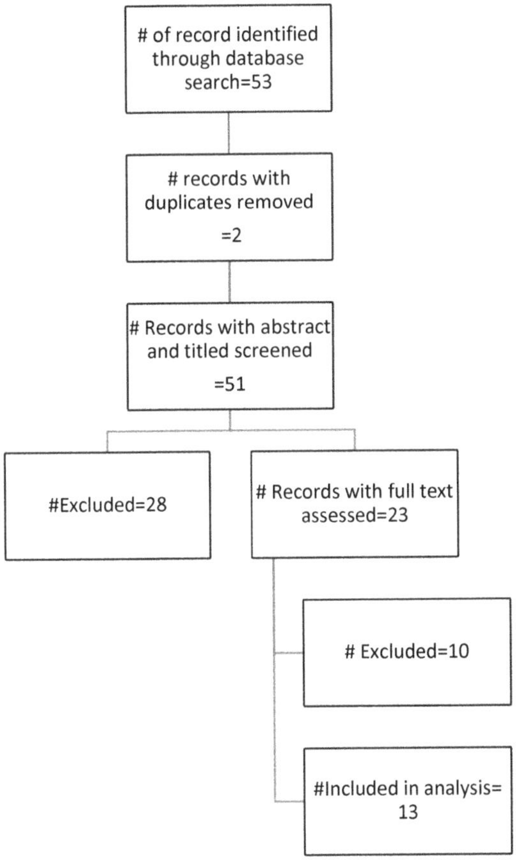

Figure 1. Literature search results.

Table S1 (included in the Supplementary Materials) summarizes the characteristics of the studies analyzed. Ten (76.9%) studies analyzed mental health outcomes in relation to DPs, and three (23.1%) studies compared intake of different FGs between depressed and non-depressed cohorts.

Table S2 (included in the Supplementary Materials) lists the top three fiber ranking FGs in each study and their consumption ranking within each dietary pattern. The total number of FGs/items included in the study, and the relative placement of the top three fiber FGs (percentile placement) are also demonstrated. Additionally, the significant mental health findings from Table S1, is simplified to worsened, unchanged, and improved categories for each DP.

For example, in study #3 [40] of the 33 FGs included, the highest-ranking fiber FGs are seaweeds, mushrooms, and beans. Three dietary patterns, healthy, Japanese, and Western were identified in this study. In the healthy DP, seaweeds ranked fifth (5/33 = 15.2%), mushrooms third (9.1%), and beans ranked fourth (12.1%), suggesting that in the healthy DP, the top three fiber ranking FGs were commonly consumed. By comparison, in the Western DP, the same three FGs were the least consumed FGs.

Statistical tests assessing the relationship between the consumption ranking, consumption ranking percentiles, and overall mental health changes within each DP, were analyzed using Spearman's correlation. Table 5 illustrates this analysis. A strong inverse correlation was found between the consumption ranking of the first [r = −0.41 (95%CI: −0.66 to −0.06) p-value: 0.019] and third [−0.46 (95%CI: −0.696 to −0.122) p-value = 0.008] and average ranking of all top three [rho = −0.419 (95%CI (−0.67 to −0.078), p-value: 0.015] fiber FGs in relation to mental health outcomes. The same finding was observed for the percentile ranking and average top three percentiles (See Table 6). The second highest fiber FGs did not bear any significant relation to mental health outcomes.

Table 5. Relationship between consumption ranking and consumption ranking percentage of high fiber food groups and mental health outcomes.

Confidence Intervals of Spearman's Rho				
Top 3 FG	**Spearman's Rho**	**95% Confidence Intervals (2-Tailed) [a,b]**		**p-Value [c]**
		Lower	**Upper**	
1st Ranked	−0.407	−0.664	−0.064	0.019
2nd Ranked	−0.063	−0.407	0.296	0.727
3rd Ranked	−0.455	−0.696	−0.122	0.008
Average of 1st, 2nd, and 3rd	−0.419	−0.672	−0.078	0.015
1st % Ranking	−0.501	−0.726	−0.181	0.003
2nd % Ranking	−0.095	−0.433	0.267	0.599
3rd % Ranking	−0.454	−0.695	−0.120	0.008
Average of 1st, 2nd, and 3rd %s	−0.556	−0.760	−0.253	0.001

a. Estimation is based on Fisher's r-to-z transformation. b. Estimation of standard error is based on the formula proposed by Fieller, Hartley, and Pearson. c: Two-tailed significance. Dependent variable: overall mental health outcome, independent variables: ranking and ranking percentile of highest fiber FGs within each DP.

Table 6. Intake of top 3 fiber containing foods/food groups, between depressed and non-depressed patients.

			Depressed	**Non-Depressed**	**Antidepressant Treated**
Study #	**# of Food Groups/Items**	**Top 3 Fiber FGs**	**Top 3 Rank (z-Score)**	**Top 3 Rank (z-Score)**	**Top 3 Rank (z-Score)**
Galbally, 2021 [36]	9	Cereals	5 (−0.80)	6 (−0.85)	6 (−0.79)
		Fruit	3 (0.51)	3 (0.79)	3 (0.66)
		Bread	4 (0.00)	4 (−0.05)	4 (−0.05)
Avalos, 2020 [43]	12	Whole Grains	4 (0.44)	4 (0.63)	
		Fatty Acids	5 (0.05)	5 (0.17)	
		Greens and Beans **	12 (−1.30)	11 (−1.15)	
		Total Fruits **	10 (−0.96)	9 (−0.83)	

Table 6. *Cont.*

Study #	# of Food Groups/Items	Top 3 Fiber FGs	Depressed Top 3 Rank (z-Score)	Non-Depressed Top 3 Rank (z-Score)	Antidepressant Treated Top 3 Rank (z-Score)
Shi, 2020 [35]	14	Staple Foods-Wheat	11 (−1.25)	11 (−1.21)	
		Other Vegetables **	1 (3.28)	1 (3.89)	
		Light Vegetables **	4 (0.98)	4 (1.34)	

Z-scores calculated using the means and standard deviations in the depressed groups; ** indicate significant difference in consumption between cohorts.

4. Discussion

The correlation between the microbiome and neuropsychiatric disease has been demonstrated in the literature and is largely accepted in the scientific community. Numerous studies have linked poor diets to poor mental health outcomes, and since the gut microbiome is greatly impacted by diet composition, it is of interest to understand the role it may have in modifying mental health outcomes.

Plant fibers are indigestible carbohydrates that can only be metabolized by specific species of gut microbiota via anaerobic fermentation, the primary product of which is SCFA. It is well established that different fibers can alter the microbiome profile (and output) and exert effects on the host. The type of effect depends on the physiochemical properties of the ingested fiber [44].

The therapeutic potential of fiber in mental health, however, has received little attention. No studies at the onset of this review had investigated the relationship between maternal fiber intake, gut microbiome, and perinatal mental health outcomes. The few relevant studies on this topic are limited to maternal nutritional status, macronutrient intake, dietary patterns, and dietary quality and the subsequent impact on, primarily, depression.

This study is the first to focus on fiber intake and perinatal maternal anxiety and depression. The major challenge for this review was the absence of fiber data, and the need to use proxy variables to assess fiber exposure in each study. We used a ranking system in each study, by which we identified the highest fiber FGs, and ranked their consumption within each of the dietary patterns in that study. We then simplified the mental health outcomes in each study and assessed this in relation to the consumption ranking of the top three fiber FGs within each dietary pattern. In doing so, we reframed the findings for the dietary patterns/intakes to fiber intake. Analyzing this relationship yielded the results that higher consumption of the highest fiber FGs was negatively correlated with mental health outcomes.

Without a list of food items for the studied FGs, standardized serving sizes, and the intercultural/continental variations in both, many arbitrary assumptions needed to be made. This may be one reason why the ranks for fiber FGs vary amongst the studies. A country with a higher consumption of white rice will have a lower fiber ranking in their grains/cereals FG than a country with a higher consumption of whole grain breakfast cereals. Likewise, a country with a heavy consumption of beans in their traditional dishes will have a higher fiber ranking for their prepared-dish FG than one with a higher noodle consumption.

To account for the vast variation in serving sizes, we also ranked food groups by their fiber per 100 g serving. The sum rank of both (FS and fiber/100 g) were used to ultimately decide which three FGs had the highest fiber content (Table 6). Given the scarcity and cumbersome nature of searching published literature, government, and retail websites just to identify popular brands and FGs in each country, we are confident that our approach is unique and helps consolidate gaps in the literature, regarding the consumption of dietary fiber in different DPs, and the correlation to mental health outcomes in mothers.

These assumptions and estimates of the most frequently consumed food items as well as serving sizes are the primary limitation of this study. Other limitations include the timing, frequency, and tools used to capture dietary intake and mental health outcomes in each cohort. Our approach to categorize mental health outcomes facilitated our ability to synthesize the existing literature. However, it prevents a more precise examination of magnitude or clinically meaningful associations between mental health outcomes and interventions with fiber-based dietary components.

The timing of assessments may be critical in the outcomes observed. For example, the risk of depression and anxiety may be higher in the early weeks postpartum than six months postpartum, and studies that did not assess outcomes in the first three months postpartum may have missed those early episodes [45,46].

Having a history of mental health disorders is a significant predictor of perinatal anxiety and/or depression, yet most studies did not assess or report this history in their cohort [46]. The use of antidepressants and psychotherapy, which can modulate disease courses, was also not consistently assessed or reported.

In the studies involving dietary patterns, most often the highest quartile was compared to the lowest quartile, yet some studies used one identified DP as the reference DP (i.e., Study 6 [33] and Study 24 [38]) to which others were compared to. This type of comparison may introduce confounders given the overlap between dietary patterns, and the lack of evidence for the sub/superiority of the reference DP.

Finally, the role of diet in mental health is increasingly seen as a synergistic play between macronutrients, minerals, vitamins and antioxidants, and foods typically higher in fiber tend to be more nutrient dense. Thus, the reported inverse association in this study, between the consumption of high fiber foods and mental health, is not of great novelty or may be confounded by other aspects of nutrition in food consumption. However, a focus on fiber intake specifically and mental health outcomes, may be warranted, as the primary modulator of gut microbiome, and the irrefutable link to anxiety and depression. A large observational study published in April 2022 identified fiber, some vitamin Bs, and magnesium as the primary drivers of mental well-being during pregnancy [47]. The mechanism by which the microbiome is involved requires further investigation.

Future studies should aim to quantify fiber intake during pregnancy and postpartum from all sources, including snacks, replacement meals (nutritional bars, supplements), and prebiotic supplements, using repeated assessments throughout the perinatal period. It will be of great interest to use a clinical population at risk of perinatal anxiety and depression, and to collect stool and blood samples in parallel to dietary assessments, to understand the impact on the microbial profile and output. Finally, mental health assessments should be conducted at least once every 3 months from early pregnancy until 12 months postpartum to ensure the capturing of all critical phases of the perinatal period, i.e., nausea and vomiting in the early trimester, weight gain, physical discomfort and sleep issues in later trimesters, delivery, breastfeeding, and recovery in the first month postpartum, etc.

Fiber intake is low in pregnancy across most pregnant populations. In Canada, prenatal fiber intake in one large cohort (N = 861) was a median 23.5 g/day, ~17% below the recommended 28 g/day [48]. If the therapeutic potential of fiber and prebiotic foods and supplements in mental health is established, diet alone can provide an accessible, effective, safe and affordable option to women everywhere, particularly those at risk of experiencing PDA. Future research, including clinical trials, is warranted.

Supplementary Materials: The following supporting information can be downloaded at: https://www.mdpi.com/article/10.3390/nu16152484/s1, Table S1: Characteristics of the studies included; Table S2: Consumption ranking, and percentile ranking, of the top 3 Fiber Food Groups in each Dietary Pattern & Simplified Mental Health outcomes.

Author Contributions: Conceptualization, N.E. and T.T.; methodology, N.E., F.G., T.T., A.C., R.K., R.L. and V.F.; formal analysis, N.E.; writing—original draft preparation, A.C. and R.K.; writing—review and editing, N.E., T.T., F.G., A.C., R.K. and K.C.; supervision, N.E. and K.C. All authors have read and agreed to the published version of the manuscript.

Funding: This research received no external funding.

Data Availability Statement: The raw data supporting the conclusions of this article will be made available by the authors on request.

Acknowledgments: We would like to acknowledge the work of our research volunteer students Angelica Brigino, Shabnam Rahdar, and Sholeh Ghayoori at CCNM involved in data extraction, and identification of high fiber food groups in the respective countries of each study.

Conflicts of Interest: The authors declare no conflicts of interest. The funders had no role in the design of the study; in the collection, analyses, or interpretation of data; in the writing of the manuscript; or in the decision to publish the results.

References

1. Wang, Z.; Liu, J.; Shuai, H.; Cai, Z.; Fu, X.; Liu, Y.; Xiao, X.; Zhang, W.; Krabbendam, E.; Liu, S.; et al. Correction: Mapping global prevalence of depression among postpartum women. *Transl. Psychiatry* **2021**, *11*, 640. [CrossRef]
2. Government of Canada SC. The Daily—Maternal Mental Health in Canada, 2018/2019. Published 24 June 2019. Available online: https://www150.statcan.gc.ca/n1/daily-quotidien/190624/dq190624b-eng.htm (accessed on 6 February 2024).
3. Bowen, A.; Muhajarine, N. Prevalence of Antenatal Depression in Women Enrolled in an Outreach Program in Canada. *J. Obstet. Gynecol. Neonatal Nurs.* **2006**, *35*, 491–498. [CrossRef]
4. Gheorghe, M.; Varin, M.; Wong, S.L.; Baker, M.; Grywacheski, V.; Orpana, H. Symptoms of postpartum anxiety and depression among women in Canada: Findings from a national cross-sectional survey. *Can. J. Public Health* **2021**, *112*, 244–252. [CrossRef] [PubMed]
5. Falah-Hassani, K.; Shiri, R.; Dennis, C.-L. The prevalence of antenatal and postnatal co-morbid anxiety and depression: A meta-analysis. *Psychol. Med.* **2017**, *47*, 2041–2053. [CrossRef]
6. Earls, M.F.; The Committee on Psychosocial Aspects of Child and Family Health. Incorporating Recognition and Management of Perinatal and Postpartum Depression Into Pediatric Practice. *Pediatrics* **2010**, *126*, 1032–1039. [CrossRef] [PubMed]
7. Slomian, J.; Honvo, G.; Emonts, P.; Reginster, J.-Y.; Bruyère, O. Consequences of maternal postpartum depression: A systematic review of maternal and infant outcomes. *Women's Health* **2019**, *15*, 1745506519844044. [CrossRef]
8. Lee, Y.-L.; Tien, Y.; Bai, Y.-S.; Lin, C.-K.; Yin, C.-S.; Chung, C.-H.; Sun, C.-A.; Huang, S.-H.; Huang, Y.-C.; Chien, W.-C.; et al. Association of Postpartum Depression with Maternal Suicide: A Nationwide Population-Based Study. *Int. J. Environ. Res. Public Health* **2022**, *19*, 5118. [CrossRef] [PubMed]
9. Leight, K.; Fitelson, E.; Kim, S.; Baker, A.S. Treatment of post-partum depression: A review of clinical, psychological and pharmacological options. *Int. J. Women's Health* **2010**, *3*, 1–14. [CrossRef]
10. Chabrol, H.; Teissedre, F.; Armitage, J.; Danel, M.; Walburg, V. Acceptability of psychotherapy and antidepressants for postnatal depression among newly delivered mothers. *J. Reprod. Infant Psychol.* **2004**, *22*, 5–12. [CrossRef]
11. Grzeskowiak, L.E.; Saha, M.R.; Nordeng, H.; Ystrom, E.; Amir, L.H. Perinatal antidepressant use and breastfeeding outcomes: Findings from the Norwegian Mother, Father and Child Cohort Study. *Acta Obstet. Gynecol. Scand.* **2022**, *101*, 344–354. [CrossRef]
12. Slykerman, R.F.; Hood, F.; Wickens, K.; Thompson, J.M.D.; Barthow, C.; Murphy, R.; Kang, J.; Rowden, J.; Stone, P.; Crane, J.; et al. Probiotic in Pregnancy Study Group. Effect of Lactobacillus rhamnosus HN001 in Pregnancy on Postpartum Symptoms of Depression and Anxiety: A Randomised Double-blind Placebo-controlled Trial. *EBioMedicine* **2017**, *24*, 159–165. [CrossRef]
13. Desai, V.; Kozyrskyj, A.L.; Lau, S.; Sanni, O.; Dennett, L.; Walter, J.; Ospina, M.B. Effectiveness of Probiotic, Prebiotic, and Synbiotic Supplementation to Improve Perinatal Mental Health in Mothers: A Systematic Review and Meta-Analysis. *Front. Psychiatry* **2021**, *12*, 622181. [CrossRef]
14. Mörkl, S.; Wagner-Skacel, J.; Lahousen, T.; Lackner, S.; Holasek, S.J.; Bengesser, S.A.; Painold, A.; Holl, A.K.; Reininghaus, E. The Role of Nutrition and the Gut-Brain Axis in Psychiatry: A Review of the Literature. *Neuropsychobiology* **2020**, *79*, 80–88. [CrossRef] [PubMed]
15. Miller, A.H.; Maletic, V.; Raison, C.L. Inflammation and Its Discontents: The Role of Cytokines in the Pathophysiology of Major Depression. *Biol. Psychiatry* **2009**, *65*, 732–741. [CrossRef]
16. Peirce, J.M.; Alviña, K. The role of inflammation and the gut microbiome in depression and anxiety. *J. Neurosci. Res.* **2019**, *97*, 1223–1241. [CrossRef]
17. Jiang, H.; Ling, Z.; Zhang, Y.; Mao, H.; Ma, Z.; Yin, Y.; Wang, W.; Tang, W.; Tan, Z.; Shi, J.; et al. Altered fecal microbiota composition in patients with major depressive disorder. *Brain Behav. Immun.* **2015**, *48*, 186–194. [CrossRef]
18. Jiang, H.-Y.; Zhang, X.; Yu, Z.-H.; Zhang, Z.; Deng, M.; Zhao, J.-H.; Ruan, B. Altered gut microbiota profile in patients with generalized anxiety disorder. *J. Psychiatr. Res.* **2018**, *104*, 130–136. [CrossRef] [PubMed]
19. Cherak, S.J.; Fiest, K.M.; VanderSluis, L.; Basualdo-Hammond, C.; Lorenzetti, D.L.; Buhler, S.; Stadnyk, J.; Driedger, L.; Hards, L.; Gramlich, L.; et al. Nutrition interventions in populations with mental health conditions: A scoping review. *Appl. Physiol. Nutr. Metab.* **2020**, *45*, 687–697. [CrossRef] [PubMed]
20. Aucoin, M.; LaChance, L.; Naidoo, U.; Remy, D.; Shekdar, T.; Sayar, N.; Cardozo, V.; Rawana, T.; Chan, I.; Cooley, K. Diet and Anxiety: A Scoping Review. *Nutrients* **2021**, *13*, 4418. [CrossRef]
21. Swann, O.G.; Kilpatrick, M.; Breslin, M.; Oddy, W.H. Dietary fiber and its associations with depression and inflammation. *Nutr. Rev.* **2020**, *78*, 394–411. [CrossRef]

22. Ramezani, F.; Pourghazi, F.; Eslami, M.; Gholami, M.; Khonsari, N.M.; Ejtahed, H.-S.; Larijani, B.; Qorbani, M. Dietary fiber intake and all-cause and cause-specific mortality: An updated systematic review and meta-analysis of prospective cohort studies. *Clin. Nutr.* **2024**, *43*, 65–83. [CrossRef]
23. Karlsson, F.; Tremaroli, V.; Nielsen, J.; Bäckhed, F. Assessing the Human Gut Microbiota in Metabolic Diseases. *Diabetes* **2013**, *62*, 3341–3349. [CrossRef]
24. Gorczyca, K.; Obuchowska, A.; Kimber-Trojnar, Ż.; Wierzchowska-Opoka, M.; Leszczyńska-Gorzelak, B. Changes in the Gut Microbiome and Pathologies in Pregnancy. *Int. J. Environ. Res. Public Health* **2022**, *19*, 9961. [CrossRef]
25. Pantazi, A.C.; Balasa, A.L.; Mihai, C.M.; Chisnoiu, T.; Lupu, V.V.; Kassim, M.A.K.; Mihai, L.; Frecus, C.E.; Chirila, S.I.; Lupu, A.; et al. Development of Gut Microbiota in the First 1000 Days after Birth and Potential Interventions. *Nutrients* **2023**, *15*, 3647. [CrossRef]
26. Chia, A.-R.; Chen, L.-W.; Lai, J.S.; Wong, C.H.; Neelakantan, N.; van Dam, R.M.; Chong, M.F.-F. Maternal Dietary Patterns and Birth Outcomes: A Systematic Review and Meta-Analysis. *Adv. Nutr. Int. Rev. J.* **2019**, *10*, 685–695. [CrossRef]
27. Sikorski, C.; Yang, S.; Stennett, R.; Miller, V.; Teo, K.; Anand, S.S.; Paré, G.; Yusuf, S.; Dehghan, M.; Mente, A. Changes in energy, macronutrient, and food consumption in 47 countries over the last 70 years (1950–2019): A systematic review and meta-analysis. *Nutrition* **2023**, *108*, 111941. [CrossRef]
28. Canada, H. Nutrition Labelling: Nutrition Facts Table. Published 26 July 2004. Available online: https://www.canada.ca/en/health-canada/services/food-nutrition/nutrition-labelling/nutrition-facts-tables.html (accessed on 7 March 2024).
29. Poutanen, K.S.; Fiszman, S.; Marsaux, C.F.M.; Pentikäinen, S.P.; E Steinert, R.; Mela, D.J. Recommendations for characterization and reporting of dietary fibers in nutrition research. *Am. J. Clin. Nutr.* **2018**, *108*, 437–444. [CrossRef]
30. Smith, M.R.; Micha, R.; Golden, C.D.; Mozaffarian, D.; Myers, S.S. Global Expanded Nutrient Supply (GENuS) Model: A New Method for Estimating the Global Dietary Supply of Nutrients. *PLoS ONE* **2016**, *11*, e0146976. [CrossRef]
31. Vilela, A.A.F.; Pinto, T.d.J.; Rebelo, F.; Benaim, C.; Lepsch, J.; Dias-Silva, C.H.; Castro, M.B.T.; Kac, G. Association of Prepregnancy Dietary Patterns and Anxiety Symptoms from Midpregnancy to Early Postpartum in a Prospective Cohort of Brazilian Women. *J. Acad. Nutr. Diet.* **2015**, *115*, 1626–1635. [CrossRef]
32. Vilela, A.A.F.; Farias, D.R.; Eshriqui, I.; Vaz, J.d.S.; Franco-Sena, A.B.; Castro, M.B.T.; Olinto, M.T.A.; Machado, S.P.; da Silva, A.A.M.; Kac, G. Prepregnancy Healthy Dietary Pattern Is Inversely Associated with Depressive Symptoms among Pregnant Brazilian Women. *J. Nutr.* **2014**, *144*, 1612–1618. [CrossRef]
33. Paskulin, J.T.; Drehmer, M.; Olinto, M.T.; Hoffmann, J.F.; Pinheiro, A.P.; Schmidt, M.I.; Nunes, M.A. Association between dietary patterns and mental disorders in pregnant women in Southern Brazil. *Rev. Bras. Psiquiatr.* **2017**, *39*, 208–215. [CrossRef] [PubMed]
34. Baskin, R.; Hill, B.; Jacka, F.N.; O'Neil, A.; Skouteris, H. Antenatal dietary patterns and depressive symptoms during pregnancy and early post-partum. *Matern. Child Nutr.* **2017**, *13*, e12218. [CrossRef]
35. Shi, D.; Wang, G.-H.; Feng, W. Nutritional assessments in pregnancy and the risk of postpartum depression in Chinese women. A case-control study. *Medicine* **2020**, *99*, e21647. [CrossRef] [PubMed]
36. Galbally, M.; Watson, S.J.; Boyce, P.; Anglin, R.; McKinnon, E.; Lewis, A.J. Maternal diet, depression and antidepressant treatment in pregnancy and across the first 12 months postpartum in the MPEWS pregnancy cohort study. *J. Affect. Disord.* **2021**, *288*, 74–82. [CrossRef]
37. Cao, L.; Liu, Y.; Liang, X.; Zheng, Y.; Li, W.; Yan, J.; Huang, G. Association between dietary patterns during the third trimester and the risk of postpartum depression in China. *J. Affect. Disord.* **2020**, *264*, 370–375. [CrossRef]
38. Huang, P.; Wei, D.; Xiao, W.; Yuan, M.; Chen, N.; Wei, X.; Xie, J.; Lu, J.; Xia, X.; Lu, M.; et al. Maternal dietary patterns and depressive symptoms during pregnancy: The Born in Guangzhou Cohort Study. *Clin. Nutr.* **2021**, *40*, 3485–3494. [CrossRef] [PubMed]
39. Okubo, H.; Miyake, Y.; Sasaki, S.; Tanaka, K.; Murakami, K.; Hirota, Y.; The Osaka Maternal and Child Health Study Group. Dietary patterns during pregnancy and the risk of postpartum depression in Japan: The Osaka Maternal and Child Health Study. *Br. J. Nutr.* **2011**, *105*, 1251–1257. [CrossRef] [PubMed]
40. Miyake, Y.; Tanaka, K.; Okubo, H.; Sasaki, S.; Furukawa, S.; Arakawa, M. Dietary patterns and depressive symptoms during pregnancy in Japan: Baseline data from the Kyushu Okinawa Maternal and Child Health Study. *J. Affect. Disord.* **2018**, *225*, 552–558. [CrossRef] [PubMed]
41. Teo, C.; Chia, A.-R.; Colega, M.T.; Chen, L.-W.; Fok, D.; Pang, W.W.; Godfrey, K.M.; Tan, K.H.; Yap, F.; Shek, L.P.-C.; et al. Prospective Associations of Maternal Dietary Patterns and Postpartum Mental Health in a Multi-Ethnic Asian Cohort: The Growing up in Singapore towards Healthy Outcomes (GUSTO) Study. *Nutrients* **2018**, *10*, 299. [CrossRef]
42. Miura, K.; Takamori, A.; Hamazaki, K.; Tsuchida, A.; Tanaka, T.; Origasa, H.; Inadera, H.; The Japan Environment and Children's Study Group. Dietary patterns during pregnancy and health-related quality of life: The Japan Environment and Children's Study. *PLoS ONE* **2020**, *15*, e0236330. [CrossRef]
43. Avalos, L.A.; Caan, B.; Nance, N.; Zhu, Y.; Li, D.-K.; Quesenberry, C.; Hyde, R.J.; Hedderson, M.M. Prenatal Depression and Diet Quality During Pregnancy. *J. Acad. Nutr. Diet.* **2020**, *120*, 972–984. [CrossRef] [PubMed]
44. Cronin, P.; Joyce, S.A.; O'Toole, P.W.; O'Connor, E.M. Dietary Fibre Modulates the Gut Microbiota. *Nutrients* **2021**, *13*, 1655. [CrossRef] [PubMed]
45. Nakić Radoš, S. Anxiety During Pregnancy and Postpartum: Course, Predictors and Comorbidity with Postpartum Depression. *Acta Clin. Croat.* **2018**, *57*, 39–51. [CrossRef] [PubMed]

46. Kee, M.Z.L.; Ponmudi, S.; Phua, D.Y.; Rifkin-Graboi, A.; Chong, Y.S.; Tan, K.H.; Chan, J.K.Y.; Broekman, B.F.; Chen, H.; Meaney, M.J. Preconception origins of perinatal maternal mental health. *Arch. Women's Ment. Health* **2021**, *24*, 605–618. [CrossRef] [PubMed]
47. Yelverton, C.A.; Rafferty, A.A.; Moore, R.L.; Byrne, D.F.; Mehegan, J.; Cotter, P.D.; Van Sinderen, D.; Murphy, E.F.; Killeen, S.L.; McAuliffe, F.M. Diet and mental health in pregnancy: Nutrients of importance based on large observational cohort data. *Nutrition* **2022**, *96*, 111582. [CrossRef]
48. Dubois, L.; Diasparra, M.; Bédard, B.; Colapinto, C.K.; Fontaine-Bisson, B.; Tremblay, R.E.; Fraser, W.D. Adequacy of nutritional intake during pregnancy in relation to prepregnancy BMI: Results from the 3D Cohort Study. *Br. J. Nutr.* **2018**, *120*, 335–344. [CrossRef]

MDPI AG
Grosspeteranlage 5
4052 Basel
Switzerland
Tel.: +41 61 683 77 34

Nutrients Editorial Office
E-mail: nutrients@mdpi.com
www.mdpi.com/journal/nutrients

www.ingramcontent.com/pod-product-compliance
Lightning Source LLC
Chambersburg PA
CBHW061629210926
51850CB00009B/2482
* 9 7 8 3 7 2 5 8 4 7 2 9 7 *